T0331919

Debates in Values-Based Practice: Arguments For and Against

VALUES-BASED PRACTICE is a series from Cambridge University Press on values and values-based practice in medicine. Edited by Bill Fulford and Ed Peile, volumes in the series will speak to clinicians, policy makers, managers, patients and carers.

Other volumes in this new series include

Essential Values-Based Practice: Fulford, Peile and Carroll
ISBN: 9780521530255
Values-Based Commissioning of Health and Social Care: Heginbotham
ISBN: 9781107603356
Values-Based Interprofessional Collaborative Practice: Thistlethwaite
ISBN: 9781107636163

Debates in Values-Based Practice: Arguments For and Against

Edited by

Michael Loughlin
Professor of Applied Philosophy, Department of Interdisciplinary Studies,
Manchester Metropolitan University, Manchester, UK

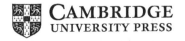
CAMBRIDGE
UNIVERSITY PRESS

CAMBRIDGE
UNIVERSITY PRESS

University Printing House, Cambridge CB2 8BS, United Kingdom

One Liberty Plaza, 20th Floor, New York, NY 10006, USA

477 Williamstown Road, Port Melbourne, VIC 3207, Australia

314-321, 3rd Floor, Plot 3, Splendor Forum, Jasola District Centre, New Delhi - 110025, India

103 Penang Road, #05-06/07, Visioncrest Commercial, Singapore 238467

Cambridge University Press is part of the University of Cambridge.

It furthers the University's mission by disseminating knowledge in the pursuit of education, learning and research at the highest international levels of excellence.

www.cambridge.org
Information on this title: www.cambridge.org/9781107038936

First published 2014

A catalogue record for this publication is available from the British Library

Library of Congress Cataloging in Publication data
Debates in values-based practice : arguments for and against / edited by
Michael Loughlin, Professor of Applied Physiology, Department of Interdisciplinary Studies,
Manchester Metropolitan University, Manchester, UK.
    pages   cm. – (Values-based practice)
Includes index.
ISBN 978-1-107-03893-6
1. Medicine – Practice.   2. Medical ethics.   3. Medicine – Decision making.
I. Loughlin, Michael, editor of compilation.
R728.D397   2014
610.1–dc23
                                                                    2014006989

ISBN 978-1-107-03893-6 Hardback

....

Every effort has been made in preparing this book to provide accurate and
up-to-date information which is in accord with accepted standards and practice
at the time of publication. Although case histories are drawn from actual cases,
every effort has been made to disguise the identities of the individuals involved.
Nevertheless, the authors, editors and publishers can make no warranties that the
information contained herein is totally free from error, not least because clinical
standards are constantly changing through research and regulation. The authors,
editors and publishers therefore disclaim all liability for direct or consequential
damages resulting from the use of material contained in this book. Readers
are strongly advised to pay careful attention to information provided by the
manufacturer of any drugs or equipment that they plan to use.

Contents

Section 3: Conclusions

Contributors

Natalie Banner
Wellcome Research Fellow, Centre for Humanities and Health, King's College London, London, UK

Robyn Bluhm
Associate Professor, Department of Philosophy and Religious Studies, Old Dominion University, Norfolk, VA, USA

Bob Brecher
Professor of Moral Philosophy, Centre for Applied Philosophy, Politics and Ethics, University of Brighton, Brighton, UK

Gideon Calder
Professor of Social Ethics, University of South Wales, Newport, UK

K. W. M. Bill Fulford
Fellow, St Catherine's College, and Member of the Philosophy Faculty, University of Oxford, Oxford, UK and Emeritus Professor of Philosophy and Mental Health, University of Warwick, Warwick, UK

Mona Gupta
Assistant Professor, Department of Psychiatry, Université de Montréal, and Psychiatrist, Centre Hospitalier de l'Université de Montréal (Saint-Luc), Montréal, Québec, Canada

Richard Hamilton
The University of Notre Dame, Sydney, NSW, Australia

Phil Hutchinson
Senior Lecturer (Philosophy), Department of Interdisciplinary Studies, Manchester Metropolitan University, Manchester, UK

Elselijn Kingma
Lecturer, Department of Philosophy, University of Southampton, Southampton, UK

Harry Lesser
Honorary Research Fellow (Philosophy), University of Manchester, Manchester, UK

Wendy Lipworth
National Health and Medical Research Council Postdoctoral Research Fellow, University of New South Wales and University of Sydney, Sydney, NSW, Australia

Miles Little
Emeritus Professor, Centre for Values, Ethics and the Law in Medicine, School of Public Health, University of Sydney, Sydney, NSW, Australia

Michael Loughlin
Professor of Applied Philosophy, Department of Interdisciplinary Studies, Manchester Metropolitan University, Manchester, UK

Andrew Miles
World Health Organisation Collaborating Centre for Public Health Education and Training, Faculty of Medicine, Imperial College, London, UK

Kathleen Montgomery
Edward A. Dickson Emerita Professor, Emerita Professor of Organizations and Management, and Professor of the Graduate Division, University of California, Riverside, CA, USA

Ed Peile
Emeritus Professor of Medical Education, University of Warwick Medical School, Warwick, UK

Rupert Read
Reader in Philosophy, University of East Anglia, Norwich, UK

Alistair Stewart
Consultant Psychiatrist, Royal Oldham Hospital, Oldham, UK

Tim Thornton
Professor of Philosophy and Mental Health, School of Health, University of Central Lancashire, Preston, UK

Mark R. Tonelli
Professor of Medicine and Adjunct Professor of Bioethics and Humanities, University of Washington, Seattle, WA, USA

Ross E. G. Upshur
Professor, Department of Family and Community Medicine, Canada Research Chair in Primary Care Research, University of Toronto, Toronto, Ontario, Canada

Sridhar Venkatapuram
Lecturer in Global Health and Philosophy, Department of Social Science, Health and Medicine, King's College London, London, UK

Editorial introduction

Michael Loughlin

Values-based practice (VBP) is an approach to managing conflict in values, initially developed by Professor K. W. M. Fulford in the context of the philosophy of psychiatry (Fulford, 2004) but designed to be applicable to a wide range of practice contexts in medicine, health and social care (Fulford *et al.*, 2012). It is founded on a recognition of a fundamental feature of the human condition: that all human practices are in some sense based on values[1] but that, for much of human history and for the foreseeable future, we are confronted with a plurality of values – people bring with them different commitments, goals, desires, interests and perspectives (including moral perspectives) when forming judgements about what it is reasonable to do in any given context.

Yet despite these sincere and often legitimate differences, people are required to work together to form common strategies for identifying and responding to practical problems. VBP is designed as an alternative to resolving differences by simple recourse to existent power structures – where some in positions of authority simply rule, then others follow the rule – or to some of the quasi-legal frameworks developed in contemporary bioethics. As a consequence, its advocates contend, its potential implications for practices within organisations are profound. It emphasises the development of reasoning and communication skills to enable all parties to a decision to recognise and respect divergent values, and to discuss their resolution in complex and potentially unique contexts. It has already won recognition in the British National Health Service, informing the Values Framework of the National Institute for Mental Health in England (2004). But the approach is by no means without its critics. Serious concerns about VBP have been raised by commentators in philosophy, psychiatry, public health and bioethics,[2] who subject to critical scrutiny its assumptions about value, rational decision-making, evidence, the political and organisational context of health care decisions and its relationship to dominant ideological assumptions and the economic status quo. In the process, these critics raise important and fundamental questions about how we characterise the problems currently facing health services, and how we think about rational decision-making and the limits upon it in the context of contemporary organisations.

This book aims to give voice both to proponents of VBP and to those raising serious concerns about its development and application. It also identifies two strands of thinking

---

[1] Though see below – even this apparently innocuous claim might need clarification if it is not to risk begging some important questions raised by critics of one of the forms of VBP discussed in this volume.

[2] Cf. *Journal of Evaluation in Clinical Practice*, 17(5), incorporating a full section on VBP (pp. 976–1001) with contributions from Fulford (2011), Thornton (2011), Gupta (2011), Brecher (2011) and Hutchinson (2011). For a discussion of the debate see also p. 844 of the editorial (Loughlin *et al.*, 2011) and for Fulford's response and further criticism see Fulford (2013) and Cassidy (2013).

representing different forms of VBP. While both recognise shared values in many practical contexts, Fulford and colleagues note that the essential values-component of decisions emerges primarily when differences in values come into play, and VBP is proposed as a practical approach to identifying and managing these differences. Another form of VBP is also designed to have practical applications, but it emphasises the need for shared values as a basis for coherent social practices, and is associated with a form of 'modest foundationalism' identified in the work of Professor Miles Little and colleagues working on values-based medicine (VBM) at the Centre for Values, Ethics and the Law in Medicine in the University of Sydney's School of Public Health (Little *et al.*, 2012; Little, 2013). This approach identifies foundational values and their different interpretations as having an explanatory role in practical dialogue, arguing that medicine survives as a social practice because it serves the foundational human values of survival, security and flourishing.

The book is called *Debates in Values-Based Practice* and is structured accordingly. In each of its two sections, a version of VBP is introduced by its leading proponent in the opening chapter, then subjected to a series of detailed analyses and responses – some supportive and others critical – in the ensuing chapters. The proponent is then invited to respond, to consider clarifying, or indeed modifying, the position in the light of the diverse and incisive arguments presented by the commentators. In addition to these concluding chapters for each section, the book contains a final chapter in which the designers of VBP and VBM attempt to draw together the key outcomes of their respective sections to discuss what they see as the crucial lessons to be learned, as well as the contrasts and comparisons between their approaches that the preceding debate has identified and challenged.

So the text can, of course (like any edited collection), be 'dipped into' – the reader may preferentially select specific chapters to suit her own interests, and each chapter is written in such a way that its intelligibility does not depend on having read the others. However, the book will be of greatest value to the reader who can follow the whole debate through its various stages. In so doing the reader is able to get a full sense of the different dimensions to the problems discussed and the (often unexpected) relationships between them. In particular, these exchanges bring out effectively the relationship between urgent practical questions concerning how we respond to the current problems facing contemporary health services, and fundamental and characteristically *philosophical* questions: about how we conceptualise 'value' and the relationship between value judgements and evidence concerning 'the facts'; and how we understand the relationships between health care provision and the broader economic, social and political environment, both nationally and globally. Differences are evident in the authors' philosophical starting points and the ways in which they characterise the true nature of the practical problem, and consequently the form that a proper solution would take. By the end of it, whatever her position on VBP, the reader will have acquired an overview, a map of the intellectual territory traversed in these exchanges. She can form her own conclusions about the validity of the criticisms and the adequacy of the responses, in the process gaining insight into a very current, very lively, on-going academic exchange about a set of issues whose urgent practical import seems undeniable.

My purpose in editing the volume was simply to bring together VBP's most prominent champions with those I regard as its most astute and insightful critics, and really just to 'see what happens'. The result is a text that I hope will appeal to a diverse group of readers – a comprehensive investigation of the intellectual foundations and practical implications of VBP in the context of contemporary global health services. Primarily, the text should appeal to the growing numbers of academics working in ethics and applied philosophy (including health care ethics and medical epistemology), management and organisational theory, social policy, political philosophy and practice-based research. It will also be of interest to managers and practitioners in health organisations facing radically different internal and external environments, whose professional development requires them to seek out a fuller understanding of the problems that shape the work environment. But it has something to say to anyone with an interest in the on-going debate about values in health care, whether that interest is held as a patient (or potential patient), a member of the working population whose taxes fund health services or indeed anyone concerned with making a serious study of the problems of reasoning and decision-making in the modern world.

I have deliberately avoided using this introduction to the volume as an opportunity to state my own conclusions about VBP/VBM, as I think the value of the book is the insight it gives the reader into this on-going debate, and as noted the reader can judge the adequacy of the key protagonists' positions for herself. The brief overview of the arguments below is simply my effort to identify some patterns that emerge as the discussion progresses. It is obviously no substitute for the eloquent expression of those arguments by the contributing authors. The debate about VBP and (most importantly) the issues and conflicts it sets out to address, is by no means settled, and while this volume is a significant contribution to that discussion, none of its contributors would regard this as its conclusion – a point surely confirmed by the open-ended nature of the 'concluding' chapter.

Practice, philosophy and the meaning of 'mutual respect'

So, then, what do proponents of VBP claim on its behalf? What are their assumptions and the alleged advantages of VBP to practitioners and patients? What motivates its critics and opponents? What do the two 'strands' of VBP/VBM have in common and what is the significance of their differences? What is the relationship between these and other academically inspired 'movements' aimed at improving practices within health care? Do we really need another approach or 'movement' to facilitate improvements in practice?

In the opening chapter of this volume, Bill Fulford explains and defends VBP, summarising 'the facts' regarding its development, intellectual starting point and applications. The chapter is very much his statement of what VBP 'is and isn't', reiterating the position in the way that Sackett *et al.* (1996) famously sought to 'clarify' evidence-based medicine (EBM) in response to diverse questions and criticisms. So Fulford restates the 'essentials' of VBP, including the foundational 'premise of mutual respect', the emphasis on learnable clinical skills, the relationship with EBM and the grounding of it all in 'a branch of analytic philosophy called ordinary language philosophy applied to the language of values'. This philosophical basis is contrasted to 'prescriptive' ethics, as its 'modest aim' is to clarify meanings, such that the premise of mutual respect is 'semantic' not 'moral': VBP provides a 'process' for balanced decision-making to serve the 'liberal' aim that competing voices be heard, a stance Fulford contrasts to 'the abuses of absolutism'. His chapter is very strongly supported by Ed Peile's ensuing discussion of values-based clinical reasoning. Writing as a doctor and medical educationalist, Peile argues that VBP 'stands or falls on its usefulness' and defends the utility of VBP, stressing the centrality of the 'two feet principle' – that clinical decisions stand on the 'two feet' of evidence and values. Presenting a brief historical review of research into clinical reasoning, Peile explains and defends a crucial implication of this principle, and one welcomed enthusiastically in the chapters to follow even by authors otherwise critical of VBP: that values have an ineliminable role not only in the management of medical conditions, but also in their diagnosis.

Elselijn Kingma and Natalie Banner endorse Peile's assessment of the value of VBP as lying in 'its pragmatic as opposed to its philosophical aspects'.[3] They argue that the 'learnable skills' Fulford and Peile identify are extremely valuable, most notably the ability to recognise that '*particular features* of individual cases are deeply relevant to what is the right clinical path', such that 'even what appear to be minor or inconsequential aspects of situations can make all the difference in the decisions that should be made'; and, further, that 'particular features *differ radically* between different people'. The sort of training Fulford and Peile advocate should assist practitioners in identifying 'unexpected differences in desires, preferences, relationships, circumstances, emotions, evaluations of outcomes, responses to the world, interpretations of the world. . .' and in taking all of these factors into account in practical deliberations. However, they regard Fulford's claims about the philosophical basis for VBP as misleading and counter-productive. His efforts to 'ground' VBP in a form of 'ordinary language philosophy' that is contrasted to 'prescriptive value-theory' are, they argue, not only unnecessary, but actually detract from its practical value, because they commit VBP to philosophical claims that are deeply problematic.

The authors argue these points with great clarity, but one of these commitments is particularly worthy of attention here because it is taken up and examined in detail in several of the chapters to follow. The premise of 'mutual respect' plays a pivotal role in Fulford's account of VBP, acting as a constraint on which values may be included in the VBP process: values such as 'racism' are incompatible with mutual respect and are thus excluded. But when questions are raised about what other values are excluded, besides the rather obvious one of racism, the inherent unclarity of the term 'mutual respect' becomes apparent. Is the defender of female genital mutilation (FGM) excluded for having a value incompatible with mutual respect for women, or is the critic of FGM excluded for failing to show 'respect' for the cultural values of its defenders? Or are both these values to be treated as 'equal' in the VBP process, and each 'respected'? (In which case, a feminist might wonder why Fulford regards racist cultural values as 'beyond the pale' but does not feel the same way about sexist cultural values.) To explain what exactly we *mean* by mutual respect requires, Kingma and Banner contend, engaging in the sort of 'prescriptive' evaluative exercise Fulford claims VBP can avoid. It is as though he wants to present VBP as a kind of value-neutral mechanism, grounded in a philosophy that derives merely from an understanding of the meanings of ordinary words but which has, nonetheless, substantial implications. They note that it is unclear where this underlying value 'comes from': it seems to be a substantive value (as it is able to be formally incompatible with other prescriptive value-positions, such as racism) yet Fulford treats it as an 'analytic' premise, as though it derives from the meaning of ordinary language terms.

---

[3] This phrase is taken from their chapter, not Peile's: he would no doubt baulk at the words 'as opposed to' as it is not the goal of his chapter to critique Fulford's philosophical arguments, but simply to recommend VBP by focusing on its practical benefits.

The three chapters to follow present explanations of these features of Fulford's VBP with reference to the influence of an ideological framework identified variously as a form of 'radical liberalism' (in Chapter 4 by Tim Thornton), as 'neoliberal' (in Chapter 5 by Bob Brecher) and as a 'liberal deliberative democracy' (in Chapter 6 by Phil Hutchinson and Rupert Read). Thornton (along with Hutchinson and Read) welcomes enthusiastically VBP's 'radical' insight that diagnosis is a value-laden enterprise and not a 'merely factual matter', and (like Kingma and Banner) he praises its recognition of the centrality of the distinctive and particular features of real situations in decision-making, in opposition to a movement he represents as attempting to reduce decision-making to a deductive process based on principles. But Fulford's VBP contains, in addition, the idea that conflicts of values should be resolved not by 'a rule prescribing "right" outcome, but by processes designed to support a balance of legitimately different perspectives (the "multi-perspective" principle).' Thornton questions the status of this claim. While certain values (again, the only one explicitly identified is 'racism') are ruled out, and others are apparently ruled in, what matters in VBP is not finding the correct outcome but simply following the right process – within the range of 'legitimate' values (many of which may be mutually incompatible in practice) none is treated as objectively right or wrong, and the right outcome is, it would seem, whichever outcome emerges from the process. So why 'should' conflicts be resolved in this way? Does the word 'should' here have any prescriptive 'teeth'? In Chapter 1, Fulford asserts that it *does not*, nor can it, if VBP is to avoid 'the abuses of absolutism' – a term he appears to equate with what others might call moral objectivism, the view that moral claims can be correct or incorrect. Thornton argues persuasively that this version of VBP 'faces a dilemma when it comes to accounting for its own normative status'. Either it fails to account for the value of the process it prescribes, or it must 'violate its own principles' by accepting that moral judgements 'answer to real moral features of the world: the moral particulars realised in specific cases'.

Similarly, Brecher remarks that Fulford's dismissal of 'moral objectivism' as 'authoritarian' is self-defeating, because the rejection of the meta-ethical doctrine which allows for the possibility of making correct value judgements undermines every such judgement, including the condemnation of both authoritarianism and racism. This dismissal is, however, in line with Fulford's wilfully vague use of 'values', where the term is used as a cover word for 'needs, wishes, preferences' as well as for commitment to substantive evaluative positions including racism and anti-racism. For Brecher (reinforcing the concerns of Kingma and Banner) this vagueness allows VBP's exponents to present its underpinning values as 'in some sense neutral', 'self-evident' or 'sheer common sense', and therefore requiring no defence. This in turn allows them to regulate all other values, which by implication have the status of mere subjective opinion. In contrast to Kingma and Banner, Brecher doubts that VBP will have practical benefits. Citing earlier work in which he argued that the true role of 'ethical practice guidelines' was to formalise practical problems and so diminish the moral agency of practitioners, in the process transferring responsibility to practitioners for structural problems and thereby rationalising prevailing arrangements (Brecher, 2004), he depicts VBP as yet another mechanism invented by academics to allow organisations to 'manage' clashes of value. The management of clashes stands in contrast to the 'resolution', in any meaningful sense, of real problems, and such approaches typically 'undermine the critical moral reflection that is the essence of genuine moral deliberation'.

Hutchinson and Read argue that Fulford's VBP derives 'from a particular brand of liberal political theory: liberal deliberative democracy'. They regard this as a huge advance on alternative philosophical frameworks that have shaped approaches to problem-solving in health organisations in the past, but they note that ultimately Fulford's approach remains firmly within the 'dominant liberal paradigm'. The liberal conception of value reduces genuinely evaluative claims to mere 'expressions of individual preference', confusing the contentious with the purely subjective and translating the acknowledgement of value-pluralism into an implicit value-relativism. Citing Thornton approvingly, they state that liberalism 'somehow seems to think it has a right to help itself to a "master-value", which Fulford characterises in the rhetorically appealing language of "mutual respect". That really *is* a value, unlike the "values" that people hold.' They conclude that VBP is founded in a procedural conception of justice, claiming a spurious 'neutrality' between different value-perspectives while in fact involving a particular, and controversial, evaluative position. For these authors, the only way to 'resolve' value-conflicts is to acknowledge their status as real conflicts and then to try to work out which position in any particular conflict is the right one. They recommend a teleological approach to understanding value in health, which takes seriously the ancient concept of 'human flourishing' as the proper goal of clinical practice, and they readily acknowledge that this approach is contentious and requires argument – it does not assume the status of some sort of 'master-value' or neutral structure, beyond reasonable criticism.

We will return to this debate when considering Bill Fulford's response, which rightly focuses on the meta-ethical issue of the status of value judgements and the 'fact-value gap'. But it strikes me that one difference between the defenders and critics of VBP's liberalism may be the perspective authors implicitly assume when framing a 'practical' problem. If one starts one's thinking from the point of view of an individual, confronted with various possible value-positions and constrained by broader organisational, social, legal and other factors, then the first job of practical reasoning is to determine which value-position on the issue at hand is the right one. That will tell you which features of the situation, including the values of various parties, are 'problematic'. Consider the example of FGM, mentioned by Kingma and Banner. As an individual, confronted with a situation in which FGM features as an issue, I cannot begin to assess what the 'pragmatic' strategy is until I have worked out whether I regard FGM as a wholly unacceptable violation of the rights of women or as a cultural practice I may not 'like' but need to 'respect'. (Obviously I am not suggesting these are the only possible evaluations here.) Once I have determined my moral starting point, I must build in knowledge of the facts about my context – in what sort of society am I practising, are the laws and social conventions with me or against me? what are the beliefs and attitudes of the parties involved? and all manner of specific features of the situation at hand – in order to come to a view as to what course of action is the best one in context. The fact that some parties' values on this issue differ radically from my own is obviously a very important thing to know but it is not, in itself, an argument for regarding something I view as an atrocity as any more acceptable.

To generalise the point: for any 'conflict of values', it is only when one has formed a view as to where one stands that one can decide what is truly pragmatic, and which strategies represent the best ways to pursue what is the right outcome given the constraints of the context. One can then consider the possibility that sometimes the context makes a morally acceptable solution impossible – Brecher's point, noted above, that some problems are structural and beyond the scope of individual practitioners to resolve. Thus, rigorous moral reasoning can enable us to identify problems requiring *political* solutions, in the form of radical organisational or social change.

However, if one approaches practical problems not from the perspective of an individual (as it were, in the first-person singular) but rather from what might be termed the 'first-person plural' perspective[4] of a policy-maker for an organisation or society, or the sort of working group Fulford discusses in Chapter 1 (deciding on its 'framework of shared values' within a remit set by its role 'at a particular time and within a defined context') then the fact that 'we' differ, often radically, in our value judgements, means that 'which position is right?' is automatically ruled out as a 'practical' question. The issue becomes which organisational and social structures and procedures we need to manage our differences as effectively as possible, and which differences we are going to allow to remain 'in play' (cf. Fulford's discussion in Chapter 1 of drawing up the Guiding Principles for the 2007 Mental Health Act, 'consensus' and 'dissensus'). From that perspective, the focus on 'process' over 'outcome' can indeed seem self-evident, as following from an understanding of the nature of practical reasoning.

Undoubtedly this reading has severe limitations, but it at least links the debates here about VBP's commitment to liberalism to the broader issues in political philosophy (such as the debate between Rawls and his critics, to which Brecher and Hutchinson and Read allude) from which the terminology of 'liberalism' derives its meaning.[5]

Virtue, expertise and the social causes of illness

Mona Gupta's chapter takes us in a rather different direction, raising crucial questions about the relationship between VBP, EBM and clinical ethics. Picking up on Fulford's use of the terminology of decision-making 'tools', Gupta questions the extent to which VBP represents a clear and distinctive alternative to already established approaches in clinical ethics. She challenges Fulford to explain in more detail how precisely VBP operates 'in parallel with' EBM, looking at cases where this idea seems particularly problematic and noting VBP's apparent failure to interrogate the values underpinning EBM, which should not be seen as a value-neutral mechanism discovering 'the facts'. The chapter is pivotal in linking issues about the distinctiveness of VBP (raised by Kingma and Banner) with questions about 'upstream' values that 'lie behind frontline care, such as policy choices about the social determinants of health, or decisions about which agendas to serve in medical research' and possible directions in the future evolution of VBP (questions explored in ensuing chapters by Venkatapuram and Bluhm, as well Fulford and Little in their summary chapters). Following the chapter by Hutchinson and Read, her discussion of different ethical theories brings out a sense in which ideas set up in opposition in their chapter (their favoured, teleological approach, based on the idea of cultivating virtue and Fulford's emphasis on 'process' over 'outcome', the focus on 'how' rather than 'what' to do) could, in principle, be reconciled.

In Chapter 8, which develops a detailed analysis of a particular case involving a home birth, Richard Hamilton brilliantly draws together a number of concerns from the

---

[4] A phrase I have lifted from Fulford's summary chapter for Section 1.

[5] As noted, it is not the purpose of this editorial introduction to pronounce on the issues debated by the contributors, but I attempted to say something about background assumptions determining whom work in applied philosophy is 'for' in Chapter 6 of Loughlin (2002).

preceding chapters, exposing the weaknesses of paternalist, consumerist and principilist approaches to medical ethics, commending VBP's emphasis on a 'team-based model of decision-making' but defending 'an alternative Aristotelian model of collaborative medical decision-making'. Like Hutchinson and Read, Hamilton prefers an approach privileging the idea of cultivating virtue over 'respecting values'. In line with the criticism that VBP's radical liberalism actually undermines the most important advantages (both theoretical and practical) that VBP has to offer, he notes that there is 'a world of difference between insisting that the right answer to any moral problem is occasion sensitive and only available to the practically wise, and Fulford's "no right answer thesis".' Stripped of its 'unfortunate meta-ethical baggage', Fulford's VBP has the potential to cultivate practical wisdom, thus making an important contribution to improving medical decision-making.

Such claims might suggest that VBP can help to promote something like 'ethical expertise' or at least improved 'competence' in decision-making. Yet as Gideon Calder notes, the former idea seems wholly at odds with Fulford's 'democratic' and 'anti-authoritarian' leanings, and even the notion of ethical 'competence' is rendered deeply problematic by VBP's radical liberalism. In an impressively detailed analysis of different possible interpretations of ethical expertise and ethical competence, Calder aims to discover a version of ethical 'know-how' compatible with VBP and the idea that 'the handling of values' is a skill we can learn and, by implication, get better at as time goes on. Like *any* framework for practice VBP must, Calder argues, 'define what counts, or does not, as practice befitting the framework – and define competence as what counts as "good enough" in this respect'. The framework must be set up 'so that it is accessible and inclusive with regard to people arriving with different kinds of "baggage" in terms of their own values'. But there is a tension between this priority and 'the requirement to establish the values on which VBP itself depends. It is a tension between process and substance.' And it is on the side of VBP's radical liberalism that, Calder suggests, 'something has to give'.

This concern is reflected in Harry Lesser's call for VBP to specify more clearly which values need to be identified *in order to be rejected*. In a chapter rich in descriptions of cases and narratives, he notes that there are many values, held by patients, medical staff and other stakeholders, that are clearly 'unacceptable' and that to identify them we need a conception of the 'whole purpose of treatment' that, by implication, is not reducible to the expressed values of the parties involved. Lesser complicates the picture further with an extensive discussion of values that may not be openly expressed because they are unconscious, suggesting that people's accounts of their own values cannot be treated as authoritative. Echoing the concerns about structural problems raised by Brecher, he notes that the organisational context may impose values on practitioners that are 'social and political' in nature, including economic and legal restraints, and far from it being a requirement that we respect these constraints, it may sometimes be our duty to subvert them. This is a point developed extensively by Sridhar Venkatapuram, who notes that 'producing a site of exemplary deliberation and value management could be quite difficult if the surrounding environment is amoral or where values are deeply in conflict and contested'. Referring to the substantial and growing evidence-base regarding the social causes of illness, he challenges VBP to address directly the social and economic forces that determine health and shape the environments in which care is delivered and decisions about care are made. While 'concern about the surrounding social values that shape the clinical encounter is valid anywhere VBP is applied', he points out that it is particularly pertinent when we consider the issue of 'global health': in the context of the developing world, the relationships between economic inequalities, levels of social development and the choices open to participants in the medical process are most apparent and most shocking.

Chapter 12 by Alistair Stewart draws together the questions and problems about when disagreements about value are 'legitimate', the role of political factors, the sense in which people's values are or are not knowable and sustainable and the value-laden nature of illness raised by authors throughout Section 1 of the book. Like Peile, Stewart writes as a practitioner, asking how precisely VBP contributes to his understanding of the problems he faces in his practice as a psychiatrist.

The sheer scope of the questions and criticisms raised across the section left Bill Fulford with a huge task in terms of providing a meaningful response within the limitations of its concluding chapter. Critics may feel that they have not been given a full answer to their wide-ranging and detailed criticisms, and to some extent Fulford would agree, as he does not see the role of his response as providing a resolution of all of the key controversies discussed in the section. He is concerned to address misconceptions about the nature of his project, including the idea that VBP is being advocated as some sort of 'competitor' to 'other ways of working with values in health care'. While he shares many of the commentators' concerns about overly simplistic or 'cut-price' versions of clinical ethics, Fulford stresses that he is not proposing VBP as a competitor to clinical ethics, but rather as a way of supplementing the best work in the area. He reiterates the partnership between VBP and evidence-based medicine, arguing that criticisms of EBM raised by authors in the section do apply to a 'cut-price' version of EBM – but he does not believe that the movement's founders, much less its prominent contemporary protagonists, are logically committed to this 'cut-price' version.[6]

Related to his explanation of the ways in which VBP works in partnership with both clinical ethics and EBM is his account of the development of the 'Lucerne protocol' – a reference to the time and place where his ideas on values, evidence and practice came together in the formulation of the position he was to characterise as VBP. Fulford endorses the view expressed by Hutchinson and Read that medicine as a practical discipline is not 'philosophy free', because practical disciplines are 'shaped by largely implicit conceptual frameworks'. He argues that making the frameworks explicit can allow us to work with them more effectively, and sometimes to change them. It was this conviction that led him to use ordinary language philosophy to clarify the relationship between evidence and values in health care. He outlines one particular line of reasoning to illustrate the dangers in the approach of Kingma and Banner, of disengaging the practical benefits of VBP from its philosophical underpinnings. His own application of ordinary language philosophy led him to appreciate both the role and limitations of casuistry in medical ethics. While the authors are right to point to the power of case-based reasoning, agreement about specific cases may reflect 'shared albeit implicit values', such that 'without an awareness of values the very effectiveness of casuistry in

---

[6] Several of Peile's examples (Chapter 2) are meant to illustrate the claim that VBP and EBM work together in practice, the former 'balancing' the latter. In particular, his illustration of the RCOG statement on C-sections implies that 'sometimes individual patient values must be given more weight than scientific evidence'. It is interesting to contrast this statement to Hamilton's example in Chapter 8, of the AMA statement in respect of an Australian woman requesting home birth.

driving agreement on cases puts it at risk of self-confirming bias'. So VBP needs cased-based reasoning, but case-based reasoning needs VBP if it is to avoid the pitfall of self-confirming bias.

He accepts that this is by no means the final word in the debate, and he offers what he calls 'promissory notes' regarding future work, that give us a sense of the future evolution of VBP in the light of the debates in this collection. In particular, more attention needs to be given to questions about the political and social factors framing decision-making in health (though he notes work already done on 'socio-collective' forms of VBP), on the concepts of expertise and competence in VBP, and on the debate about the meaning of 'mutual respect'. He describes this as his 'biggest personal learning point from the commentaries' and indicates that it is still his view that the premise ('mutual respect for differences of values') can be derived analytically from 'moves and counter-moves in theoretical ethics on the nature of values in general usually called the "is-ought" debate' – a claim he returns to in the book's concluding chapter, co-authored with Miles Little.

Modest foundations

Miles Little's chapter on 'values, foundations and being human' opens Section 2 with an account of the thinking behind VBM, an approach developed as an extension of Fulford's work on VBP and grounded in axiology – the philosophical study of value. For Little, values are not preferences, but preferences may express values, and his key claim is that there are fundamental human values which form the basis of all coherent social practices. He identifies these 'foundational' (F) values as 'survival, security and flourishing'. Medicine survives as a social practice because it serves the foundational values. These values may be instantiated in different ways in different cultural contexts (he cites the differences between the health systems in the UK and the USA as one example) but he argues that these systems represent different practical expressions of the foundational values, and the different expressions can be socially analysed as reflecting different 'axioms': beliefs and commitments regarding the best ways to ensure 'maximum rates of survival, secure resources for those in trouble, and the capacity to restore the disabled to the potential to flourish'.

His position is called 'modest foundationalism': F-values are not foundational in the sense of being logically or epistemologically necessary, but rather they are 'end-points of iterative enquiry, a series of questions that keep asking for justifications until there is no answer except something like "Because that is the way humans are", or "Because societies can't function any other way."' Citing the great empiricist philosopher David Hume, Little notes that a line of enquiry about the value of a thing must end somewhere, in something that simply is desired for its own sake. So his conception of value is 'naturalistic'. F-values are 'descriptive and pre-normative'. This seems to contrast significantly with the position of Fulford, who has consistently rejected 'naturalism' and 'descriptivism'. We have seen that Fulford's only 'foundational' premise was, he maintained, 'analytic' in nature, not grounded in any empirical claims about what people 'just do' value. And if these F-values are shared by all human beings, from Albert Schweitzer to Josef Mengele, and underlie all human systems and practices, from the NHS to the slave trade, from the provision of child-care and old-age pensions to senilicide and infanticide, then how do they serve to explain, let alone help us resolve, the real differences about value that give rise to normative conflict?

For Little and his colleagues, the understanding that shared values underlie even serious and substantive differences can help us understand other parties and may contribute to a resolution or reframing of debates. The two chapters that follow his, both co-authored by Little's close collaborators Wendy Lipworth and Kathleen Montgomery, provide illustrations of the approach, firstly to analyse debates about the pharmaceutical industry and secondly about the emergence and shape of the medical profession. Divergent practices were, in their empirical work, discovered to be underpinned by 'more convergent, or at least recognisable, axioms', and awareness of this 'shared normative background' could, in principle, make discourse 'less antagonistic and more sophisticated'. In another apparent departure from the position of Fulford (but in line with Little's use of 'flourishing') the authors seem sympathetic to the 'virtues' approach to ethics, advocated by some of the critics of VBP contributing to Section 1, and which they found to be key to understanding the discourse of their subjects.

In a detailed and tightly argued chapter, Ross Upshur draws on his own extensive scholarship in medical epistemology to raise incisive questions about what, precisely, Little means by the terminology of 'foundations' and 'axioms'. Upshur has consistently argued that medicine does not need a 'base', 'rooted either in values or evidence'. He regards the language of 'foundations', even when qualified by the term 'modest', as at best misleading – implying a link to a 'totalising' explanatory project that is unsustainable given the evolution of medical practice – or as actually misguided. While there are a number of important 'regulatory ideals' regarding the significance of evidence, respect for certain values, respect for persons and respect for the choices and interests of patients, talk of 'basing' or 'founding' all practice in any of these ideals implies we can find, or should strive to find, some overall systematic account of their relationship that will be valid for all future practice. There is no reason to assume that this intellectual project could have any pragmatic or indeed explanatory value, as medicine is informed by a growing range of epistemic and normative sources, particularly 'given the forces of globalisation and the advent of concern for ecology and public health. . . These epistemic and normative sources are by no means completely aligned, aimed at the same ends or at the same stage of historical evolution.' Nor is there any reason ever to expect them to be. Upshur finds the idea of 'pre-normative' foundations deeply problematic given the vast diversity of human practices, and defends a fallibilist account of clinical reasoning that resonates with the casuist account, to be defended in detail by Mark Tonelli later in Chapter 19.

Aspects of that account are also evident in Andrew Miles' argument that while medicine must be 'informed' by a broad range of sources, including various conceptions of 'evidence' and 'values', it is a mistake to treat any of these sources as foundational, and that VBM is therefore a distraction from the project of integrating 'science and art, fact and value. . . in the service of medicine and humanity'. He regards his own conception of 'person-centred clinical care' as non-foundational, explaining this claim with reference to a meticulous discussion of the history of different forms of 'foundationalism' in philosophy, and coming to the conclusion that we can do no more (and no less) than conceptualise medicine as 'a human endeavour which draws necessarily on the multiplicity of medicine's knowledge sources, without being referentially harnessed to any single, privileged foundation'. Little's 'modest' version of foundationalism cannot, in principle, inform practice, as 'there is no non-arbitrary way of bridging the gap between the foundational values identified and specific decisions about real cases'. We can of course 'note' that different persons interpret F-values via different 'axioms', but these differences may be radical indeed, and the approach leaves us with no way to say which practical interpretation is correct. So how it fosters rational dialogue, mutual understanding or any substantive conclusion is very unclear.

Mark Tonelli's chapter opens with a brief explanation of the casuistry he has defended for many years. In contrast to EBM, which he characterises as representing a more deductive approach, 'where the results of clinical research serve as the major premises from which conclusions about particulars are derived', casuistic reasoning focuses on the particular, and 'begins by asking whether and how a particular case differs from a stand-ard, paradigmatic case'. Tonelli applauds the fact that both the forms of VBP/VBM discussed in this volume attempt to incorporate casuistry, but he laments the fact that, in Fulford's version, reasoning about values is treated as distinct from reasoning about evidence, 'with casuistry only applying to the former'. This perpetuates a false 'fact-value dichotomy' that distorts reasoning in real cases, where there is no necessarily clear divide between factual and evaluative aspects of a situation: 'casuistic reasoning on the part of clinicians can and should incorporate all factors relevant to a particular case in order to arrive at a recommendation or action, not just the values involved'. So by presenting VBP and EBM as addressing respectively each of the 'two feet' of clinical reasoning, casuistry is limited artificially to the 'values' foot. A more serious problem is presented by VBM's commitment to F-values, because casuistry, 'while clearly incorporating values, has no particular use for the foundational variety' and any attempt 'to place some values above others in a *universal* fashion... undermines the very notion of care focused on the individual.'

Robyn Bluhm's discussion of patient autonomy also finds the different versions of VBP/VBM inadequate, in isolation, to support a proper respect for autonomy, by which she means an idea of patient autonomy that goes beyond simplistic conceptions of informed consent on the one hand, and the unsustainable idea of privileging a patient's preferences over all other concerns. (She explains in some detail why these versions of 'autonomy' are inadequate.) Citing criticisms from Thornton and Brecher about Fulford's 'inclusive' use of 'value' to incorporate the preferences of a very broad range of parties, and a lack of clarity regarding the process employed to 'balance' all of these values, she then raises concerns that echo those of Miles regarding the gap between Little's account of F-values and decisions about real cases in health care. However, her conclusion is far more positive for VBP and VBM than those of the three chapters preceding her own: she finds that *in combination* the approaches of Fulford and Little complement each other in a way that enables them to incorporate a defence of the rich, philosophically adequate account of patient autonomy she presents. She explains how Fulford's VBP process, if modified by the incorporation of Little's foundational values, can provide a practical method for ensuring that a theoretically adequate conception of patient autonomy can be protected in clinical decisions.

In his summary chapter for Section 2, Miles Little obviously welcomes Bluhm's contribution and the empirical work of Lipworth and Montgomery in illustrating impor-tant practical applications of VBM. Rather interestingly, given the arguments about VBP and liberalism in Section 1, his response to Tonelli appeals to an idea associated with great liberal political thinkers such as John Rawls, that of 'wide reflective equilibrium'. For Little, VBM situates casuistry within a 'broader domain' incorporating 'previous moral experience, ethical learning, intuition, the details of context and the formal use of ethical structures (including casuistic reasoning) as fuel for reflective consideration.' So in keeping with the methodology of his whole approach, Little is keen to point out the ways in which he and Tonelli are actually in agreement, and his more extensive response to Upshur similarly notes that he and Upshur are 'much closer in our positions than a reader of both chapters might assume'. Both Upshur's criticisms, and those of Miles, seem to assume that Little is 'doing epistemology' and that his use of the terms 'axioms' and 'foundations' must be read as *in some sense* an extension of the use of these expressions in the context of a justificatory exercise. But, he reiterates, his F-values are 'pre-normative': 'I am not trying to construct a rigid base or foundation for medicine's *knowledge*, nor for the details of its practice, nor its bioethics.' These 'foundations' are *'explanatory* in an aetiological or evolutionary sense. They are not prescriptive.'

This brings out another significant parallel between the debates of the two sections. Fulford's critics were puzzled by his insistence on a foundational premise that he deemed 'semantic' or 'analytic' – implying no substantive position in 'prescriptive ethics'. Little also denies that his 'foundations' have what Thornton would call 'prescriptive teeth', though for a different reason: that they represent not analytic but descriptive claims, albeit of a very general nature, regarding 'the way humans are'. These and other fundamental issues are returned to in the chapter Fulford and Little co-author, billed not strictly as a 'conclusion' but as their 'concluding reflections' on the debate thus far.

Reflections, comparisons and prospects for evolution

That final chapter presents a comparison of the two approaches in the light of contributions to the book, reflecting on their similarities and differences and looking for 'practical pay-offs'. It is not like the conclusion of any other philosophy edition I have read. Consistent with their avowed methods, the authors do not attempt to 'resolve' all of the problems identified in the preceding chapters. While they bring out many significant points of comparison between the approaches, they also recognise a fundamental and irresolvable difference between the way they respond to what is termed in philosophy 'the fact-value gap'. As their whole approach is geared towards providing a basis for decision-making that throws light on the relationship between value judgements and the facts, one might assume that a fundamental difference in how they construe this relationship would raise serious problems for their claims about the compatibility/complementarity of their approaches. But instead they argue that 'the open and unresolved nature of the is-ought debate' is reflected in their differences and that it 'translates via their respective starting points into their complementary practical roles as decision support tools in clinical care'. Like the participants in the VBP process, they map out their shared framework assumptions, the complementary applications of their differences in emphasis and the elements of 'dissensus' that they are happy to live with, because in doing so they can find ways to address some of the practical problems the contributions to the volume have exposed. In particular, Little's foundational approach will, it is suggested, help Fulford's VBP to incorporate the sort of global concerns that need to be addressed if VBP is to maintain its relevance in the light of considerations of the social and economic causes of morbidity and mortality globally. But they reflect on other potential developments in the evolution of their combined approaches and they conclude by celebrating 'the new community of ideas' brought together in this book, seeing the process of debate as inherently valuable in stimulating new ways of thinking about the real and important problems the respective chapters address.

References

Brecher, R. (2004) Against professional ethics. *Philosophy of Management*, **4**, 3–8.

Brecher, R. (2011) Which values? And whose? A reply to Fulford. *Journal of Evaluation in Clinical Practice*, **17**, 996–998.

Cassidy, B. (2013) Uncovering values-based practice: VBP's implicit commitments to subjectivism and relativism. *Journal of Evaluation in Clinical Practice*, **19**, 547–552.

Fulford, K. W. M. (2004) Ten principles of values-based medicine. In Radden, J. (editor), The Philosophy of Psychiatry: A Companion, pp. 205–234. New York: Oxford University Press.

Fulford, K. W. M. (2011) The value of evidence and evidence of values. *Journal of Evaluation in Clinical Practice*, **17**, 976–987.

Fulford, K. W. M. (2013) Values-based practice: Fulford's dangerous idea. *Journal of Evaluation in Clinical Practice*, **19**, 537–546.

Fulford, K. W. M., Peile, E. and Carroll, H (2012) *Essential Values-Based Practice: clinical stories linking science with people.* Cambridge: Cambridge University Press.

Gupta, M. (2011) Values-based practice and bioethics. *Journal of Evaluation in Clinical Practice*, **17**, 992–995.

Hutchinson, P. (2011) The philosopher's task: VBP and 'bringing to consciousness'. *Journal of Evaluation in Clinical Practice*, **17**, 999–1001.

Little, M. (2013) Ex nihilo nihil fit? Medicine rests on solid foundations. *Journal of Evaluation in Clinical Practice*, **19**(3), 467–470.

Little, M., Lipworth, W., Gordon, J., Markham, P. and Kerridge, I. (2012) Values-based medicine and modest foundationalism. *Journal of Evaluation in Clinical Practice*, **18**(5), 1020–1026.

Loughlin, M. (2002) *Ethics, Management and Mythology.* Abingdon: Radcliffe Press.

Loughlin, M., Bluhm, R., Buetow, S., Goldenberg, M., Upshur, R., Borgerson, K. and Entwistle, V. (2011) Virtue, progress and practice. *Journal of Evaluation in Clinical Practice*, **17**, 839–846.

National Institute for Mental Health in England (2004) *The National Framework of Values for Mental Health.* London: Department of Health.

Sackett, D. L., Rosenberg, W. M. and Gray, J. A. (1996) Evidence-based medicine: what it is and what it isn't. *British Medical Journal*, **312**(7023), 71–72.

Thornton, T. (2011) Radical, liberal values-based practice. *Journal of Evaluation in Clinical Practice*, **17**, 988–991.

CHAPTER 1 begins on following page

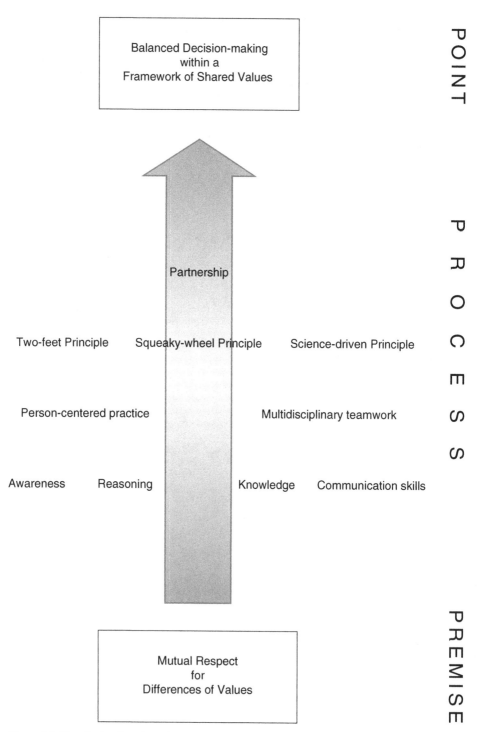

Figure 1.1 Map of values-based practice.

Values-based practice: the facts

K. W. M. (Bill) Fulford

Values-based practice is a new skills-based approach to health care decision-making where complex and conflicting values are in play. The flow diagram in Figure 1.1 shows how, starting from a premise of mutual respect, the ten key elements of values-based practice come together to support balanced decision-making within frameworks of shared values.

Values-based practice is only one tool among others in medicine's tool kit for working with values. Besides ethics and law, such tools include decision analysis (Hunink *et al.*, 2001) and health economics (Brown *et al.*, 2005). Values-based practice, in building primarily on learnable clinical skills, adds to the tool kit a particular focus on and ways of working with the diversity of *individual* values.

In this chapter I outline briefly the skills for values-based practice, the nature of professional relationships within values-based practice, the links between values-based and evidence-based practice, and the concept of dissensus at the heart of partnership in values-based decision-making. I then turn to theory: values-based practice as I will show owes many of its defining characteristics to its origins in a branch of analytic philosophy called ordinary language philosophy applied to the language of values. In a brief concluding section I indicate the importance of values-based practice for medicine as a science at the cutting edge.

The skills for values-based practice

Crucial to the practical effectiveness of values-based practice has been the development of training materials for frontline staff. The first training manual, appropriately titled *Whose*

Debates in Values-Based Practice, ed. Michael Loughlin. Published by Cambridge University Press. © Cambridge University Press 2014.

Values? (Woodbridge and Fulford, 2004), was launched by the then Minister of State with responsibility for mental health, Rosie Winterton, at a conference in London in 2005. *Whose Values?* was the basis for a series of national policy, training and service developments in the UK and there were similar initiatives in a number of other countries (Fulford *et al.*, 2004).

The starting point for training in values-based practice is raised awareness of values and it is on this that I focus here, although with a few comments also on reasoning, knowledge and communication skills (see Table 1.1 and Figure 1.1). In everyday practice, values-based decision-making depends on a well joined up and unselfconscious use of the skills (and indeed other elements) of values-based practice working together as a whole. Raised awareness however is always the starting point.

Training in awareness of values has two main learning outcomes: an understanding of the diversity of values (including but extending well beyond ethical values); and the often surprising nature of the values people actually hold (this includes our own values as well as those of others).

Diversity of values

A word association exercise is a good way to get started. Table 1.2 shows one set of responses to an exercise of this kind with a group of trainee psychiatrists. The group had been asked to 'write down three words or short phrases that mean "values" to you'. As Table 1.2 indicates, everyone produced a different triplet of words! In feedback and discussion the list of associations the group had produced together helped them to see just what a wide and diverse range of things are covered by values – ethical values, certainly, but also needs, wishes, preferences, and indeed anything positively or negatively weighted as a guide to action (Fulford *et al.*, 2012, Chapter 1).

The diversity of values notwithstanding, many values are shared. In this exercise trainees will usually spot this for themselves. Thus in Table 1.2, the values of 'autonomy' and 'best interests' both come up more than once. Recognising such shared values then leads naturally into talking about the relationship between ethics and values-based practice. For shared values are readily identified as the *ethical* values that in values-based practice together provide a framework for partnership in decision-making (see below). The trick though is to see that these same shared framework ethical values are both individually complex and collectively conflicting – best interests for example means widely different things to different people (it is in this sense a complex value); and best interests is often in conflict with autonomy of patient choice.

One response to the complex and conflicting nature of values is to develop ever more elaborate ethical codes. Values-based practice offers a different response. Values-based practice starts from the idea that, while ethical codes provide a vital framework for practice, the complex and often conflicting nature of the values such codes embody has the consequence that the clinical skills and other elements of values-based practice are required in coming to *balanced decisions in individual cases* (Fulford *et al.*, 2012, Chapter 2 – see below, 'Dissensus and partnership', for an example).

Surprising values

Having 'got' diversity the next step is to 'get' surprise. One way to 'get' surprise is illustrated by Figure 1.3. This is taken from a training workshop with a mental health

Table 1.1 A summary of values-based practice (VBP)

Elements of VBP	Brief explanations
Premise	The basis for balanced decision making in VBP is the premise of **mutual respect for differences of values**
Ten-part process	VBP supports balanced decision making through **good process** rather than prescribing preset right outcomes. The process of VBP includes four areas of **clinical skills**, two aspects of **professional relationships**, three principles **linking VBP with EBP**, and **partnership in decision making** based on 'dissensus'
The four skills areas are	
(1) Awareness	The first and essential skill for VBP is raised awareness of values and of the often surprising diversity of individual values
(2) Reasoning	Values reasoning in VBP may employ any of the methods standardly used in ethics (principles reasoning, case-based reasoning, etc.) but with an emphasis on opening up different perspectives rather than closing down on 'solutions'
(3) Knowledge	A key skill for VBP is knowing how to find and use knowledge of values (including research-based knowledge) while never forgetting that each individual is unique (we are all an 'n of 1')
(4) Communication	VBP communication skills, include skills (1) for eliciting values, in particular StAR values (Strengths, Aspirations and Resources), and (2) for conflict resolution
The two aspects of professional relationships are	
(1) The extended MDT	The role of the MDT (multidisciplinary team) in values-based practice is extended from its traditional range of different professional skills to include also a range of different value perspectives
(2) Patient-values-centered care	In VBP, patient-centered care means focusing primarily on the patient's values though other values (including those of the clinician) are important too
The three principles linking VBP with EBP are	
(1) 'Two feet' principle	The 'two feet' principle of VBP is that all decisions are based on values as well as evidence even where (as in diagnostic decisions) the values in question may be relatively hidden
(2) 'Squeaky wheel' principle	The 'squeaky wheel' principle of VBP is that we tend to notice values when they are conflicting and hence causing difficulties (based on the saying 'it's the squeaky wheel that gets the grease')
(3) 'Science driven' principle	The 'science driven' principle of VBP is that the need for VBP is driven by advances in medical science (this is because such advances open up new choices and with choices go values)
Partnership in decision making	
. . . based on dissensus	Consensual decision making involves agreement on values, with some values being adopted and others not. In dissensual decision making by contrast, different values remain in play to be balanced sometimes one way and sometimes in others according to the particular circumstances of a given case
Outputs	Rather than giving us answers as such, VBP aims to support **balanced decision making within frameworks of shared values** appropriate to the situation in question

Table 1.2 What are values?

Faith	How we treat people
Internalisation	Attitudes
Acting in best interests	Principles
Integrity	Autonomy
Conscience	Love
Best interests	Relationships
Autonomy	
Respect	Non-violence
Personal to me	Compassion
Difference … diversity	Dialogue
Beliefs	Responsibility
Right/wrong to me	Accountability
What I am	Best interests
Belief	What I *believe*
Principles	What makes me tick
Things held dear	What I won't compromise
Subjective merits	'Objective' core
Meanings	Confidentiality
Person-centred care	Autonomy
A *standard* for the way I conduct *myself*	Significant
Belief about how things *should* be	Standards
Things you would not want to change	Truth

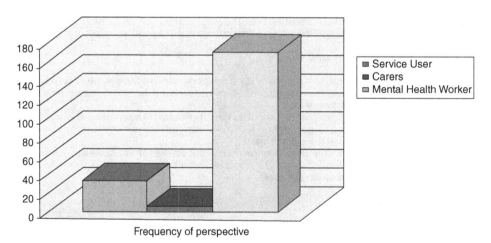

Figure 1.2 values explanation with chart

Figure 1.2 The perspectives expressed in a case review meeting.

team in London (Fulford and Woodbridge, 2008). It shows the values implicit in the comments of team members in a case review meeting. The team in question had asked for training in values-based practice because of their shared commitment to a person-centred approach. This was the team's shared core value in fact. Yet as Figure 1.2 shows, the values actually expressed by team members in their meeting (and thus likely-as-not in their practice as well) were very largely their own rather than those of their clients.

This came as a considerable surprise to the team. But precisely *because* it came as such a surprise it proved a strong basis on which to build their training in values-based practice.

Reasoning, knowledge and communication skills

Reasoning, knowledge and communication skills are of course not unique to values-based practice. Values-based practice, however, brings a particular and unique slant to each of them. The result is a two-way relationship in which values-based practice depends (in part) on reasoning, knowledge and communication skills, while, conversely, reasoning, knowledge and communication skills are all in different ways enriched by values-based practice.

Thus, in the case of reasoning skills, values-based practice employs any and all of the established methods of ethical reasoning (such as principles reasoning, casuistry or case-based reasoning, utilitarianism and deontology). It is in this sense that values-based practice depends in part on ethical reasoning skills. Values-based practice in turn, however, enriches ethical reasoning by using it not to derive ethical conclusions as such but rather to explore the 'space of values', i.e. the range of often very diverse values bearing on a given situation (Fulford *et al.*, 2012, Chapter 5).

Knowledge acquisition and values-based practice are in a similar way mutually reinforcing. On the one hand, the skills of knowledge acquisition required for values-based practice are essentially the same as in any other area: they include everything from day-to-day experience through to full-on evidence-based medicine. True, retrieving knowledge of values from electronic databases requires nuanced use of search terms (Petrova *et al.*, 2011). But the skills of knowledge acquisition are essentially the same. On the other hand though, values-based practice brings to knowledge acquisition a unique slant in setting a definite limit on what can be known. In values-based practice, generalised knowledge, however reliable and complete, can never trump the actual values of a given individual in a given situation. In values-based practice then, the individual is always an '*n* of 1' (Fulford *et al.*, 2012, Chapter 6).

This is one reason why communication skills are so essential to values-based practice: if the individual is always an '*n* of 1' then the skills for eliciting values are essential if decision-making is to be based on the actual rather than imagined values in play. Another reason is the sometimes conflicting nature of values (as above) with its consequent requirement for skills of conflict resolution (Fulford *et al.*, 2012, Chapter 7).

Again though, the relationship is two-way. For what matters in practice is not communication skills as such but what they are used to communicate. In the UK, for example, medical students are taught to enquire about ideas, concerns and expectations (ICE). In practice students (and indeed more experienced clinicians) tend to focus only on the negatives. This is natural enough given that patients by definition present with 'problems'. In coming to a balanced view, however, as the basis for an effective management plan it is important to look also at the positives, at the strengths, aspirations and resources of the person concerned (National Institute for Mental Health in England (NIMHE) and the Care Services Improvement Partnership, 2008). Values-based practice then, in adding strengths, aspirations and resources to ICE, gives us ICE-StAR (Fulford *et al.*, 2012, Chapter 7).

Professional relationships in values-based practice

In the past, professional relationships in health care were predominantly doctor centred. Contemporary health care practice is characterised instead by a person-centred approach supported by multidisciplinary teamwork (see e.g. Thistlethwaite, 2012). Both of these approaches, as Figure 1.1 and Table 1.1 indicate, are important in values-based practice though in each case with a particular and distinctive edge, captured in the concepts respectively of 'person-*values*-centred care' and of the '*extended* multidisciplinary team'.

The importance of person-*values*-centred care in values-based practice follows directly from the individuality of values. If each of us is an *n* of 1, then person-centred care is nothing if it is not person-*values*-centred care. Person-centred care has a number of different meanings in modern health care: it includes genetically targeted treatments for example. The distinctive edge that values-based practice brings is to show that whatever else the 'person' in person-centred care means it must include care that is responsive to (though not of course entirely determined by) the values (positive and negative) of the person in question as a unique individual: hence the central significance of the *values* added to 'person-centred-care' in the 'person-*values*-centred care' of values-based practice (Fulford *et al.*, 2012, Chapter 8).

It is to the delivery of person-*values*-centred care that the '*extended* multidisciplinary team' of values-based practice is essential. Multidisciplinary teams bring a variety of distinct areas of knowledge and skills to the complex challenges of modern patient care. Values-based practice extends the importance of the multidisciplinary team to include also the distinct *values* of different team members. It is in this specifically *values* sense that the multidisciplinary team of values-based practice is an '*extended* multidisciplinary team'.

The extent of differences in team values is illustrated by Table 1.3. This is based on research by the British social scientist, Anthony Colombo, in which he explored the values implicit in the work of community-based multidisciplinary mental health teams (Colombo *et al.*, 2003). Asked directly, team members, from whatever professional background, will express a shared commitment to a balanced 'bio-psycho-social' perspective. In Colombo's research, however, the perspectives implicit in team members' actual working practices strongly reflected their respective professional backgrounds. Table 1.3 shows the findings for psychiatrists and social workers: psychiatrists adopted a medical perspective (the 'bio' in the 'bio-psycho-social' model) with almost no overlap at all with the psychosocial perspective of social workers.

Making such implicit differences of perspective explicit is important for communication and shared decision-making. Their full significance, however, only became apparent when Colombo went on to show that patients too showed a *similar range of perspectives* as professionals.

The extent of the similarities between the perspectives of team members and those of patients can be seen by comparing the perspectives of psychiatrists and social workers in Table 1.3 with those of the two groups of patients shown in Table 1.4. As can be seen, patients in this study divided naturally into two groups expressing respectively medical and psychosocial perspectives essentially similar to those of psychiatrists and social workers. Hence the importance of different team values – for a shared *perspective* facilitates shared *understanding*. So the different value perspectives of team members

Table 1.3 Perspectives of psychiatrists (P) and social workers (S) (shared cells highlighted)

Elements	Models – psychiatrists					Political
	Medical (organic)	Social stress	Cognitive behaviour	Psycho-therapeutic	Family (interaction)	
1 Diagnosis/description	P					
2 Interpretation of behaviour	P					
3 Labels	P					
4 Etiology	P					
5 Treatment	P					
6 Function of the hospital	P	P				P
7 Hospital and community	P					
8 Prognosis	P					
9 Rights of the patient	P					
10 Rights of society	P					
11 Duties of the patient	P		P			
12 Duties of society	P					

Elements	Models – social workers					Political
	Medical (organic)	Social stress	Cognitive behaviour	Psycho-therapeutic	Family (interaction)	
1 Diagnosis/description				S		
2 Interpretation of behaviour				S		
3 Labels				S		
4 Etiology				S		
5 Treatment		S			S	
6 Function of the hospital	S	S				S
7 Hospital and community		S		S		
8 Prognosis				S		
9 Rights of the patient	S	S				S
10 Rights of society	S					
11 Duties of the patient			S			
12 Duties of society		S				

Table 1.4 Perspectives of two groups of patients

Elements	Models – Group 1 (similar to psychiatrists)					Political
	Medical (organic)	Social stress	Cognitive behaviour	Psycho-therapeutic	Family (interaction)	
1 Diagnosis/description	Pt-Med					
2 Interpretation of behaviour			Pt-Med	Pt-Med		
3 Labels	Pt-Med					
4 Aetiology	Pt-Med					
5 Treatment	Pt-Med					
6 Function of the hospital	Pt-Med	Pt-Med				Pt-Med
7 Hospital and community		Pt-Med		Pt-Med		
8 Prognosis	Pt-Med					
9 Rights of the patient	Pt-Med					Pt-Med
10 Rights of society		Pt-Med				
11 Duties of the patient		Pt-Med	Pt-Med			
12 Duties of society	Pt-Med		Pt-Med			Pt-Med

Elements	Models – Group 2 (similar to social workers)					Political
	Medical (organic)	Social stress	Cognitive behaviour	Psycho-therapeutic	Family (interaction)	
1 Diagnosis/description				Pt-SW		
2 Interpretation of behaviour				Pt-SW		
3 Labels			Pt-SW	Pt-SW		
4 Aetiology				Pt-SW		
5 Treatment		Pt-SW		Pt-SW		
6 Function of the hospital	Pt-SW					Pt-SW
7 Hospital and community		Pt-SW		Pt-SW		
8 Prognosis				Pt-SW		
9 Rights of the patient	Pt-SW	Pt-SW				Pt-SW
10 Rights of society		Pt-SW				
11 Duties of the patient		Pt-SW	Pt-SW			
12 Duties of society		Pt-SW				Pt-SW

help to ensure that their knowledge and skills are matched more accurately to the distinct needs of individual patients, thus ensuring the delivery of care that is genuinely person-*values*-centred (Fulford *et al.*, 2012, Chapter 9).

Values-based and evidence-based practice

A common misunderstanding about values-based practice is that it is a counterbalance or (somehow) is even in opposition to evidence-based practice. Well, it is not. Values-based practice is a *partner* to evidence-based practice: it connects best evidence, derived from research and clinical experience, with the particular values, positive as well as negative, of the individual. Values-based practice, then, as the subtitle of the launch volume to this series puts it, *links science with people* (Fulford *et al.*, 2012).

Three key principles of values-based practice highlight its partnership with evidence-based practice (Figure 1.1). The first of these, the '*two feet*' principle, spells out that *all* decisions are based on facts *and* values. This was well recognised by those in the vanguard of evidence-based practice. David Sackett, for example, in his foundational book actually defined evidence-based medicine as including values. Evidence-based medicine, he wrote (Sackett *et al.*, 2000, p. 1), is about the integration of three elements: (1) the familiar best research evidence, and also (2) clinical expertise and, crucially, (3) patients' values. Values-based practice incorporates the values of all stakeholders rather than just patients. But there could hardly be a more authoritative endorsement of the need for a 'two feet' 'evidence *plus* values' approach to health care decision-making.

Values however are not always obvious: like the air we breathe we only notice values when they cause trouble. This is the point behind the second principle, the '*squeaky wheel*' principle – 'it's the squeaky wheel that' in the American saying, 'gets the grease!' But extending the metaphor, we should remember that while the wheel may not get noticed until it squeaks, it is nonetheless there all the time and that without it the vehicle would be unable to move at all. Correspondingly then, when someone has for example a cardiac arrest and the 'crash team' dives into resuscitation mode, those involved will be thinking not values but evidence – evidence-based resuscitation. This is because everyone's shared priority in this situation is effective resuscitation. In other words, effective resuscitation is the *shared value* driving everyone concerned. But the crash team does not notice this shared value driving everything they do precisely because it is a *shared* value and hence unproblematic in practice (as a shared value it is not 'squeaking', as it were).

Cardiac arrest and other acute high-tech medical interventions are emblematic of the successes of medical science. This is where the third principle linking values with evidence, the '*science driven*' principle, comes into play. It is natural to associate science with evidence: after all, the need for evidence-based medicine is driven by the growing volume of medical research and the increasingly complex and sometimes conflicting evidence-base for medicine that is thus generated. But it is science too that drives the need for values-based practice. For the impact of science in medicine is to open up new choices, and with choices go values. Reproductive medicine is a clear example of the way in which the new choices opened up by the remarkable developments in assisted fertility since the first 'test tube baby', Louise Brown, have pushed complex and conflicting values into the limelight (Fulford *et al.*, 2012, Chapter 12). The future then of medical science is not more facts and fewer values but, so the '*science driven*' principle reminds us, more facts *and more values too*.

Dissensus and partnership in values-based practice

Another common misunderstanding about values-based practice is that its open and inclusive nature means 'anything goes'. Well, again, it does not. In the first place the values-based premise of mutual respect precludes by definition values that are disrespectful – racism, paradigmatically, together with any form of discrimination, is beyond the values-based pale for this reason. The exclusion of discrimination by values-based practice was made explicit by the UK's National Institute for Mental Health (NIMH) in its National Framework of Values (National Institute for Mental Health in England, 2004; reproduced in full in Fulford, 2011).

A second and no less important reason why it is simply not true that 'anything goes' is that values-based practice, as already indicated, is about balanced decision-making *within frameworks of shared values*. The shared values in question are not 'foundational' in any absolute sense: they are contingent – agreed locally and for the time being for particular ranges or kinds of decision being made by a given group working at a particular time and within a defined context. Shared framework values then, in values-based practice, are derived by consensus: people get together and agree what values they share and what values they do not share. Decision-making *within* a given framework of shared values, however, is made rather by what in values-based practice is called *dissensus*.

With dissensus we come to the heart of partnership in values-based decision-making (Fulford *et al.*, 2012, Chapter 13). Consensus means including some values and excluding others: people, as just noted, get together and agree which values are in and which are out. Dissensus by contrast means different values remaining in play to be balanced, sometimes one way and sometimes other ways, according to the particular circumstances presented by individual decisions.

A worked example of how consensus and dissensus come together in values-based practice is provided by the way the Guiding Principles to the UK's Mental Health Act 2007 were incorporated into the training materials developed to support implementation (Care Services Improvement Partnership (CSIP) and the National Institute for Mental Health in England (NIMHE), 2008). It will be worth looking at this in a little more detail since the Act, covering as it does compulsory psychiatric treatment, is a hotspot for values-based practice if ever there was one. So if dissensus works here it should work anywhere!

Broadly, the approach adopted was that the Act is the starting point, it sets the agenda, it tells us what to do (so no 'anything goes' there); the accompanying Code of Practice gives further information about how to apply the law in general (again, very far from 'anything goes'); and the Guiding Principles (which are specified in the Code of Practice) guide us in applying the law in each individual case. The key insight from values-based practice behind this approach was to see that the Guiding Principles were in effect a *framework of shared values*. This is because the Guiding Principles had been derived by consensus (they represented the points of agreement) from an extensive and otherwise highly contentious public consultation held in the run-up to the Act. As points of agreement therefore, the Guiding Principles amounted to a framework of shared values which, since they were already incorporated in the Code of Practice, provided a framework of shared values for balanced decision-making set firmly within (note again '*not* anything goes') the specific provisions of the Act.

The Guiding Principles are represented diagrammatically in Figure 1.3 (which is taken from the training materials) as a kind of 'round table' within which, drawing on the skills

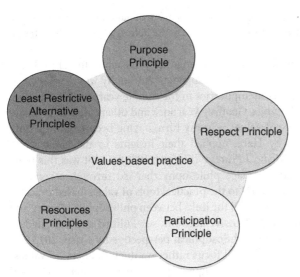

Figure 1.3 The guiding principles as a framework of shared values.

and other elements of values-based practice, balanced decisions are made. Reducing risk, for example, included under the 'purpose' Guiding Principle, has always to be balanced against, among other considerations, the Guiding Principle of enhancing 'participation' (roughly, autonomy). In the circumstances presented by a given case, the balance between risk and participation may come out one way while in other circumstances it may come out differently (worked examples are given in the training materials, see 'Further information' below). But the point is that *both* values (and by extension the values making up the round table as a whole) *remain fully in play* from one occasion to the next as a resource for balanced case-by-case decision-making. This then is *dissensus*. The Guiding Principles are not merged or selected between or subsumed one to another. Instead they remain each of them in play, thus providing collectively a framework of shared values that guides balanced decision-making in the particular circumstances presented by each successive occasion of the use of the Act.

It is perhaps worth adding that this dissensual way of working within frameworks of shared values is not unprecedented. Lord Woolf, at the time one of the UK's most senior lawyers, argued for a similar approach to human rights legislation. His point, writing as a lawyer, was that the Human Rights Act should not be understood, as it is perhaps widely understood among lawyers, as a kind of checklist of rights to be 'ticked off' individually. It should be understood rather as providing a framework of values within which balanced judgements have to be made according to the individual circumstances of each particular case (Lord Woolf, 2002).

Theory and practice

Values-based practice, although derived in part empirically (as in the study of Colombo *et al.* (2003), discussed above), is essentially a product of philosophy. The principal philosophical root of values-based practice is in a branch of analytic philosophy called 'ordinary language philosophy' or 'linguistic analysis'. Ordinary language philosophy is particularly apt for practical application in an area like health care because as its name implies it focuses on ordinary (i.e. non-philosophical) uses of language as a guide to meanings (Fulford, 1990). It focuses, that is to say, where the action is. And values-based practice is very much where the action is.

There is a direct line of descent from ordinary language philosophy to values-based practice (Fulford and van Staden, 2013). Ordinary language philosophy was developed by J. L. Austin and his (mainly) Oxford contemporaries in the middle years of the twentieth century; R. M. Hare, one of Austin's pupils, Geoffrey Warnock and others applied ordinary language philosophy to the language of values. I in my turn, having been taught by both Geoffrey and Mary Warnock and by Hare, applied their insights to the language of medicine in my *Moral Theory and Medical Practice* (Fulford, 1989); and it was this book as a theoretical exercise in ordinary language philosophy that led through a series of intermediate stages (e.g., Fulford *et al.*, 2002) to the practical tools of values-based practice.

I do not have space here to explore in detail the links between philosophical theory and values-based practice (for a more comprehensive account, see Fulford and van Staden, 2013, with a commentary from a different philosophical perspective by Crisp, 2013). In the final part of this introductory chapter I will focus rather on the influences on values-based practice of just two features of ordinary language philosophy, its methodological starting point in ordinary language use, and its self-set limitations.

Use as a guide to meaning

Ordinary language philosophy starts from the observation that for many of our higher level or more general concepts we are better at using than defining them. The concept of time is a standard philosophical example. As was first pointed out by St Augustine in his *Confessions* (Chadwick, 1992) we all *use* the concept of time without difficulty and yet if we are asked to *define* it, after a moment's reflection we find ourselves well-and-truly stumped. Lower level concepts by contrast can be defined readily enough: a watch for example is defined straightforwardly along the lines of 'a small instrument normally worn on the wrist and used for measuring time.' Notice however that this definition only works *as* a definition (it only conveys the meaning of 'watch') because without being able to *define* it we are already able to *use* the concept of time with understanding.

Ordinary language philosophy trades on our ability to use higher level concepts by adopting a 'look-and-see' methodology. Instead of sitting in a study somewhere and reflecting on the meaning of a given concept, ordinary language philosophy starts by looking at how the concept in question is actually used in a range of ordinary (i.e. non-philosophical) contexts. Austin called this quasi-empirical methodology 'philosophical field work' (cited by Warnock, 1989, p. 25). And many of the training exercises used in values-based practice, directly reflecting its origins in ordinary language philosophy, are (in all but name) exercises in philosophical field work.

The 'three words' exercise, described earlier, is a case in point. Rather than trying to define 'values', this exercise taps directly into how the concept is used by the trainees themselves. Another field-work training exercise runs thus: trainees are asked to come prepared with an example of any written material that they or others use in their day-to-day practice – this might be a letter from a doctor, for example, or a clinical practice guideline, or perhaps a statement of local policy. In the workshop, trainees are then asked to look through this written material highlighting any values-related words. Their initial reaction is usually to complain that their particular text is not 'about values' – yet by the end of the exercise, and through subsequent discussion, they find that values of many kinds, both explicit and implicit, are woven right through the very warp and weft of their chosen text.

These and similar exercises thus build directly on the importance that the Oxford School attached to our *use* of concepts. For much of the time we are generally unaware of the many values on which we draw in our work. These values are important but, to repeat my earlier analogy, like the air we breathe we only notice them when they cause difficulties. So one powerful way to open our eyes to the values influencing us, is to see how they are reflected in the language that we use for real in our everyday work.

Self-set limitations

Powerful as it may be in certain contexts, ordinary language philosophy has always been careful to set clear limits on what it can and cannot do. One clear limit is the extent of its writ. Thus, the premise of values-based practice in mutual respect, consistently with its origins in ordinary language philosophy, is a semantic and not (as such) moral premise. So this raises legitimate questions about what Thornton has called the 'prescriptive force that gives it (values-based practice) teeth' (Thornton, 2011, p. 991). To which the answer is that values-based practice makes no claims to prescriptive force. Setting itself indeed directly against the abuses of absolutism, the ambition of values-based practice is limited to the modest aim of providing a process that those concerned in a given decision on a given occasion may find helpful (especially if used in conjunction with other relevant 'tools') in coming to a balanced decision about what to do. This (to some) dangerously liberal idea carries with it the also modest (yet I believe *truly* dangerous) ambition that competing voices are (really) heard (Fulford, 2013).

Austin himself was at pains to emphasise the modest ambitions of ordinary language philosophy. On one occasion for example, he noted that while ordinary language is necessarily always the first word, it 'is *not* the last' (Warnock, 1989, p. 27, emphasis in the original). Ordinary language philosophy then, following Austin, may indeed help to give us a more complete view of the meanings of a given concept. But the view it gives has no pretensions to being a final or complete or definitive view. We saw this reflected in the 'three words' training exercise (above). This exercise is certainly effective in producing a more complete view of the meaning of 'values'. The list of words in Figure 1.3 would make an excellent contents list for a book on values. And similarly rich lists are produced by groups of any stripe, large or small, old or young, such is the power of philosophical field work. But these lists never give a final or complete or definitive account of the meaning of values. Indeed it is very much at the heart of what values-based practice is all about to eschew claims to final or complete or definitive views and the cramping orthodoxies such claims seek to justify (Fulford, 2008, 2013).

All of which is not to say that local knowledge – limited and contextual knowledge – of values is beyond us. Far from it, the importance of the skills of knowledge acquisition in values-based practice, noted earlier, directly reflects the responsiveness of values-based practice to the real rather than fancied values in play in a given situation (Fulford, 2008). Ultimately, the knowledge in question is subordinate to individual values: the individual is as I put it earlier, always an *n* of 1. This is one reason, as we have seen, why communication skills (the skills for eliciting values) are irreducible. But research knowledge too, knowledge of the *kind* of values likely to be in play in this or that *kind* of situation may be (so long as it is not allowed to trump the *n* of 1) enormously helpful in coming to understand the values that actually *are* in play – knowing what to look out for is half (though again only half) the battle.

The dependence of values-based practice on a two-way relationship with other disciplines (empirical as well as philosophical) reflects a third self-set limitation of ordinary language philosophy. Austin again, though in this instance rather more long-windedly, spelled this out: he described ordinary language philosophy as being no more than 'something about one way of possibly doing one part of philosophy' (Warnock, 1989, p. 6). So, we need other ways as well. Austin indeed, building on this point, extended the idea of philosophical field work by suggesting that philosophers might profitably team up with others with different skills sets, philosophical and, yes, empirical (Warnock, 1989, pp. 9–10). We might therefore nowadays call this 'philosophical field *team*work'.

There is much scope for Austin's philosophical field *team*work when it comes to research on values. The social and psychological sciences offer a rich range of methods as Colombo *et al.*'s (2003) study described above illustrates – this work indeed directly combined empirical social science methods with those of ordinary language philosophy (Fulford and Colombo, 2004). Other highly productive philosophical methods for studying values include phenomenology (for example, Stanghellini, 2004), hermeneutics (Widdershoven and Widdershoven-Heerding, 2003) and discursive philosophy (Sabat, 2001). A recently launched pilot study of the impact of a values-based approach to assessment in mental health, the '3 Keys Programme' (National Institute for Mental Health in England (NIMHE) and the Care Services Improvement Partnership, 2008) is using an action research paradigm to support a 'co-production' model of research. Co-production means service users having an equal voice with service providers. As a research paradigm, therefore, co-production shares with values-based practice the modest yet dangerous ambition that competing voices really *are* heard.

Conclusions

In this chapter I have set out briefly the facts about values-based practice as it has been developed to date. Derived from ordinary language philosophy via philosophical value theory applied to the language of medicine, values-based practice provides a process (no more and no less) that supports balanced clinical decision-making in individual cases within frameworks of shared values.

The process of values-based practice is based on four key areas of learnable clinical skills (awareness, reasoning, knowledge and communication skills); it depends on and in turn contributes to both person-centred care and multidisciplinary teamwork (respectively through person-*values*-centred care and the *extended* disciplinary team); it includes three distinct principles linking it with evidence-based practice (the 'two feet' principle, the 'squeaky wheel' principle, and the 'science driven' principle); and it relies on dissensus as the basis of partnership in clinical decision-making within (consensually derived) frameworks of shared values.

Values-based practice is no panacea. Consistently with the philosophical field teamwork of ordinary language philosophy, values-based practice is a partner to and works best in partnership with not only evidence-based practice but also the many other tools available to medicine for working with values: ethics and medical law, decision analysis, health economics, and the like. Each of these has its proper scope and application. The proper scope and application of values-based practice is individual values. Starting from its (semantic) premise of mutual respect and working within (locally derived) frameworks of shared values, the process of values-based practice links science (represented by evidence-based practice) with the unique values of the individual people (clinicians as well as patients) involved in particular clinical decisions.

In a period of unprecedented advances in medical science it might seem surprising that a discipline as product oriented and clinically focused as values-based practice should have its origins in philosophy and in analytic philosophy at that. Yet on inspection there is nothing surprising about this at all. For it is very much the mark of a science at the cutting edge that it should make progress not by observations alone but by observations combined with radical new ways of understanding what those observations mean – think here physics and in particular think theoretical physics. And if medicine is a science at the cutting edge it has the further complication of being a science not merely (as physics is a science) of bodies but of people. This is indeed precisely *why* values-based practice links science *with* people. Without evidence-based practice, medicine will fail to maintain its position as a science at the cutting edge. Without values-based practice, medicine risks as they say falling over onto the bleeding edge.

Further information

Further details of each of the elements of values-based practice together with extensive clinical examples covering a range of clinical areas are given in the launch volume to this series, Fulford, Peile and Carroll's (2012) *Essential Values-Based Practice: clinical stories linking science with people.* For details of the philosophical theory underpinning values-based practice see Fulford and van Staden's (2013) 'Values-based practice: topsy-turvy take home messages from ordinary language philosophy (and a few next steps)' in Fulford *et al.*'s edited collection *The Oxford Handbook of Philosophy and Psychiatry.* A website hosted jointly by Warwick Medical School and Cambridge University Press gives much further information including full text versions of many key documents such as 'Whose Values?' and the '3 Keys to a Shared Approach in Mental Health Assessment' (www.go.warwick.ac.uk/values-basedpractice or just Google 'values-based practice').

Sources and acknowledgements

Figures 1.1 and 1.2 are taken from Fulford, Peile and Carroll (2012). Figure 1.3 was first published in Fulford and Woodbridge (2008). Tables 1.2 and 1.3 are based on data from Colombo *et al.* (2003). Figure 1.4 is from Care Services Improvement Partnership (CSIP) and the National Institute for Mental Health in England (NIMHE) (2008). I am grateful to those concerned for permission to reproduce these figures here.

References

Brown, M. M., Brown, G. C. and Sharma, S. (2005) *Evidence-Based to Value-Based Medicine.* Chicago, IL: American Medical Association Press.

Care Services Improvement Partnership (CSIP) and the National Institute for Mental Health in England (NIMHE) (2008) *Workbook to Support Implementation of the*

Mental Health Act 1983 as Amended by the Mental Health Act 2007. London: Department of Health.

Chadwick, H. (1992) *St Augustine Confessions* (translation). Oxford: Oxford University Press.

Colombo, A., Bendelow, G., Fulford, K. W. M. and Williams, S. (2003) Evaluating the influence of implicit models of mental disorder on processes of shared decision making within community-based multi-disciplinary teams. *Social Science & Medicine*, **56**, 1557–1570.

Crisp, R. (2013) Commentary: values-based practice by a different route. In Fulford, K. W. M., Davies, M., Gipps, R., Graham, G., Sadler, J., Stanghellini, G., and Thornton, T. (editors), *The Oxford Handbook of Philosophy and Psychiatry*, pp. 411–412. Oxford: Oxford University Press.

Fulford, K. W. M. (1989, reprinted 1995 and 1999) *Moral Theory and Medical Practice*. Cambridge: Cambridge University Press.

Fulford, K. W. M. (1990) Philosophy and medicine: the Oxford connection. *British Journal of Psychiatry*, **157**, 111–115.

Fulford, K. W. M. (2008) Values-based practice: from the real to the really practical. In Thornton, T. (editor), special issue on evidence-based and values-based practice. *Philosophy, Psychiatry and Psychology*, **15**(2), 183–185.

Fulford, K. W. M. (2011) The value of evidence and evidence of values: bringing together values-based and evidence based practice in policy & service development in mental health. *Journal of Evaluation in Clinical Practice*, **17**(5), 976–987.

Fulford, K. W. M. (2013) Values-based practice: Fulford's dangerous idea. *Journal of Evaluation in Clinical Practice*, **19**(3), 537–546.

Fulford, K. W. M. and Colombo, A. (2004) Six models of mental disorder: a study combining linguistic-analytic and empirical methods. *Philosophy, Psychiatry and Psychology*, **11**(2), 129–144.

Fulford, K. W. M. and van Staden, W. (2013) Values-based practice: topsy-turvy take home messages from ordinary language philosophy (and a few next steps). In Fulford, K. W. M., Davies, M., Gipps, R., Graham, G., Sadler, J., Stanghellini, G. and Thornton, T. (editors), *The Oxford Handbook of Philosophy and Psychiatry*, Chapter 26, pp. 385–412. Oxford: Oxford University Press.

Fulford, K. W. M. and Woodbridge, K. (2008) Practising ethically: values-based practice and ethics: working together to support person-centred and multidisciplinary mental health care. In Stickley, T. and Basset, T. (editors), *Learning About Mental Health Practice*, Chapter 5, pp. 145–160. John Wiley & Sons.

Fulford, K. W. M., Dickenson, D. and Murray, T. H. (editors) (2002) *Healthcare Ethics and Human Values: An Introductory Text with Readings and Case Studies*. Oxford: Blackwell Publishers.

Fulford, K. W. M., Stanghellini, G. and Broome, M. (2004) What can philosophy do for psychiatry? Special article. *World Psychiatry (WPA)*, October, 130–135.

Fulford, K. W. M., Peile, E. and Carroll, H. (2012) *Essential Values-Based Practice: clinical stories linking science with people*. Cambridge: Cambridge University Press.

Hunink, M., Glasziou, P., Siegel, J. *et al.* (2001) *Decision Making in Health and Medicine: Integrating Evidence and Values*. Cambridge: Cambridge University Press.

National Institute for Mental Health in England (2004) *The National Framework of Values for Mental Health*. London: Department of Health. (Reproduced in full in Woodbridge and Fulford, 2004, and in Fulford, 2011.)

National Institute for Mental Health in England (NIMHE) and the Care Services Improvement Partnership (2008) *3 Keys to a Shared Approach in Mental Health Assessment*. London: Department of Health.

Petrova, M., Sutcliffe, P., Fulford, K. W. M. and Dale, J. (2011) Search terms and a validated brief search filter to retrieve publications on health-related values in Medline: a word frequency analysis study. *Journal of the American Medical Informatics Association*, doi:10.1136/amiajnl-2011-000243.

Sabat, S. R. (2001) *The Experience of Alzheimer's Disease: Life Through a Tangled Veil*. Oxford: Blackwell Publishers.

Sackett, D. L., Straus, S. E., Scott Richardson, W., Rosenberg, W., and Haynes, R. B. (2000) *Evidence-Based Medicine: How to Practice and Teach EBM*, 2nd edition. Edinburgh: Churchill Livingstone.

Stanghellini, G. (2004) *Deanimated Bodies and Disembodied Spirits. Essays on the psychopathology of common sense*. Oxford: Oxford University Press.

Thistlethwaite, J. E. (2012) *Values-Based Interprofessional Collaborative Care: Working Together in Healthcare*. Cambridge: Cambridge University Press.

Thornton, T. (2011) Radical, liberal values-based practice. *Journal of Evaluation in Clinical Practice*, **17**, 988–991.

Warnock, G. J. (1989) *J. L. Austin*. London: Routledge.

Widdershoven, G. and Widdershoven-Heerding, I. (2003) Understanding dementia: a hermeneutic perspective. In Fulford, K. W. M., Morris, K. J., Sadler, J. Z. and Stanghellini, G. (editors), *Nature and Narrative: An Introduction to the New Philosophy of Psychiatry*, Chapter 6, pp. 103–112. Oxford: Oxford University Press.

Woolf, L. (2002) *Lecture to the British Academy*, 15 October 2002, quoted in Hansard 28/10/2002 col 607.

Woodbridge, K., and Fulford, K. W. M. (2004) *Whose Values? A workbook for values-based practice in mental health care*. London: Sainsbury Centre for Mental Health.

Values-based clinical reasoning

Ed Peile

Introduction

This chapter is written by a non-philosopher. I approach the debate from a pragmatic standpoint. I am a doctor and a medical educationalist. For me, values-based practice (VBP) stands or falls on its usefulness. In the clinical consultation between doctor and patient, does VBP improve the patient experience of health care? If the answer to this question is more positive than negative, then VBP is here to stay, and needs our best efforts to improve both concept and application.

Clinical decision-making and *clinical* reasoning are contextualised by their descriptor term. What difference does the clinical context make? We need first to understand what distinguishes a clinical decision from, for example, a military decision? Why is clinical reasoning any different from the reasoning we conduct as we consider the on-line purchasing options for a particular commodity? *Essential Values-Based Practice* makes clear that 'Actions in a clinical context are guided not only by evidence, *but also by values*. Clinical decisions thus stand on two-feet' (Fulford *et al.*, 2012, p. 8). It is thus important to consider the 'two feet principle', which is axiomatic in the case for the utility of values-based practice in medicine. Whereas, arguably, any decision involves some, usually inexplicit, consideration of evidence and values, it is the professional obligation to consider explicitly both the relevant scientific evidence and the values of the individual patient that distinguishes clinical reasoning.

Clinical reasoning has been intensely researched over the past forty years. The research endeavour has been of particular interest to medical educators, such as myself. If we can understand what goes on in the black box of clinical reasoning, chances are we will be able

Debates in Values-Based Practice, ed. Michael Loughlin. Published by Cambridge University Press. © Cambridge University Press 2014.

to differentiate between effective and ineffective reasoning, and what is more teach the essentials to novices and improvers in the clinical professions, thereby accruing benefit for patients. So runs the argument. The briefest consideration will expose some of the complexities that have been glossed over. What determines whether reasoning is effective? If reasoning is not only context specific but also case specific, might it not also be specific to the individual reasoner, and thereby defy attempts to deconstruct and generalise? What does patient benefit look like? Whilst the more philosophical questions are too ambitious for me to attempt in this chapter, I see a necessity to conduct a brief historical review of research into clinical reasoning, looking at the implications for values-based clinical reasoning.

Central to the chapter is a closer inspection of how values relate to reasoning. This begins with a look at how principles reasoning can be combined with case-based reasoning in the clinical setting to yield a values-based reasoning process. Moving to clinical decision-making, an attempt to elucidate what a 'good' decision looks like seems inescapable if we are to avoid uninterrupted circular arguments.

I move on to look more closely at the arena of clinical reasoning, looking at how both evidence and values are pertinent not only to a consideration of possible treatment options but also to diagnosis, and indeed the whole clinical encounter including the ways in which we 'take a history', 'conduct a clinical examination', or 'order investigations'. At the centre of the argument is the patient. If values-based practice confers no patient benefit, then the debate on VBP is lost to those who argue against it. Patient-centredness is a difficult concept to pin down. Following a brief review of some writing on the topic, I introduce the concept of person-values-centred practice.

Analysis of VBP process elements demonstrates that values-based reasoning is inextricably linked to values-awareness and values-communication skills, for example. In the penultimate section, I return to the implications for medical education, which discipline I see (unsurprisingly) as crucial in the transition from theoretical research to advancing clinical practice.

The chapter concludes by looking at how clinical reasoning which adopts the 'two feet principle' can lead to balanced decision-making within a shared framework of values.

Clinical reasoning and clinical decision-making

'Clinical reasoning describes the cognitive processes that *clinicians* use to understand the significance of patient data, to identify and diagnose actual patient problems, to make clinical decisions to assist in problem resolution and to achieve positive patient outcomes' (Fonteyn and Ritter, 2008, p. 236). I substituted the word '*clinicians*' here – it read '*nurses*' in the original. The point is made that I, writing from my medical background, only feel qualified to discuss clinical reasoning from a doctor's and patient's viewpoint, yet I emphasise at the outset that clinical reasoning applies to all clinicians (Higgs *et al.*, 2008).

In what way does the 'clinic' semantic qualifier affect reasoning and decision-making processes? What does the 'clinic' context convey? (The locus 'clinic' throughout this chapter is intended to include not only clinics – surgeries (UK), physicians' offices (USA), but also wards, theatres and operating rooms, emergency departments and patients' homes.) The most important aspect is that the clinical context includes one or more patients. The reasoning is about the patient(s) and the decisions are about the patient(s). This can be expanded to affirm that, ideally, clinical decisions are made for, with, and about the patient(s).

Already, there are multiple axes to consider regarding the forms of reasoning which take place in a clinical consultation. The power dimension, for example, concerns the locus of control which may be situated anywhere on a spectrum from paternalistic doctoring to a patient-knows-best assumption. Related to this are other considerations around autonomy, as the clinical encounter includes reasoning and decision-making where the patient is unconscious, deemed to have no capacity to make personal decisions, or under-age. There are particular sets of stakeholders in decisions about an individual's health: as well as patient and clinician, others such as parents, carers and loved-ones may have legitimate interests, as may the clinician's colleagues (in respect of equity, workload, policy observance and mutual support), the community (in respect of public health dimensions), health managers and politicians (in respect of resource management). The clinician wanting to practise in a values-based way must take account of all of the values of all these stakeholders in different consultations. This is over and above the normal considerations of societal ethos and ecological responsibility.

Contrast the clinical context with, say, the military context and the commercial context for reasoning and decision-making. Considerations of whether and how to mount an attack, or which product to purchase, likewise involve the interests of many stakeholders. They are also multi-dimensional in reasoning processes, with the pragmatics needing to be balanced against ethical considerations. What makes clinical reasoning different is the requirement to address the needs of the individual patient in that particular situation – '*In whatever house where I come I will enter only for the good of my patients*' (Hippocrates) – and simultaneously to balance in the decision-making the interests of community and society in ways which are tightly prescribed by professional rules. A degree of altruism is expected of doctors in their clinical decision-making, but this is not a complete distinction as self-sacrificing bravery may be involved in a military decision. It is really that serving the interests of the individual patient is something of an end-in-itself. Even within clinical practice, however, the balance is changing. Perhaps the most significant change in clinical practice in the early years of this millennium has been the encouragement, and indeed requirement, that doctors and other clinicians increase their attention to public and community health and to equitable use of finite service resources in clinical decision-making. There is a cost. No longer can the doctor reassure the patient that 'you are my sole consideration'. This may never have been a truth, but it is less true now than fifty years ago. The demography of a population living longer, the availability of more potent and more expensive remedies, and the consequent resource pressures have impacted on health delivery in different systems around the world. As a consequence, the relationship between doctor and patient has changed significantly. The doctor's dedication of time and personal attention to the patient engendered reciprocal love and respect by way of reward. As the format of the caritas has changed to become more technical-rational, team-based, and time-limited so this tacit contract has changed. Patients, aware of the doctor's duty to ration treatment and to promote treatments (like immunisation for herd immunity) on the basis of achieving the greatest good for the greatest number, are not unreasonably more suspicious about the extent to which their own individual interests will be advanced in their consultation.

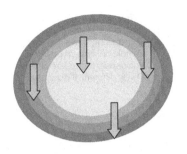

Figure 2.1 Acquiring information for clinical decision-making: expanding the sphere of what is known about the patient's problem.

• History

• Examination

• Investigation

What happens in a typical consultation? Of course there is no such thing as a typical consultation – even meeting the banal request for relief of cough or sore throat results in a completely different consultation every time as the particular circumstances are weighed up. I cannot think of two identical consultations in the twenty-five thousand I must have conducted. There are, however, some common elements.

The first step usually involves assembling the necessary management information. History-taking describes the communication skill of eliciting all the relevant information in the patient narrative. Clinical examination begins with noting the patient's demeanour and extends in many cases to personal and intimate 'laying on of hands' to prod and poke, listen and inspect, using craft-based techniques. There are cultural differences even at this stage. French internal medicine practitioners will place more reliance on physical examination and less on history-taking than their British counterparts. Further investigation may be required by way of blood or urine tests or radiographic imaging. Graphically, the expanding sphere of knowledge is illustrated in Figure 2.1.

The initial purpose of acquiring the information is to achieve diagnosis, being discernment of the condition. The word derives from Greek διά (meaning apart) and γιγνώσκειν (meaning perceive). A Babylonian *Diagnostic Handbook*, written more than a thousand years before Christ, describes diagnosis of disease based on empiricism, logic and rationality (Horstmanshoff *et al.*, 2004).

Medical students are taught that diagnosis precedes management. This is not the case in some 50% of consultations in General Practice (Heneghan *et al.*, 2009). 'Gut feelings' have been described as a non-analytic processing of the available information promoting action as the GP perceives 'something to be wrong' (Stolper *et al.*, 2011). Alertness to turbulence in the smooth flow of information is recognised as an expert skill (Balla *et al.*, 2012).

Thus a model of clinical reasoning has to take account of the fact that progression towards an acceptable diagnosis and progression towards an acceptable management decision may proceed simultaneously or independently. I conceive this as a 'squaring down process' with the two halves of the square (Figure 2.2 and Figure 2.3) coming together.

Both foci of clinical reasoning (diagnosis and management) involve iterative reference to scientific knowledge (the evidence-base) and to the values at play in the individual situation (the values-base).

Evidence and values can be seen as the two forces driving refinement and selection of differential diagnosis and management possibilities. This is represented in Figure 2.4.

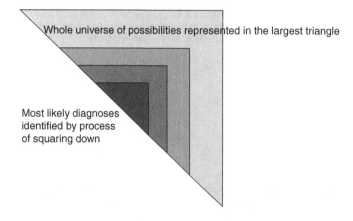

Figure 2.2 The clinician's frame: diagnosis as a process of squaring down from the whole universe of possible diagnoses to those retained as likely differential diagnoses.

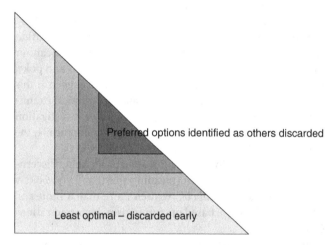

Figure 2.3 The clinician's frame: management options refine as the least optimal ones are discarded in the process of squaring down.

Two feet principle

Thus, evidence and values form the two feet on which clinical decision-making is based. The two feet principle (Fulford *et al.*, 2012) emphasises that professional judgement is a matter of ascertaining as much as possible of the relevant information about the values and the scientific evidence pertinent to the particular situation of that individual patient's situation and weighing that up in respect of decisions about the differential diagnosis and the management options, as represented in Figure 2.5.

The premise of the two feet principle is that the best clinical decisions are based both on the best available scientific evidence and on the values relevant to the individual patient situation. In the words of Sackett *et al.* (2000), 'By *patient values* we mean the unique preferences, concerns and expectations each patient brings to a clinical encounter and which must be integrated into clinical decisions if they are to serve the patient.' 'When these three elements (best evidence, clinical experience and patient values) are integrated,

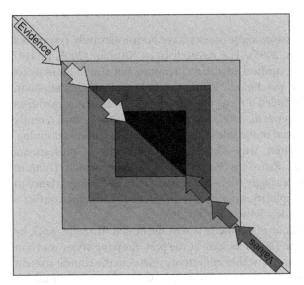

Figure 2.4 Forces at work on refinement and selection: evidence and values driving the squaring down process.

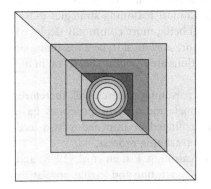

Figure 2.5 The round peg in the square hole: a basis for balanced clinical decision-making.

Where does it fit?
=
Professional
Judgement

clinicians and patients form a diagnostic and therapeutic alliance which optimises clinical outcomes and quality of life.'

The relevance of values to management options is not difficult to appreciate. The clinician debating the merits of cancer treatments or therapeutic approaches to depression can seldom if ever conduct an effective reasoning and decision-making process in ignorance of the pertinent patient values. By contrast, it may be less obvious why diagnosis is likewise a clinical decision resting on the 'two feet principle'. It may be tempting to consider that clinical processes to determine, for example, whether a breathless patient has pneumonia or restrictive lung disease, or a feverish child with a rash has measles or chickenpox, can take place in a values-free zone. Not so: in the first case there are issues of occupation and hobby to consider, which though fact based are value laden in the implications. In the second case there could be issues about missed vaccination, which may be guilt associated for the carer. We will return to this topic later.

History of clinical reasoning

Over the past forty years, clinical reasoning processes have been intensively researched (Dowie and Elstein, 1988; Norman, 2005). The research is, as Norman (2005, p. 418) identifies, to be found mainly in the medical education literature, but also in journals on sociology and cognitive and clinical psychology. Whilst psychological research attention (Elstein and Bordage, 1988) has included a focus on matters such as semantic qualifiers (Bordage and Lemieux, 1991; Bordage *et al.*, 1997; Norman and Eva, 2003), until recently there has been very little attention paid to the role of the values-base in clinical reasoning. A notable exception is Donald Schön, who addressed the generality of professional reasoning in his seminal book *The Reflective Practitioner: How Professionals Think in Action* (Schön, 1983). He said, 'Increasingly we have become aware of the importance to actual practice of phenomena – complexity, uncertainty, uniqueness, and value-conflict – which do not fit the model of Technical Rationality' (p. 39).

The point that Schön makes about phenomena is well illustrated in recent work by Sladek *et al.* (2008) and Stolper *et al.* (2011) looking at the part 'thinking styles' and 'gut feelings' play in clinical reasoning, and how this subjectivity relates to the clinical content of consultations. Research goes some way to explaining how this happens. Problems perceived by doctors to be somatic focus their attention more on the disease than on the person, whereas the converse is true if their immediate characterisation is that the problem is a psychosocial one (Andre *et al.*, 2012). Clinical reasoning strategies differ, with immediate, intuitive reasoning (type 1 reasoning) being more commonly deployed for somatic conditions, whereas the doctor becomes more analytical (type 2 reasoning) if psychosocial or mixed psychosocial and somatic conditions are recognised early on in the consultation (Andre *et al.*, 2012).

My perspective in reviewing the history of clinical reasoning research will, therefore, be on how, as the models based on cognitive, rational, and analytic processes have advanced, the prevalent thinking is likely to have facilitated or impeded a 'two feet' approach incorporating values-basing into the clinical reasoning process.

Early research focused on hypothetico-deductive reasoning. Elstein *et al.* (1978) and Barrows *et al.* (1982) elaborated a process of hypothesis generation and testing, consisting of five basic stages:

(1) identification of the clinical information that is relevant to diagnosis;
(2) interpretation of its meaning;
(3) generation of hypotheses which provide a coherent explanation of the patient's problem;
(4) testing and refining of those hypotheses through further data collection;
(5) establishment of a working diagnosis.

As far as values-based practice is concerned, everything turns on the middle step of hypothesis generation. If the first two steps include skilled assimilation of values data, then the scope for hypothesis generation and testing could transcend the level of assumptions and guesswork which are not conducive to VBP.

Researchers turned away from hypothetico-deductive reasoning because the determinant of success was the content knowledge of the clinician problem-solver and success in problem-solving was very 'content specific', meaning that success on one problem did not predict success on another. That the content knowledge was testable in this way indicates to me that knowledge of values was not an important component in this early research.

Norman (2005) relates that researchers moved on to study expert recall of patient data in the next phase of research into clinical reasoning. It soon emerged that it was difficult to relate 'success' in clinical reasoning to the amount of knowledge that experts could recall, and researchers moved on to look at the kinds of knowledge that experts stored and how they stored and retrieved it – what Norman calls the 'mental representations'. This appears to open up scope for values-based practice to contribute to the efficacy of clinical reasoning. If values dimensions are contextualising cases in ways that assist knowledge retrieval and knowledge organisation, then the case for values strengthens. But is there any evidence of this? Limiting their synthesis to cognitive research, Schmidt et al. (1990) constructed a stage theory of clinical reasoning which posited that experienced physicians operate on knowledge structures called 'illness scripts' which emerge from continuous exposure to patients. They describe these 'illness scripts' as containing 'relatively little knowledge about patho-physiological causes of symptoms but a wealth of clinically relevant information about disease, its consequences, and the context in which it develops.' They go on to say that these scripts range from representations of categories of disease to 'representations of individual patients seen before'. They emphasise their 'presupposition' that physicians actually use the memories of previous patients while diagnosing a new case (Schmidt et al. 1990, p. 613).

With a focus on the individual patient and on the content of disease, it is tempting to infer that 'illness scripting' incorporates values-based practice into the clinical reasoning process. I think we need to be cautious about this. Although the focus on the individual is encouraging, the process of referencing one patient to another is contrary to much of the process of values awareness, which acknowledges the uniqueness of each individual's values set (Fulford et al., 2012). Subsequent work by Schmidt and Rikers (2007) examined in more detail the encapsulation of 'illness scripts', but did not focus on relevance of values dimensions.

Building on the schemata of 'illness scripts', a form of scheme-inductive reasoning has been described, whereby the clinical problem-solver works to dichotomous decision points (does it fit into this category or that category?). Using such 'chunking' propositions can be an effective strategy in excluding conditions to the point of likely diagnosis (Coderre et al., 2003). I see scheme-induction as antithetical to values-based processes. 'If you are not this, then you must be that', simply does not work for the complexity of human values.

Research advanced with techniques such as script concordance tests (Sibert et al., 2002; Charlin and van der Vleuten, 2004; Bland et al., 2005), and key features and feature lists (Page et al., 1995; Kulatunga-Moruzi et al., 2004); and think-aloud protocols (Patel et al., 1986; Boshuizen and Schmidt, 1992). It was the work with think-aloud protocols that drew attention to the importance of pattern recognition in clinical reasoning. Pattern recognition supposes that clinicians structure and store their knowledge in such a way that they can quickly 'match' previous examples to cues in a new clinical situation. Pattern recognition is thus a non-analytic form of reasoning. It is widely used by experts and novices alike (Coderre et al., 2003). They differ in the patterns they recognise, and there is a concern that novices may recognise an irrelevant pattern connecting cases, for example, 'they are both red-heads' instead of 'they both had crushing central chest pain'. However, Brooks et al. (1991) demonstrated progressive pattern recognition in dermatology as students saw more cases, and this has been amplified in later work (Norman *et al.*, 2007). Training in pattern recognition can be tracked and assessed (Dunn and Woolliscroft, 1997).

The impact on values-based practice of clinicians developing accuracy in pattern recognition has not been tested formally. I can see both positive and negative implications for values awareness. On the positive side, awareness benefits from a deep focus on what makes people different. On the negative side, patterns are a form of generalisation – this person had one set of beliefs and preferences, so it is likely that the other person who is in a similar situation will have the same set of beliefs and preferences. An example arose after I had asked a medical student to take a history from a man with prostate cancer. When I questioned the student afterwards, our dialogue went like this:

Tutor: Did the patient have any concerns about how treatment might affect his sexual function?

Student: Oh, patients with prostate cancer don't worry about sexual function.

Tutor: How do you know?

Student: Well, we saw a patient last week, and he said that was the last of his worries.

Eva (2004) advanced the case for a combined model of clinical reasoning wherein 'the analytic and non-analytic models are combined to interact with both the mental representation of the case being presented and the hypotheses that are raised, but to different degrees depending on the context' (Eva, 2004, p. 102).

Reasoning and values

Clinical reasoning within the consultation may or may not be concerned with achieving accurate diagnosis, which is the gold standard of much of the research discussed above. Indeed, reasoning may or may not concern formal treatment options. Many consultations are fundamentally more about reassurance or the relief of distress, than reasoning through to precise diagnosis or a defined treatment plan. Reasoning tasks depend on the clinical role. Marinker (1994) characterised the diagnostic task of the specialist as 'to reduce uncertainty, to explore possibility and to marginalise error.' This he contrasted with the diagnostic task of the general practitioner which he perceived as 'to accept uncertainty, to explore probability and to marginalise danger.'

It takes two (or more) to consult. Patients vary widely in their expectations of the clinical consultation. Some want full participation, and may indeed start from a position of technical expertise in the micro-domain of their condition that exceeds that of the professional. Others want to devolve the clinical decisions to their trusted clinician, and to avoid the onus of choice. As values-based practice is premised on a mutual respect for the diversity of values, clinicians need to develop the skills to ascertain patient values and to get in touch with their own beliefs and preferences in order to understand those at play in any consultation. Then they need to apply the skills of values-reasoning. Only then can balanced decision-making processes take place within a shared framework of values.

The philosophical basis of values-based practice is explored in detail elsewhere in this volume (Chapter 1), and here it is important only to recognise that the 'prescriptive' nature of values (Hare, 1952) founds our recognition that values are 'action-guiding' alongside evidence (Fulford *et al.*, 2012).

Two types of reasoning are commonly mentioned in respect of clinical decision-making. The first is principles reasoning, and here the exemplar is that expounded by Beauchamp and Childress (1994). So widely taught is the *Principles of Biomedical Ethics* that it would be difficult to find a doctor who graduated in the UK in the past 10–20 years who is not at least familiar with the concepts of autonomy, beneficence, non-maleficence and justice. It is important, however, to remember that elucidation of principles which encompass the ethical dimensions of dilemmas in clinical practice, and encouragement to base reasoning upon these principles, does not assure good process or good outcome. As Limentani (1999) points out, principles are not a complete or self-standing means of establishing ethical practice. In the words of Beauchamp and Childress (1994, p. 67), 'Principles guide us to actions, but we still need to assess a situation and formulate an appropriate response'. Protagonists and antagonists of *Principles of Biomedical Ethics* agree on the absence of 'explicit decision rules' (Gillon, 1995; Holm, 1995). Decision rules are not the answer. Values are too complex for algorithms. The reasoning process recommended in *Essentials of Values-Based Practice* combines principles-based reasoning with case-based reasoning, or casuistry (Fulford *et al.*, 2012). (See also Chapter 19.)

The clinician is encouraged to reflect on 'In what way is this case similar to or different from other cases I have seen?' before asking 'Does this change the way I think about this case?' We can see how this fits into the frameworks of clinical reasoning defined by researchers. Non-analytical problem recognition is important for case-based reasoning, as is a structure for mental representations around values issues. In situations where values are complex or conflicting, scheme inductive reasoning around ethical principles is a vital component, as is reference to the professional codes and decision rules.

Clinical decision-making: what does a 'good' decision look like?

As clinical decision-making is the objective of clinical reasoning, it is important to understand criteria for judging clinical decisions. Firstly, decisions can only be judged with regard to the time the decision is made. Bearing in mind that the best decision may have the worst outcome, we need not to be blinded by outcomes in judging processes through the retrospectoscope. Were the right steps taken to obtain the appropriate amount of evidence (about science and about values)? Was a shared framework of values constructed (tacitly or explicitly)? Were proper processes used to balance the decision-making?

There is much that is subjective in these questions as framed, and indeed those who wish to examine the quality of clinical decision-making need constantly to remind themselves that it is doubtful whether there is such a thing as the 'right' outcome. Every time we are faced with league tables, based on measuring the measurable of operative deaths or trolley waits, we need to ask ourselves, 'What is important, but not measured here?' More often than not, in my experience, the answer concerns a values dimension. Whitney *et al.* (2004) designed a typology that covers the spectrum between shared decision-making, informed consent and simple consent.

Jack Dowie, who is an advocate of the analytic hierarchy process for shared decision-making (Dolan, 2008), has spent a professional lifetime looking at clinical decision analysis (Dowie and Elstein, 1988). In contemporary presentations (e.g. Dowie, 2009) he discusses his recent analyses of decision-making where he introduces modern forms of analysis (analysia) that balance beliefs (evidence) with preferences (values).

Values and evidence

Earlier in this chapter I referred to the two feet principle as the view that values and evidence act as the two feet on which sound clinical decision-making is based. I want now to look at the interaction between evidence and values in more detail. Firstly, it is important to clarify that the terms are not mutually exclusive. There is an evidence-base around values. Petrova (2012) has elucidated processes for searching electronic databases for references to values in health care. Likewise, the scientific evidence-base relevant to a particular clinical problem may be value laden: particularly in psychosomatic domains, for example, the doctor may wish to access information about coping mechanisms to help in determining appropriate management options.

The scientific database for medicine contains only a very small proportion of qualitative explanatory research in comparison to the vast preponderance of empirical quantitative research (Gagliardi and Dobrow, 2011). This highlights one of the major epistemological differences between the scientific evidence implicit in evidence-based practice and the values of values-based practice. The former is usually derived from population studies; the latter always concerns the individual, hence why Sackett *et al.* (2000) talk about the 'the unique preferences, concerns and expectations of the patient'.

Diagnosis is not a values-free domain. 'To an unprejudiced eye, pathology – mental or physical – is an evaluative notion' (Chapter 4). Consider the alternative value-laden diagnoses which the doctor may offer to a patient, shown in Table 2.1.

In terms of treatment, a very clear example of how population evidence and individual values must interact in clinical decision-making is contained in the statement put out by the Royal College of Obstetricians and Gynaecologists (2011) commenting on the draft guidance issued by the National Institute for Health and Care Excellence on Caesarean sections (Box 2.1). Note the last line, implying that sometimes individual patient values must be given more weight than scientific evidence.

Table 2.1 Which diagnosis best fits with the values at play in this particular consultation?

Depressed?	or	Stressed?
Obese?	or	Overweight?
Dying?	or	Seriously ill?
ME (myalgic encephalomyelitis)	or	Post-viral syndrome

Box 2.1 RCOG statement on draft NICE Caesarean section guidelines (2011)

C-sections are a safe medical procedure but as with any intervention, there are risks involved. All doctors must ensure that women are informed about the risks and/or benefits of procedures undertaken and the alternative options. Women must have access to good quality information so that they can make informed decisions.

There are well defined *indications* for Caesarean section for both elective and emergency and these should form the basis of clinical practice.

Health care providers have the *responsibility* to ensure the safest, most cost-effective method of delivery for women and babies accepting that very occasionally women will request an elective C-section in the absence of conventional obstetric indications.

Patient centredness

Since McWhinney (1989) developed the concept of patient centredness, which had been introduced by his group three years earlier (Levenstein *et al.*, 1986), much has been written on the topic, particularly in respect of family practice. Elwyn *et al.* (2000) defined the competences of involving patients and Dolan (2008) described a framework called the analytic hierarchy process intended to promote shared decision-making and enhance communication in the consultation. Duggan *et al.* (2006) analysed key concepts of patient centredness in terms of consequentialist, deontological and virtue-based ethical theories, concluding that moral value was demonstrated in each.

Donald Berwick proposed a definition of 'patient-centred care':

> The experience (to the extent the informed, individual patient desires it) of transparency, individualization, recognition, respect, dignity, and choice in all matters, without exception, related to one's person, circumstances, and relationships in health care. (Berwick, 2009, p. 559)

Mead and Bower (2002) identified five 'conceptual dimensions' of patient centredness. In their terms, a patient-centred consultation has a biopsychological perspective, it involves sharing power and responsibility, and it builds a therapeutic alliance between patient and doctor. The other two dimensions concern the individual consulters: the patient-as-a-person dimension involves understanding the individual's experience of illness, whereas the doctor-as-a-person dimension considers the contribution that the individual doctor makes to the relationship.

The contribution of values-based practice is to develop person centredness in situations where there is potential conflict between patient values and clinician values (Fulford *et al.*, 2012). The premise of mutual respect when combined with a shared aim of balanced decision-making (through dissensus-based partnership) is fundamental to patient-values-centred practice. The inclusion of the values word here is important. It indicates that by centring on values and working with processes that admit of dissensus, one can avoid the *Scylla* danger of doctor paternalism and the *Charybdis* peril of abdicating professional responsibility to 'patient choice'.

Balanced decision-making implies that there is a balance between the weighting given to scientific evidence and the weighting given to values in the decision-making process, and also that values of clinician, patient and other stakeholders are fairly balanced. Venkatapuram (2011) in his exploration *Health Justice* demonstrates that such balance is not easy on a global scale. Heginbotham (2012) likewise demonstrates some of the difficulties of clinical decision-making within any single health economy in respect of resource allocation.

Values-based practice elements relevant to clinical reasoning

Throughout this chapter I have mentioned VBP elements which have relevance to clinical reasoning. Table 2.2 lists the elements in the order in which they are discussed by Fulford *et al.* (2012).

The way in which these elements build on the basic VBP premise of 'mutual respect for the diversity of values', in the drive to achieve the point (aim) of 'balanced decision-making within a shared framework of values' is illustrated in Figure 2.6.

Table 2.2 Relevance of VBP elements to clinical reasoning

1. Awareness of values	Clinicians need to be aware of their own values as well as the patient values at play in the particular consultation
2. Reasoning about values	A combination of principles reasoning and case-based reasoning is most likely to be effective when values are complex and conflicting
3. Knowledge about values	Clinicians who have extended their knowledge and understanding of values-science are better skilled to incorporate values in clinical decision-making
4. Values communication skills	Eliciting information about patient strengths, ambitions and resources, in addition to their ideas, concerns and expectations, helps to inform clinical reasoning
5. Person-*values*-centred practice	Patient centricity involves complex balancing acts if clinicians are to avoid both paternalism and abdication of professional responsibility; values-centricity helps
6. Extended multidisciplinary team	Involving colleagues, not just for their professional skills but also for their values-perspectives, helps to broaden the base for values-based reasoning
7. The two feet principle	The best clinical decisions rest on the 'two feet' of evidence-based practice (EBP) and values-based practice (VBP)
8. The squeaky wheel principle	In balanced clinical reasoning, the noise of a squeaky wheel (an important values element demanding attention) must not divert attention from all other evidence
9. The science driven principle	Clinical reasoning takes place in a high-technology environment where scientific advances change the values dimensions for clinical decision-making
10. Partnership in decision-making	Whereas it is possible to work towards consensus in respect of the implications of scientific evidence, clinical reasoning sometimes requires dissensus around values

Clinical education

The best clinical decisions are based on both evidence and values. Anecdotally, educationalists find that teaching clinicians to become more evidence based is relatively simple in comparison to encouraging them to become more values based. One reason is likely to be the importance of values awareness.

Kevin Eva (2004) is sceptical about any '. . .fundamental belief that causal rules linking features (e.g. signs and symptoms) to categories (e.g. diagnoses) can be extracted from the world and that the development of expertise in clinical reasoning consists of the elaboration of rules that become more and more attuned to reality' (p. 100). Later, he claims that a growing body of evidence suggests that 'various diagnostic strategies identified in the literature on clinical reasoning are not mutually exclusive and that trainees can benefit from explicit guidance regarding the value of both analytic and non-analytic reasoning tendencies' (Eva *et al.*, 2007, p. 1152). Thus educationalists wishing to advance clinical reasoning skills have to focus on developing both technical-rational skills and professional artistry in medical learners. Norman *et al.* (2007) emphasise the interaction between dichotomised elements: 'Non-analytic reasoning is a central component of diagnostic expertise at all levels. Clinical teaching should recognise the centrality of this process, and aim to both enhance the process through the learning of multiple examples and to supplement the process with analytical de-biasing strategies' (p. 1140).

Learning and teaching values-based practice varies with the experience of the learner. Those with extensive clinical experience generally find that exploring complex examples of clinical decision-making from their own practice leads to an enthusiasm for developing

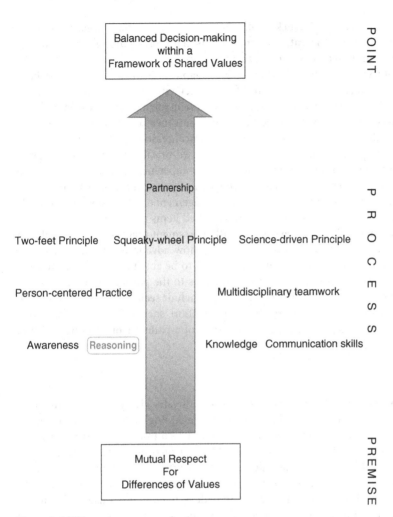

Figure 2.6 VBP premise, process and point.

further their clinical skills (e.g. communication, reasoning, and partnership-working) by implementing the processes of values-based practice. Novices, by contrast, have the opportunity to learn the extended skills *ab initio*. As soon as they start working with patients and simulated patients, they can be guided to look for the values dimensions. As they develop their understanding of evidence-based practice, ethics, and legal and professional frameworks, they put into use VBP processes so that they are helped to reach balanced decisions in individual cases.

Doctors' personal preferences and values affect the way in which they use evidence. Every consulter has their own unique preference for use of analysis and dependence on experience. Those who prefer rational modes of clinical reasoning are more guideline concordant. Doctors whose reasoning is more 'experiential' are more guideline discordant (Sladek *et al.* 2008). These authors relied on Cognitive-Experiential Self Theory (CEST) which they claim is more than simply a model of reasoning. As a personality theory, they see CEST as attempting to explain behaviour and explicitly suggesting strategies that may lead to changes in behaviour. Sladek *et al.* (2008, p. 6) claim that 'regardless of an individual's preference for the rational mode, it is their preference for experiential reasoning that may more readily influence their practice.'

Case-specificity was mentioned earlier in this chapter. Norman *et al.* (2006) have shown earlier concepts (Elstein *et al.*, 1978) of case-specificity to be over-simplifications. When it comes to assessment, expertise in clinical problem-solving varies within different 'cases' and in assessment terms it is specific to the 'items' nested within cases. In other words, clinicians differ markedly on the aspects of clinical reasoning at which they excel. Reflecting on this important finding from a values-based practice perspective, I suggest that it is vital that there are multiple items testing VBP competence in all clinical reasoning assessments. In practice I have found that assessing clinical reasoning around cases such as hypertension treatment, contraception advice, or management of depression afford ample opportunity to test VBP elements across multiple nested items in the cases.

Another of my suggestions for developing VBP assessment practice is in the realm of cultural competence (David *et al.*, 2004). To assess how advanced are skills in values awareness and values communication, it is important to be able to identify whether the clinical learner has moved past working in generalities to the point of ascertaining and reasoning with the values of the individual. Examples include seeing whether the clinician can comfortably ascertain relevant medical information such as a Roman Catholic patient's views on contraception, the sexual practices of a patient from another culture, or whether or not *this* Muslim patient takes alcohol?

Conclusion

Balanced decision-making within a shared framework of values happens when clinicians are versed in the skills of evidence-based practice, including critical appraisal of the relevant evidence, as well as in the elements of values-based practice. In patient-values-centred consultation, the clinician, being aware of his/her own values, is able to communicate skilfully with the patient about values and to ascertain the patient values. There follows a process which combines principles reasoning with case-based reasoning, and which takes account of the values of other stakeholders, making good use of the multi-disciplinary team, not only for their skills but also for their values. Aiming for consensus around the implications of the scientific evidence, the ideal clinical reasoning process can, if necessary, deploy dissensus in the construction of the shared framework of values. In this way balance can be achieved.

References

André, M., Andén, A., Borgquist, L. and Rudebeck, C. E. (2012) GPs' decision-making – perceiving the patient as a person or a disease. *BMC Family Practice*, **13**, 38.

Balla, J., Heneghan, C., Goyder, C. and Thompson, M. (2012) Identifying early warning signs for diagnostic errors in primary care: a qualitative study. *British Medical Journal Open*, **2**(5), e001539.

Barrows, H. S., Norman, G. R., Neufeld, V. R. and Feightner, J. W. (1982) The clinical reasoning process of randomly selected physicians in general medical practice. *Clinical and Investigative Medicine*, **5**, 49–56.

Beauchamp, T. L. and Childress, J. F. (1994) *Principles of Biomedical Ethics*, 4th edition (6th edition, 2009). Oxford: Oxford University Press.

Berwick, D. (2009) What patient-centred should mean: confessions of an extremist. *Health Affairs*, **28**, w555–w565.

Bland, A. C., Kreiter, C. D. and Gordon, J. A. (2005) The psychometric properties of five scoring methods applied to the script concordance test. *Academic Medicine*, **80**, 395–399.

Bordage, G. and Lemieux, M. (1991) Semantic structures and diagnostic thinking of experts and novices. *Academic Medicine*, **66**, S70–S72.

Bordage, G., Connell, K. J., Chang, R. W. *et al.* (1997) Assessing the semantic content of clinical case presentations: studies of reliability and concurrent validity. *Academic Medicine*, **72**, S37–S39.

Boshuizen, H. and Schmidt, H. (1992) Biomedical knowledge and clinical expertise. *Cognitive Science*, **16**, 153–184.

Brooks, L. R., Allen, S. W. and Norman, G. R. (1991) Role of specific similarity in a medical diagnostic task. *Journal of Experimental Psychology: General*, **120**, 278–287.

Charlin, B. and van der Vleuten, C. (2004) Standardised assessment of reasoning in contexts of uncertainty: script concordance test. *Evaluation in Health Professions*, **27**, 304–319.

Coderre, S., Mandin, H., Harasym, P. H. and Fick, G. H. (2003) Diagnostic reasoning strategies and diagnostic success. *Medical Education*, **37**, 695–703.

David, S., Scott-Taylor, J., Monroe, A. *et al.* (2004) Evaluation of an educational intervention for medical students to promote competency in social and community determinants of health. *Annals of Behavioural Science and Medical Education*, **10**, 68–73.

Dolan, J. (2008) Shared decision-making – transferring research into practice: the Analytic Hierarchy Process (AHP). *Patient Education and Counselling*, **73**(3), 418–425.

Dowie, J. (2009) *Deciding how to decide*. Available at: www.ceestahc.org/pliki/symp2009/dowie.pdf, accessed 18 April 2013.

Dowie, J. and Elstein, A. (1988) *Professional Judgement: a reader in clinical decision making*. Cambridge: Cambridge University Press.

Duggan, P. S., Geller, G., Cooper, L. A. and Beach, M. C. (2006) The moral nature of patient-centeredness: is it 'just the right thing to do'? *Patient Education and Counselling*, **62**, 271–276.

Dunn, M. and Woolliscroft, J. (1997) Assessment of a pattern-recognition examination in a clinical clerkship. *Academic Medicine*, **69**, 683–684.

Elstein, A. and Bordage, G. (1988) Psychology of clinical reasoning. In Dowie, J. and Elstein, A. (editors), *Professional Judgement: a reader in clinical decision making*. Cambridge: Cambridge University Press.

Elstein, A. S., Shulman, L. S. and Sprafka, S. A. (1978) *Medical Problem Solving: an Analysis of Clinical Reasoning*. Cambridge, MA: Harvard University Press.

Elwyn, G., Edwards, A., Kinnersley, P. and Grol, R. (2000) Shared decision making and the concept of equipoise: the competences of involving patients in healthcare choices. *British Journal of General Practice*, **50**, 892–899.

Eva, K. (2004) What every teacher needs to know about clinical reasoning. *Medical Education*, **39**(1), 98–106.

Eva, K., Hatala, R., LeBlanc, V. and Brooks, L. (2007) Teaching from the clinical reasoning literature: combined reasoning strategies help novice diagnosticians overcome misleading information. *Medical Education*, **41**(12), 1152–1158.

Fonteyn, M. and Ritter, B. (2008) Clinical reasoning in nursing. In Higgs, J., Jones, M., Loftus, S. and Christensen, N. (editors), *Clinical Reasoning in the Healthcare Professions*. Amsterdam: Elsevier.

Fulford, K. W. M., Peile, E. B. and Carroll, H. (2012) *Essential Values-Based Practice: clinical stories linking science with people*. Cambridge: Cambridge University Press.

Gagliardi, A. and Dobrow, M. (2011) Paucity of qualitative research in general medical and health services and policy research journals: analysis of publication rates. *BMC Health Services Research*, **11**, 268.

Gillon, R. (1995) Defending 'the four principles approach' to biomedical ethics. *Journal of Medical Ethics*, **21**, 323–324.

Hare, R. M. (1952) *The Language of Minds*. Oxford: Oxford University Press.

Heginbotham, C. (2012) *Values-Based Commissioning of Health and Social Care*. Cambridge: Cambridge University Press.

Heneghan, C., Glasziou, P., Thompson, M. *et al.* (2009) Diagnostic strategies used in primary care. *British Medical Journal*, **338**, b946.

Higgs, J., Jones, M., Loftus, S. and Christensen, N. (2008) *Clinical Reasoning in the Healthcare Professions*. Amsterdam: Elsevier.

Holm, S. (1995) Not just autonomy – the principles of American biomedical ethics. *Journal of Medical Ethics*, **21**, 332–338.

Horstmanshoff, H., Stol, M. and Cornelis, T. C. (2004), *Magic and Rationality in Ancient Near Eastern and Graeco-Roman Medicine*, pp. 97–98. Leiden: Brill Publishers.

Kulatunga-Moruzi, C., Brooks, L. R. and Norman, G. R. (2004) Using comprehensive feature lists to bias medical diagnosis. *Journal of Experimental Psychology, Learning, Memory & Cognition*, **30**, 563–572.

Levenstein, J. H., McCracken, E. C., McWhinney, I. R. and Stewart, M. A. (1986) The patient-centred clinical method: a model for the doctor-patient interaction in family medicine. *Family Practice*, **3**, 24–30.

Limentani, A. E. (1999) The role of ethical principles in health care and the implications for ethical codes. *Journal of Medical Ethics*, **25**, 394–398.

Marinker, M. (1994) *Bayliss Lecture*. London: Royal College of Physicians.

McWhinney, R. I. (1989) *A Textbook of Family Medicine*. Oxford: Oxford University Press.

Mead, N. and Bower, P. (2002) Patient-centred consultations and outcomes in primary care: a review of the literature. *Patient Education and Counselling*, **48**, 51–61.

Norman, G. (2005) Research in clinical reasoning: past history and current trends. *Medical Education*, **39**(4), 418–427.

Norman, G. R. and Eva, K. (2003) Doggie diagnosis, diagnostic success and diagnostic reasoning strategies: an alternative view. *Medical Education*, **37**(8), 676–677.

Norman, G. R., Bordage, G., Page, G. and Keane, D. (2006) How specific is case specificity? *Medical Education*, **40**, 618–623.

Norman, G., Young, M. and Brooks, L. (2007) Non-analytical models of clinical reasoning: the role of experience. *Medical Education*, **41**(12), 1140–1145.

Page, G., Bordage, G. and Allen, T. (1995) Developing key-feature problems and examinations to assess clinical decision-making skills. *Academic Medicine*, **70**, 194–201.

Patel, V. L., Groen, G. J. and Frederiksen, C. H. (1986) Differences between medical students and doctors in memory for clinical cases. *Medical Education*, **20**, 3–9.

Petrova, M. (2012) VaST: a manual for searching electronic databases for publications on health-related values. Available at: www2.warwick.ac.uk/fac/med/study/research/vbp/resources/manual.pdf, accessed 28 February 2013.

Royal College of Obstetricians and Gynaecologists (2011) RCOG statement on draft NICE caesarean section guidelines. Available at: www.rcog.org.uk/print/what-we-do/campaigning-and-opinions/statement/rcog-statement-draft-nice-caesarean-section-guidelines.

Sackett, D., Straus, S., Scott Richardson, W. *et al.* (2000) *Evidence-based medicine: How to practice and teach EBM*, 2nd edition. Edinburgh: Churchill Livingstone.

Schmidt, H. and Rikers, R. (2007) How expertise develops in medicine: knowledge encapsulation and illness script formation. *Medical Education*, **41**, 1133–1139.

Schmidt, H., Norman, G. R. and Boshuizen, H. P. (1990) A cognitive perspective on medical expertise: theory and implications. *Academic Medicine*, **65**, 611–621.

Schön, D. (1983) *The Reflective Practitioner: How Professionals Think in Action*. London: Temple Smith.

Sibert, L., Charlin, B., Corcos, J. *et al.* (2002) Stability of clinical reasoning assessment results with the Script Concordance test across two different linguistic, cultural and learning environments. *Medical Teacher*, **24**, 522–527.

Sladek, R., Bond, M., Huynh, L., Chew, D. and Phillips, P. (2008) Thinking styles and doctors' knowledge and behaviours relating to acute coronary syndrome guidelines. *Implementation Science*, **3**, 23.

Stolper, E., Van de Wiel, M., Van Royen, P. *et al.* (2011) Gut feelings as a third track in general practitioners' diagnostic reasoning. *Journal of General Internal Medicine*, **26**(2), 197–203.

Venkatapuram, S. (2011) *Health Justice. An Argument from the Capabilities Approach*. Cambridge: Polity Press.

Whitney, S. N., McGuire, A. L. and McCullough, L. B. (2004) A typology of shared decision making, informed consent, and simple consent. *Annals of Internal Medicine*, **140**, 54.

Chapter 3

Liberating practice from philosophy – a critical examination of values-based practice and its underpinnings

Elselijn Kingma and Natalie Banner

Introduction

Values-based practice (VBP) has been developed and promoted by Bill Fulford over the past 20 years. VBP constitutes a skill: to identify and appreciate the wide range of different values that play a role in each individual instance of medical decision-making, and to reach and implement a shared medical decision in the light of those values. But VBP is also presented in conjunction with a particular philosophical theory and method – ordinary language philosophy (OLP) – from which Fulford implies it directly follows.[1] As such, VBP is presented as opposing, and providing a distinct alternative to, what Fulford calls 'prescriptive' value theory.

In this chapter we investigate the relationship between the practical, skill-based aspects of VBP and its supposed philosophical basis. First, we argue that the practical, skills-based and educational aspects of VBP do not require the philosophical underpinnings and commitments that Fulford packages them with. Instead, most of the practical aspects of VBP are compatible with a wide range of positions on philosophical methodology and a wide range of substantive philosophical claims. Second, we argue – drawing upon a range of published objections, adding some of our own – that there are severe problems with the philosophical claims Fulford commits to. Third, we

---

[1] Fulford (2011, p. 980): 'values-based practice is derived from philosophical value theory'; its training methods 'draw directly' on the 'Oxford tradition' of Hare and an exercise in the training manual 'builds directly' on Austin's work. Later (p. 984) he says: 'These links are derived in values-based practice directly from philosophical value theory.'

Debates in Values-Based Practice, ed. Michael Loughlin. Published by Cambridge University Press. © Cambridge University Press 2014.

point out that these philosophical commitments do not in fact derive from OLP at all, which plays a much smaller role in VBP than Fulford claims. We conclude that most of the practical, skills-based and educational aspects of VBP – which seem, as far as we can judge, laudable – can be retained, but that their association with a supposed philosophical basis is disingenuous, misleading, and should be dropped.

Our conclusion is important for two reasons. First, because we are interested in truth: we want to get the relationship between our philosophical and practical claims and commitments right. Second, because it makes clear that we can criticise Fulford's philosophy, without criticising the practice he advocates. This will make VBP more easily acceptable, more robust, more transparent, and will ultimately give more credence to its valuable practical work.

VBP: divorcing its practice from its philosophy

Values-based practice: three key messages

In our opinion, the practical and educational aspects of VBP aim to hammer home three key messages for health professionals.

(1) The *particular features*[2] of individual cases are deeply relevant to what is the right clinical path,[3] and even what appear to be minor or inconsequential aspects of situations can make all the difference in the decisions that should be made.

(2) Particular features *differ radically* between different people. There are unexpected differences in desires, preferences, relationships, circumstances, emotions, evaluations of outcomes, responses to the world, interpretations of the world and the things people hold dear – as well as those they do not.[4]

(3) Values-based practice is a *skill that can and should be learned*, and should be a core part of *good clinical practice*. For, as Fulford points out, the features discussed under messages one and two may be neither transparent, nor instantly recognisable as important to the decision-making process at hand.[5]

Put together, these three key messages form the basis of VBP's skills-based approach to clinical decision-making. They are very important messages. But they are not, as we will argue, unique to what Fulford claims are the *philosophical* underpinnings of VBP.

---

[2] We hesitate to call features 'values' here – for reasons that will become clear later. As Tonelli notes (Chapter 19) all manner of particular features of a situation, whether they are best classified as 'factual' or 'evaluative', can be clinically relevant. But 'particular features' of the case can be considered as interchangeable with 'particular values in play', as a placeholder for now.

[3] Citing parallels with human rights law, Fulford (2011) describes VBP as 'a framework of values within which balanced judgements have to be made according to the individual circumstances of each particular case' (p. 983, citing Woolf). See also 'The point of Values Based Practice is to support balanced decision-making on individual cases where complex and conflicting values are in play' (Fulford, 2013, p. 537).

[4] 'the aim is to connect generalised best evidence... with the particular values – the concerns, preferences, wishes and expectations – of individual patients and their families' (Fulford, 2011, p. 977).

[5] Fulford (2013, p. 977); see also 'good clinical skills ... are required in coming to balanced judgments in individual cases' and 'Values-based practice helps to make differences more transparent, thus improving communication and shared decision-making' (Fulford, 2013, p. 977).

VBP's three messages and philosophical value theory

Particular features

Fulford claims that VBP, as one of its *theoretical* contributions, is uniquely sensitive to the relevance of particular features of cases, and to the fact that these features differ radically between people, in a way that what he dubs 'prescriptive' moral philosophy is not. In fact, these sensitivities are embedded in pretty much any respectable form of value theory.

We can illustrate this point with an example. Suppose we ask whether a person should shoot another person. On any half-decent moral theory, particular features about this case matter for what the answer will be. Is the other person slowly and painfully being tortured to death and is this the only way in which you can intervene? Is the other person threatening you and your children? Particular features of cases matter, deeply. And whilst different moral theories might still generate different answers in the above case, *all* of them will depend on and make reference to the particular facts involved.

We are happy to assert simply that if a moral theory did exist that, when applied, took no particular features of a case into account at all, it would be a bad moral theory: a theory that does not distinguish between the relevant contexts of shooting a child plucking flowers in your garden and shooting an adult firing an assault weapon into a primary school, obviously would not be a plausible moral theory at all.

So, we should be careful to distinguish between the practical emphasis VBP places on the particular features of cases in the education of physicians – which is laudable – and whether Fulford makes a novel theoretical contribution to philosophy by emphasising the relevance of particular features of cases – which he does not. We grant that theoretical moral philosophy does not tend to *emphasise* a rich set of feature descriptions. But that is for a reason: moral philosophers reason about cases that are taken to be exemplars – deliberately crafted to be simple – in order to prove or disprove certain positions that can then, hopefully, be applied to illuminate actual, richer, more complex, real-life cases.

Individual differences

It is a simple empirical fact that people differ radically – in circumstances, desires, preferences, things they hold dear – and in myriad other ways. Since, as we just argued, particular features of cases are relevant on substantive moral theory, differences in these features will be relevant too. Again, we grant that proponents of these different moral theories may not have gone to much trouble to emphasise this, whereas Fulford has made much practical progress in training programmes that help clinicians realise how much people do in fact differ, and that these differences matter.

One of Fulford's key case studies cites the example of a patient, 'Diane Abbot', who is diagnosed with bipolar disorder and has been prescribed lithium (Fulford, 2004). Although lithium works well to stabilise her mood, Abbot wishes to stop her medication because she is an artist, and the side effects of the medication, which blunt her emotional and creative responses to colour, are disastrous for her person and her work. Fulford is at pains to point out that these differences matter to her and to the decision that is made about her treatment: her diagnosis alone will not tell a clinician what to do, and the individual circumstances of the case (should) make a difference to what happens.

But again, this is a practical, indeed empirical point. It is neither a novel *theoretical contribution*, nor unique to or dependent on Fulford's specific philosophical commitments.

We have to be extremely careful in our use of language here. Most theories interested in universal values, do not use the term 'values' in anything like the inclusive sense in which Fulford uses it.[6] Suppose they uphold utility maximising, or desire-satisfaction as an important value. Given different circumstances, desires and preferences between people, these 'universal' values will still be realised in very different ways, and result in very different recommendations, for different people: chocolate for one of us, gin and tonic for another.[7] Even accounts committed to human flourishing grant that flourishing in one person will have to be realised in a very different set of actions than flourishing in a different person; flourishing in Diane Abbott requires that she can appreciate colour in all its vividness. Flourishing in others may require that to a much lesser degree.

Skills

Fulford's final message is that a sensitive engagement with values – construed broadly as the individual features with cases – can be learned and developed as a skill. That is, we hope, true, although it is a matter to be settled empirically rather than conceptually. Moreover, we agree that the importance of communication skills, and a certain amount of epistemic and moral humility, is most certainly underemphasised in medicine and medical training as a whole.

It is also, interestingly, a skill much of which would be important even if one were not committed to a VBP-type process at all but to, say, paternalism. For if one were incredibly paternalist – but properly so, i.e. one took seriously the task of judging from the third-person view what was in the patient's best interest – then one would *still* have to engage in an awful lot of the skilful work involved in bringing out the individual features of a patient and her case. A good paternalist in Diane's Abbot's case would judge that withdrawing the drug under suitably arranged circumstances was in her best interest. And to reach that position, she would have to find out an awful lot about Diane – and therefore would have to engage in many of the skills that Fulford considers essential to VBP.[8] So the practical skills Fulford emphasises are deeply important not just to VBP, but to *anyone* who tries to do the right thing on, as we argued, pretty much *any* half-decent moral theory.

So, VBP's practical messages are important, but they are compatible with a range of philosophical positions and commitments, and do not at all specifically, let alone uniquely, derive from Fulford's theoretical commitments and value theory. In emphasising these messages, Fulford makes an important contribution, but it is a practical contribution to medical education and practice, not a theoretical contribution to

---

[6] There is very substantive legitimate disagreement between Fulford and many other philosophers about what *values* are, and we will turn to that in the next section. But for *practical purposes*, that disagreement is irrelevant. Everyone agrees that many features are relevant, whether we call them values – as Fulford does – or whether we call only some values, and others 'needs', 'preferences', 'desires', 'circumstances', 'beliefs', etc. – as many other philosophers do.

[7] Whilst this is a simple example, see e.g. Papineau (2012, JECP) for a much more sophisticated account of objective agent-relative interests.

[8] A main worry about paternalism is not so much paternalism itself, but that people are *bad* paternalists: they are *bad* at judging someone else's interests, for all the reasons Fulford highlights. People differ much more than we think, and features important to clinical decision-making are rarely transparent. Many of the skills in VBP would make people much better clinicians, *even if* they remained committed to being a paternalist and intervening to make decisions on patients' behalves all the time, because they would be *better* paternalists.

philosophy – let alone one that can adjudicate between different forms of value theory or substantive moral claims.

We would much prefer it if the practical elements of VBP were promoted in clinical decision-making *without* the philosophical packaging in which Fulford now presents them. It is disingenuous to package them as novel philosophical moves, thereby falsely discrediting, as Fulford does, much substantive moral philosophy. In addition, it is surely stronger to promote the practical elements of VBP without these philosophical commitments. The present form of VBP claims to rest on a particular, and contentious, strand of philosophical thinking about values, derived from linguistic analysis. A stronger claim for the validity and utility of VBP would be something like the following: 'moral philosophy is difficult and complex, and people defend lots of different positions about how to ascertain what the good or right thing to do would be in a given situation. But we are lucky that all of this complexity rarely needs to concern us; because *whichever* of these positions turns out to be the right one, this is what we should do: all philosophical theories are committed to the deep importance of particular features of cases, and these differ between people. So on any philosophical theory, it is important that we bring out and take into account people's circumstances, preferences, wishes, desires, and so forth – as it is impossible to make a good decision without that. Often, when all those features have been brought out in the open, a good course of action can be agreed without having to agree on a specific moral theory. This is not something clinical medicine has ordinarily emphasised, but luckily, bringing out all the relevant features of a case is an important clinical skill that can be learned.'

Fulford's philosophical commitments and their problems

We now turn to some of the philosophical commitments and contributions that Fulford does make, and their problems. Given the claims in the first section, we can find these problematic and reject them, without having to reject the practice that Fulford advocates. We focus on three issues: first, Fulford's notion of values; second, his commitment to process over outcome; third, the central role of mutual respect.

What are values?

As already indicated, Fulford does make a substantive philosophical claim, which is also a legitimate point of philosophical disagreement, on what values are. Supposedly in keeping with his commitment to ordinary language philosophy, Fulford takes a very inclusive view of values: he is very explicit that circumstances, beliefs, wishes, preferences, etc., should all be considered *values*.[9] (See also Chapters 5, 6 and 8.) This is legitimately to be contrasted with many moral theories that make distinctions between

---

[9] Cf. Fulford and Colombo (2004, Figure 1, p. 141), and Fulford's claim (2011, p. 978) that the 'biopsychosocial model' is a value. This suggests that models, ways of representing the truth, are also values. Does this mean that any representation of fact goes, depending on one's values? That all belief systems are values? In a similar vein notice the circularity and unclarity in the quote: 'perhaps the most widely recognised values in healthcare are ethical values. But values are wider than ethics, extending to needs, wishes, preferences, indeed to any and all of the many and diverse ways in which people express, directly or indirectly, negative or positive evaluations and value judgments' (2011, p. 976). So values extend beyond ethics... into value judgements? What precisely does that mean?

values on the one hand, and beliefs, desires, preferences, epistemic attitudes, circumstances etc. on the other.

We make three points about this philosophical move. First, we argue that it is not justified, let alone prescribed, by OLP. Second, we lay out reasons to find Fulford's intervention unhelpful and obfuscating at both a practical and a theoretical level – meaning not only that we lack good arguments in favour of it, but also that we have ample reason to reject it. Third, we point out that although an inclusive use of the term 'values' may be contributing at a practical level to the education of physicians, that role should remain at the level of an exercise and should not be presented as a substantive philosophical claim.

OLP and the broad use of 'values'

It is worth considering Fulford's methodology when trying to ascertain where his broad use of the term 'values' comes from, and why he defends it as a practical contribution to clinical decision-making grounded in ordinary language philosophy. Inspired by the Austinian notion of philosophical fieldwork, Fulford's exploration of the term 'value' emerges from the particular view he developed about the concept of illness in earlier work (Fulford, 1989). This philosophical work focused on the notion of illness as a failure of action that prevents people from realising their valued ends, centrally undercutting the notion that illness could be defined naturalistically. Fulford's key insight here was that even supposedly 'factual' elements of illness concepts are actually imbued with evaluative judgements, and the concomitant debate over the fact/value distinction in concepts of illness is well established in philosophy.[10] So what does a linguistic analysis of illness concepts have to do with the plethora of psychological attitudes subsumed under the umbrella term 'values' as Fulford uses it? The development of VBP appears to be a different, more pragmatic route to what is essentially the same claim: that illness is inherently value laden. For Fulford, values enter our thinking about illness not because of some moral theory about what we ought to do, but rather because values enter into what people think illness is, so it is important to negotiate these values in deciding how to treat people. By conducting linguistic analyses on how ordinary people used the term 'illness', and particularly 'mental illness', Fulford drew out what the term means to different people. It transpires that a whole host of 'values' are deeply embedded in what people mean by 'illness':

> the ways we think about mental disorders. . .are determined also by values, by the *wishes* and *desires* of those concerned, by clinical *needs*, by *ethical* intuitions, and the like. . . [emphasis in original]. . . what is important about a given mental disorder may differ widely from person to person according to their particular values. (Fulford and Colombo, 2004, p. 141)

But as we can see from the quotations above, values in this sense amount to everything that people take to be important to illness *tout court*: values here encompass everything about diagnosis, treatment, management, rights and responsibilities that could be relevant in dealing with a patient. Furthermore, these are often implicit: 'raising awareness of the values that actually drive our practice as opposed to the values we believe we hold, is the first and crucial step in values-based training' (Fulford, 2011, p. 977). This seems to us to

---

[10] See, for instance, Humber and Almeder (1997), Thornton (2011).

be a significant leap away from the original exploration of the way in which evaluative terms enter into concepts of illness based on ordinary language philosophy, and one that needs defending. We recognise Fulford's insistence that mapping out the 'values' implicit in models of illness is not itself a theoretical contribution but rather a first, preparatory step towards a conceptual and empirical analysis of the relationship between illness and value, but it is perhaps *because* it is treated as an initial step that we need to be clear on quite how we have got to this starting point in the first place.

Mapping out the logical geography of 'illness' as used by ordinary people is a valuable descriptive contribution to conceptual work in the philosophy of medicine. The pragmatic claim that different people (patients or professionals) will take different things to be important to a clinical decision is likewise valuable. But linking these two claims through the expansive use of the term 'values', and the subsequent development of a normative framework to guide clinical practice, requires a substantial justification, which we cannot find in Fulford's development of VBP. This is important, because if the latter is a pragmatic (albeit plausible) claim, it ought not to give the impression of being derived from a substantial body of philosophical theory. If, on the other hand, the pragmatic claim does indeed follow from ordinary language philosophy, and ultimately leads to the development of a set of guiding principles, it is important to see what the intermediary steps in this argument are.

Arguments against the broad reading of 'values'

One concern with the slippage from an ordinary language account of the evaluative aspects of models of illness and disorder into taking values to constitute everything that may be important to a clinical decision-making process, is motivated by the concern that the expansive use of the term 'values' runs into some real problems. We find Fulford's use of the term 'values' obfuscating because *everything* seems to become a value: not just needs and preferences but also circumstances, as well as – it seems – beliefs about the external world (Fulford and Colombo, 2004, p. 141; Fulford, 2011, p. 976). This is obfuscating because Fulford's 'value' term is so broad as to become useless (see Chapter 5). And, importantly, not just useless theoretically, but even useless at a practical level, which is the level at which Fulford wants VBP to operate. We shall give two examples of this.

First, if everything different parties believe is important is intended to go into the melting pot of the decision process for negotiation, how is any distinction to be drawn between those things that really *should* be deemed important and those that may represent a minor preference or desire? For example, an oncologist's recommendation for an urgent biopsy should presumably carry a fair amount of weight, whereas her patient's disgruntlement at having to pay for the car park at the hospital when he comes in for the procedure, although relevant, should be relatively light on the scales.

Second, Fulford extends 'value-theory' into domains over which it is not at all obvious that it has jurisdiction. Does the term 'value' apply to what I *believe*? At least on the face of it, it seems that truth-apt beliefs about the external world, such as 'the grass is green', 'this is a pill containing lithium' and 'I have aliens implanted in my head' should not be treated on a VBP-able 'all are equal basis'. If they are, then psychiatry in particular, where the navigation of huge divergences in volitions, beliefs, emotions and desires is at the heart of the psychiatrist's day-to-day job, has a real problem. So Fulford really owes us some clarity here on his position: is there anything (such as a truth-apt belief) that is not a value? If so – or if not – then why? Fulford's solution to this concern is to claim that values are not chaotic, and that, like political values in a democracy, conflicts can be resolved by negotiating and balancing the values in play (Fulford and Colombo, 2004, p. 142). However, our point is not that values are many and varied and may struggle to be negotiated in the balance, but rather that in encompassing so much, the term 'values' ceases to be able to do very much work at all in his practical project that is intended to be *based* on considerations of value.

In addition to being practically unhelpful, we also find, in conjunction with others (see Chapters 5, 6, 7 and 8), that Fulford's intervention to subsume almost everything under values is prima facie unhelpful at a *theoretical* level. By distinguishing between values, preferences, needs, desires, circumstances, etc. moral philosophy has developed a fine-grained toolbox within which to do our philosophical and practical reasoning. We find that toolbox extremely helpful. It allows us to distinguish, for example, values from desires and preferences. One might desire chocolate, but disvalue that desire in the sense that one would prefer not to have it – and indeed, believe oneself to have *good reason* for the latter preference. Part of the intuitive difference between values and desires is the 'endorsement' of values as something one is genuinely committed to: should the desire for chocolate be given equal weight to the commitment to lose weight to avoid type 2 diabetes? Fulford's approach not only gives us no obvious way to debate such practical questions – the broad scope of the term 'values' actually brushes over distinctions that can help in their resolution.

Fulford is welcome to do this, but even if he can defend it, he cannot prescribe it. By his own standards, he cannot prescribe how we *ought* to use the term 'values', as that goes directly against the grain of OLP, which tells us how people use language, not how they ought to use language. He can say that some people use 'values' in an inclusive sense, but it is also true that some use 'values' in a less-inclusive sense. And they have *reasons* to make the more fine-grained distinctions within the usage of the term 'values' – as illustrated by the work moral philosophers and others have done with it, in thinking about how different factors can all be weighted in making decisions.

Minding the gap

It is fine for philosophy to use 'values' in a technical sense, distinct from some 'ordinary life' uses, but this is where we see a key tension in Fulford's attempt to produce a form of practical guidance for clinicians based on a philosophically derived framework: it draws attention to the gap between the practice and the philosophy. Fulford can use his fieldwork to get the thinking started, but not to draw any conclusions. His aim is surely not to educate people on what they should and should not call values, which goes against the grain of OLP, but to make people realise that particular elements of cases are relevant and important. Fulford can do an OLP *exercise*, then, as part of his education. But that exercise is merely illustrative, it should not be used to draw a practical, or theoretical – let alone a philosophical – conclusion about values.

Process over outcome

Fulford also claims that whether an outcome or clinical decision is right is (solely) determined by the process used to arrive at that outcome, not by features of the case. This is a substantive philosophical claim intended as a counterpoint to 'regulatory ethics', which he views as overly prescriptive and insensitive to the range of perspectives that VBP prides itself on giving voice to. We take no standpoint on either the existence or the worth of such a thing as 'regulatory ethics', nor whether VBP is superior to it. Taken on its own, the claim that good practice is solely a matter of good process is, as Thornton (2011; see also Chapter 4) rightly points out, an extremely radical claim. And, again, it is one that seems neither particularly desirable on the face of it, nor particularly well supported by Fulford.

Good process *as well as* feature-sensitivity is shared by other moral theories and is not unique to VBP. In the end, though, most moral theories recognise that there is a fact of the matter as to whether an outcome is right, that depends on more than process alone. If VBP is to be distinct then – as it claims – it is because process alone determines whether an outcome was right. So what if we take Fulford's process focus seriously? That would mean that it is an analytic truth that VBP leads to good clinical decision-making. For if one asserts that VBP is to practice good process, and a good outcome is whatever outcome results from a good process, then whatever VBP results in is good.

That seems not only to require an extreme leap of faith (where is the argument that VBP is analytically right?), but it also is not in line with how Fulford defends and presents VBP. Take, again, the case of Diane Abbott. That example is compelling *not* primarily because we recognise a good process. If so, VBP ought to be equally convincing if Fulford had never told us what outcome was reached in her case. Instead, what makes the example compelling is that we all recognise that a good outcome was achieved, *because people paid attention to Abbott's particular features* – for without that, it would not have been achieved. This gives us evidence to trust the process that Fulford presents, which promotes attention to those features – and which Fulford claims is uniquely good at achieving this outcome.

Good process, according to Fulford, involves giving all perspectives and values from different stakeholders due weight and consideration. What does it mean to do this? The problem of understanding what it means to have a good process has been examined extensively in literature on assessments of mental capacity: here, the question of what it means to use or weigh information in coming to a decision has led to powerful arguments that it is misguided to attempt to divorce the procedural elements of a decision-making process from its substantive content (Freyenhagen and O'Shea, 2013; Banner, 2012, 2013). It is arguably possible for a decision-making process to be intact, to go through all the right motions of weighing up different values and perspectives, but for these values and perspectives to be for the most part extremely bad, and result in an outcome that would also, to many observers, be undeniably bad. It is not process alone (if indeed, it is even possible to ascertain what this entails) that determines what a good outcome looks like.

This issue is further compounded by a concern raised previously, namely that an overly broad use of 'values' actually hinders rather than helps decision-making. In the stipulation to follow good process, there is no capacity for discriminating between more or less important values, considerations, beliefs, expectations, circumstances and so forth. Better communication and awareness of other people's perspectives undoubtedly will improve things, but some situations are truly a conflict of values that may not be overcome (see also Chapters 4 and 5). We see this in contentious debates around reproductive rights and the compulsory treatment of psychiatric disorders, for example: intractable conflicts in value in which we care very deeply about getting the right outcome. Thus the claim that a democratic process of balancing values (whatever this means in practice) is sufficient for good clinical practice, does not appear to have any grounding beyond mere assertion.

If, however, Fulford's claim is more modest and there are facts beyond process that determine whether an outcome is good or right, then this should be stated outright. In that case VBP derives its justification from being the best or most likely way of realising that good outcome. This may well be the case, but it is an empirical, not a conceptual, matter.

Mutual respect

Fulford makes a further substantial philosophical commitment: there is a value – mutual respect – which acts as a constraint on other values that are VBP-able. This is problematic in the context of his theory, because it seems to force him back into the kind of substantive philosophical reasoning he wants to rule out as a constraint, and only allow as an explorative measure.[11]

The constraint of mutual respect could be interpreted in multiple ways. First, as a *process* value: mutual respect means that everyone should be *heard* – which we assume does not merely mean 'allowed to open their mouths' but means something more substantial, i.e. taken seriously. That in itself is problematic. Take people who argue that foetuses should be heard, versus people who think that, really, they should not. How is this resolvable on VBP? In the context of mental health, it is questionable whether everyone's statement should be taken equally seriously – what about the delusional insistence of a patient with schizophrenia that he is a prophet from god, or being pursued by the FBI? Psychiatry is littered with grey areas, where it is by no means clear how seriously a person's professed views, beliefs and values should be taken as an expression of what they want.

Mutual respect could also be interpreted as a *substantial* value, however, and this is how Fulford seems to intend it, given his insistence that racism is precluded by VBP as incompatible with mutual respect.[12] Thus mutual respect presumably means that all people are equal or that all people should be treated equitably. That, however, again runs into problems that are difficult to resolve. First, who counts as everyone? There is controversy and substantive disagreement over the extent to which foetuses, and the severely mentally ill, count in this regard, and over what equality or equitability would *be*. Second, this actually places much more severe constraints on the VBP-able values than Fulford allows or perhaps realises. Some people, for example, reason straight from the basis of equality to, for example, the permissibility of abortion and the impermissibility of forced medical interventions on pregnant women, or a duty to donate almost all our money to the third world. At the same time, many people's attitudes – including deeply culturally sanctioned attitudes – are inherently sexist, according lesser value or weight to the desires and opinions of women, and even the importance of their health and wellbeing. In many cultures, homosexuality is viewed as pathological, and these again are deeply ingrained cultural attitudes: can homophobia and sexism be discounted as VBP-able values too? And as with racism, the expression of many such values is frequently implicit,

---

[11] There is a further worry: it is unclear where the value 'mutual respect' comes from. Fulford asserts that it comes straight from analytic philosophy. But: how? 'For the analyticity of values-based practice leads also to its unique premise in mutual respect for differences of values (again, including but not limited to ethical values)' (Fulford, 2013, p. 543). This assertion is not even explained, let alone defended.

[12] 'the premise of VBP in and of itself sets limits to the values that are VBP-able. Thus racism is incompatible with mutual respect and hence by definition is beyond the pale of VBP' (Fulford, 2013, p. 538).

hidden from view and taking the form of pernicious but undefinable bias. That leaves many people's values 'beyond the pale of VBP'.

Those latter points raise a deeper issue for Fulford. It is not merely that he has not made clear what mutual respect is exactly and *how* it is supposed to feature in the VBP process in the light of the above problem. It is that allowing a value such as mutual respect as a constraint within the process forces us back to precisely the kind of reasoning-towards-an-outcome/judgement that philosophers have traditionally engaged in, and that Fulford wants to keep *out* of VBP. For to determine what values are and are not compatible with mutual respect is precisely to engage in philosophical reasoning that is not merely explorative, but that gives answers. Such as: female genital mutilation is out (or in). And that is not just a theoretical problem for Fulford. In this case it is also a practical one: who does that reasoning? Who is the decider? What if one person says that your value is not compatible with mutual respect for women, and the other says that your statement is not compatible with mutual respect for my cultural values? Without a return to the prescriptive philosophical reasoning Fulford aims to avoid, it is very hard indeed to see how he can begin to address these questions.

The real (and rather limited) role of ordinary language philosophy

In response to critics, Fulford claims that both the foundations of VBP and his own controversial philosophical commitments – such as it being a 'liberal, electively unclear and potentially dangerous approach to clinical training and decision-making' (Fulford, 2011, p. 976) – derive from and are justified by the concepts, methodology and output of the 'Oxford School' of 'ordinary language philosophy'. In this section we argue that the OLP Fulford claims to deploy in the development of VBP does not in fact underpin the approach – or his substantive philosophical commitments – in the way that he argues. Fulford places a great deal of weight on the role his analytic approach plays in the development of VBP:

> it is from its analytic origins that much that is distinctive about VBP is derived...leads to its unique premise in mutual respect for differences of values...and from this premise flows the extent of the reliance in VBP on process over outcomes...analytic origins directly inform the specific ways in which improved skills of awareness of values are achieved. (Fulford, 2013, p. 543)

According to Fulford, then, the philosophical fieldwork inspired by Austin, exploring the implicit models of mental disorder and unearthing the multiplicity of 'values' people hold around notions of illness and its treatment, is the foundation upon which the edifice of VBP rests. This is a surprising claim, as VBP purports to be a system of guiding principles for clinical practice, and as such is normative. Thus the core problem for Fulford's claim that OLP underpins VBP is the leap from the descriptive to the prescriptive. Fulford is extremely clear that linguistic analysis provides only descriptions of how people use words, but is not prescriptive: 'the look and see philosophical fieldwork methods for raising awareness of value all merely describe; they do not prescribe' (Fulford, 2013, p. 541). How, then, can Fulford derive from linguistic analysis such guiding principles as the 'principle of mutual respect' or the 'importance of process over outcome', or indeed normatively justify a radical overextension of the term 'values', to underpin his approach?

Fulford claims that the legitimacy and distinctiveness of the whole project hinge on its methodological claim to reflect ordinary language use (exposing the values of stakeholders in health care decision-making processes) through a process of conducting Austinian philosophical fieldwork. Since that is not a normative methodology, however, it seems that Fulford *cannot* answer this question.

This does not leave VBP in as bad a position as it might seem; for as we have shown, the practical aspects of VBP are compatible with and demanded by all decent moral theories. So if OLP does not grant legitimacy there, all reasonable prescriptive theories do. These aspects can and should be retained. It does mean, however, that none of Fulford's substantive philosophical commitments discussed in the previous section – which we have already claimed were implausible or undesirable on the face of it – derive any legitimacy from OLP.

The role of linguistic analysis in VBP, then, is actually quite minor. It is, indeed, merely a first step in the project of developing an approach to clinical reasoning and decision-making. Linguistic analytic philosophy essentially justifies the methodological starting point of VBP, which is to examine the way people use the term 'value', rather than seek an explicit definition: the meaning(s) of the term are more comprehensively explored by examining the way people use the term, than the way they define it. This provides a method for demonstrating that different people mean different things by 'value', and these differences are significant for health decision-making. In other words, all Fulford gets from OLP is an *exercise*: the 'write down what you mean by values' exercise leading to the 'look how different people are and how different their use of values is'. That exercise may well be useful, can be retained and can be legitimately ascribed to Austin. But, first, it is worth noting that the same practical message can be illustrated in other ways. Second, it is important that the justification of VBP by OLP stops right then and there: at the level of giving a useful exercise that raises awareness. The justification for VBP's practical messages we have given in the first part. The justification for Fulford's substantial philosophical commitments appears non-existent.

Conclusions

Why does this matter? First, it matters because it is important to be truthful. If VBP claims to be a practical spin-off of a substantial philosophical theory of value, it had better be clear what work the philosophical theory is doing (which should be subject to close conceptual scrutiny) and what aspects of the project are not derived from the theory (and these ought to be recognised as being other than philosophically informed). If, as Fulford suggests, aspects of clinical decision-making such as the role of tacit knowledge and the irreducibility of individual judgements are indeed 'growth points' springing from the philosophical framework of VBP (Fulford, 2013, p. 542), we suspect this is a substantial overreach of its philosophical underpinnings and authority.

Second, the practical case for VBP is in fact stronger both without any contentious philosophical grandstanding, as pointed out in the first section, and without the unjustified philosophical commitments discussed in the second section. We firmly believe clinical decision-making *would* be enhanced by better communication skills, more attention paid to different perspectives and viewpoints, and, in the vein of patient-centred care, paying attention not only to the patient's symptoms but also to what he says and wants. Divorcing the unwieldy philosophy from the practice would not be a bad thing.

Third, the philosophy could be considered a mere appendix to practice, which would not in itself be problematic, were it not that this philosophical backdrop brings a questionable air of philosophical authority and credibility to what is essentially a pragmatic project driven by pragmatic considerations. There is something deeply disingenuous and indeed contradictory about Fulford's overstretched claims to philosophical authority. Despite the clear commitment of VBP to a 'democratic' process of decision-making, the issue of authority looms large for Fulford. Although perhaps intended as merely providing context and background to the philosophical theory, repeated references to the 'Oxford' school of philosophers betray a distinctly undemocratic reverence for the intellectual authority of this privileged caste of thinkers. We are not criticising their theories or the methods of linguistic analysis developed by the likes of Austin, but rather questioning the rhetoric used to justify the concepts and methods of VBP. As argued above, the key messages of VBP are all compatible with any plausible moral theory, and Fulford's substantive philosophical claims are not justified, defined or defended well, and do not derive from OLP. It is therefore neither necessary nor legitimate to appeal to a particular intellectual authority (the prestigious 'Oxford connection') in order to justify the approach Fulford advocates.

One key defender of VBP in this volume (see Chapter 2) stresses that the value of VBP lies in its pragmatic as opposed to its philosophical aspects. As we have argued throughout, VBP does indeed have much to recommend it, practically speaking. We take our conclusions to be constructive in attempts to draw out more clearly what practical value VBP may have, without the weight of unnecessary philosophical theorising that has accompanied it thus far.

References

Banner, N. F. (2012) Unreasonable reasons: normative judgements in the assessment of mental capacity. *Journal of Evaluation in Clinical Practice*, **18**(5), 1038–1044.

Banner, N. F. (2013) Can procedural and substantive elements of decision-making be reconciled in assessments of mental capacity? *International Journal of Law in Context*, **9**(1), 71–86.

Freyenhagen, F. and O'Shea, T. (2013) Hidden substance: mental disorder as a challenge to normatively neutral accounts of autonomy. *International Journal of Law in Context*, **9**(1), 53–70.

Fulford, K. W. M. (1989) *Moral Theory and Medical Practice*. Cambridge: Cambridge University Press.

Fulford, K. W. M. (2004) Ten principles of values-based medicine. In Radden, J. (editor) *The Philosophy of Psychiatry: A Companion*, Chapter 14. New York: Oxford University Press.

Fulford, K. W. M. (2011) The value of evidence and evidence of values: bringing together values-based and evidence-based practice in policy and service development in mental health. *Journal of Evaluation in Clinical Practice*, **17**, 976–987.

Fulford, K. W. M. (2013) Values-based practice: Fulford's dangerous idea. *Journal of Evaluation in Clinical Practice*, **19**, 537–546.

Fulford, K. W. M. and Colombo, A. (2004) Six models of mental disorder: a study combining linguistic-analytic and empirical methods. *Philosophy, Psychiatry, and Psychology*, **11**(2), 129–144.

Humber, J. M. and Almeder, R. P. (editors) (1997) *What is Disease?* Totowa, NJ: Humana Press.

Papineau, D. (2012) Can we be harmed after we are dead? *Journal of Evaluation in Clinical Practice*, **18**(5), 1091–1094.

Thornton, T. (2011) Radical, liberal values-based practice. *Journal of Evaluation in Clinical Practice*, **17**, 988–991.

Values-based practice and authoritarianism

Tim Thornton

Introduction

Values-based practice (VBP) is a radical view of the place of values in medical practice, which develops from a philosophical analysis of values, illness and the role of ethical principles. It denies two attractive and traditional but misguided views of medicine: that diagnosis is a merely factual matter and that the values that should guide treatment and management can be codified in principles. But, in the work of K. W. M. Fulford, it goes further in the form of a radical liberal view: that the idea of an antecedently good outcome should be replaced by that of a right process.

In this chapter I will first set out the steps needed to reach this position, and highlight its radical liberal form in the work of Fulford. I will argue, however, that the radical version faces a dilemma when it comes to accounting for its own normative status. Given that difficulty, why might one adopt the radical version? I sketch a possible motive drawing on Rorty's rejection of authoritarianism which replaces objectivity with solidarity as the aim of judgement. But I argue that, nevertheless, this does not justify the rejection of the more modest particularist version of VBP.[1]

To begin with it will be helpful to have a contrasting view in mind, whether or not it has ever been explicitly defended. (It is, in my experience, widespread among medical students at least.) On this traditional view, medical diagnosis is a matter of getting the facts

---

[1] This chapter is based on my paper 'Radical liberal values-based practice' (Thornton, 2011). I am grateful both to its publishers for permission to develop further the material published there and to K. W. M. (Bill) Fulford for his comments on that paper.

Debates in Values-Based Practice, ed. Michael Loughlin. Published by Cambridge University Press. © Cambridge University Press 2014.

right independent of any values. Values come into play – alongside good evidence-based medicine – in guiding treatment and management. And when they do, they are codified in a set of principles, a proper understanding of which forms a kind of moral calculus. The first two steps towards appreciating the radical status of VPB are recognising that it rejects both aspects of this traditional view. Values are implicated in diagnosis as well as treatment. And any moral principles to which we might appeal are insufficient. There is then a third step to which I will return shortly.

The main principles of Fulford's values-based practice are set out below (from Fulford, 2004). I will explicitly mention some of these – principles 1, 2, 5, 8 and 9 – in what follows.

Box 4.1 Ten principles of values-based practice

(1) All decisions stand on two feet, on values as well as on facts, including decisions about diagnosis (the 'two feet' principle).

(2) We tend to notice values only when they are diverse or conflicting and hence are likely to be problematic (the 'squeaky wheel' principle).

(3) Scientific progress, in opening up choices, is increasingly bringing the full diversity of human values into play in all areas of health care (the 'science driven' principle).

(4) VBP's 'first call' for information is the perspective of the patient or patient group concerned in a given decision (the 'patient-perspective' principle).

(5) In VBP, conflicts of values are resolved primarily, not by reference to a rule prescribing a 'right' outcome, but by processes designed to support a balance of legitimately different perspectives (the 'multi-perspective' principle).

(6) Careful attention to language use in a given context is one of a range of powerful methods for raising awareness of values (the 'values-blindness' principle).

(7) A rich resource of both empirical and philosophical methods is available for improving our knowledge of other people's values (the 'values-myopia' principle).

(8) Ethical reasoning is employed in VBP primarily to explore differences of values, not, as in quasi-legal bioethics, to determine 'what is right' (the 'space of values' principle).

(9) In VBP, communication skills have a substantive rather than (as in quasi-legal ethics) a merely executive role in clinical decision-making (the 'how it's done' principle).

(10) VBP, although involving a partnership with ethicists and lawyers (equivalent to the partnership with scientists and statisticians in EBM), puts decision-making back where it belongs, with users and providers at the clinical coal-face (the 'who decides' principle).

Values are involved in diagnosis as well as treatment and management

The first step to VBP is to recognise that values are involved in diagnosis as well as treatment and management. Three main arguments for this claim are available. First, it helps make sense of the recent history of debate about the status of *mental* illness in which mental illness is compared either favourably or unfavourably with physical illness. Second, to an unprejudiced eye, pathology – mental or physical – is an evaluative notion. Third, attempts to reduce the concept of illness or disease (or even disorder) to non-evaluative notions have failed for principled reasons.

Fulford's own influential argument for the first of these considerations runs as follows (Fulford, 1989). The key assumption that mistakenly drives both anti-psychiatry and biological defences of psychiatry is that *physical* illness is conceptually simple and value free. This motivates anti-psychiatrists such as Thomas Szasz to compare mental illness unfavourably with physical illness (Szasz, 1972). But it also motivates defenders of psychiatry such as Kendell and Boorse to attempt to argue that mental illness is, like physical illness, value free (Boorse, 1975; Kendell, 1975). Without the first assumption, however, neither mistaken argumentative move is necessary, nor is it justified. In setting out the consequences of this first claim – that physical illness is evaluative – Fulford draws particularly on Hare's early work, especially his *Language of Morals*, on the logical properties of value terms (Hare, 1952).

Hare pointed out that the value *judgements* expressed by (or implicit in) value *terms* are made on the basis of criteria that, in themselves, are *descriptive* (or factual) in nature. The value judgement expressed by 'this is a good strawberry', in one of Hare's examples, is made on the basis that the strawberry in question is, as a matter of fact, 'sweet, grub-free', etc. Hare then points out that where the descriptive criteria for a given value judgement are widely agreed or settled upon, it is these *descriptive* criteria that may come to dominate the use of the value term in question. This is a simple consequence of repeated association. In the case of strawberries, most people in most contexts value (prefer, like, enjoy) strawberries that are sweet and grub-free. Hence the use of 'good strawberry' comes to be associated with descriptions such as 'sweet, grub-free, etc.' to the extent that it is this *descriptive* meaning that becomes dominant in the use of the term. This contrasts with, say, pictures where there are no settled descriptive criteria for a good picture because there is no general agreement about pictorial aesthetics. Hare's general conclusion, therefore, is this: value terms by which *shared* values are expressed may come, by a process of simple association, to look like *descriptive* (or factual) terms, whereas value terms expressing values over which there is disagreement, remain overtly value laden in use.

This general claim applies equally to medical language. If illness (generically) is a value term, and if mental illness is more overtly value laden than physical illness, this is neither because (as Szasz argued) mental illness is a moral rather than a scientific concept, nor because (as Kendell and Boorse argued) psychiatric science is less advanced than the sciences in areas of physical medicine such as cardiology. Following the Oxford philosopher J. L. Austin, Fulford distinguishes between problems of definition and problems of use to suggest that, whilst at heart mental and physical illness are both equally definitionally complex, mental illness is more problematic in use because it reflects more problematic areas of human experience and behaviour, namely areas such as emotion, desire, volition and belief, in which people's values tend to be highly diverse. This line of thinking is reflected in VBP in the principle that we tend to notice values only when they are diverse or conflicting and hence are likely to be problematic (the 'squeaky wheel' principle).

Fulford then goes on to conduct an exercise in what another Oxford philosopher, Gilbert Ryle, called the 'logical geography' of medicine, of the given features of the uses of the medical concepts to justify this value-laden view of the subject. If medical terms are value terms, in Hare's sense, then many of the features of their use, including a detailed analysis of the many different kinds of disease concept, follow from the general logical properties they share with all value terms, combined, of course, with contingent features of human values (in particular the diversity of values in psychiatry).

But there is a second consideration to support an evaluative view of diagnosis. To an unprejudiced if at least enquiring eye, both the general concept of illness and specific instances of illnesses at least simply look to be evaluative. On the second point, John Sadler

(2004) has devoted considerable care to detailing and taxonomising the values involved in the DSM IV codification of mental illnesses. He claims that psychiatry is thoroughly charged with values but, at the same time, it disguises or denies the role that they play. Thus one key aim of his book is to explore the multiple roles of values in a variety of different areas. These include broad themes such as the patient and professional roles, technology, culture and politics. But it also concerns more specific areas of psychiatric interest such as sex and gender and genetics. So if Sadler's piecemeal analysis is convincing then there is reason to believe that in mental illness, at least, values are widespread in diagnosis.

But on the more general point, Fulford's picture is sustained by the idea that there is more to pathology in general than what is unusual, for example. Illness is *bad* for us. So unless there is a way to explain away that apparently evaluative or normative aspect of illness, there is good reason to believe appearances. And, arguably at least, that is the case.

Merely statistical analyses of what is usual and unusual do not seem to capture the fact that high intelligence is in itself a good thing and low intelligence is a bad thing. More sophisticated attempts to use the notion of biological function have had the more modest aim of explaining away evaluative notions from the concept of *disorder*, rather than illness or disease, conceding that the latter notions also contain the ineliminable notion of harm (Wakefield, 1999). But even with regard to that modest aim, it is far from clear that the notion of failure of function presupposed explains away, rather than smuggling in, normative notions (Thornton, 2000).

If this is right, then even if it were the case that the set of illnesses, diseases or disorders could be captured using merely factual criteria, this would only be because, contingently, we agreed about the underlying medical values. (In much the same way, if the criteria for apples which can be sold as fit for purpose are purely factual, this is because we happen to agree on which kinds of apples we like.) Such agreement may be merely culturally and temporally a local matter rather than answering to purely factual constraints about the nature of illness.

To summarise this first point, VBP is radical because it contests the idea that medical care is based on a value-free diagnosis. Values are in play in diagnosis as well as treatment or management. Hence

(1) all decisions stand on two feet, on values as well as on facts, including decisions about diagnosis (the 'two feet' principle),

(2) we tend to notice values only when they are diverse or conflicting and hence are likely to be problematic (the 'squeaky wheel' principle).

Principles are insufficient for value judgements

The second step to articulate values-based practice is the rejection of both the sufficiency and the fundamental importance of moral principles in guiding medical practice. One reason for the first element of this is not as far from medical orthodoxy as it might appear but tends to remain hidden in medical ethical teaching (Thornton, 2006). It is implicit in the most influential recent approach to medical ethics: the Four Principles approach, a deontological or principles-based approach set out at length by Tom Beauchamp and James Childress in their *Principles of Biomedical Ethics* (Beauchamp and Childress, 2001). In this book, the authors set out four general principles to guide medical ethical reasoning: autonomy, beneficence, non-maleficence and justice.

These four principles, which do not derive from any single higher principle, are supposed to capture medical ethical reasoning. However, they can conflict. Standardly, for example, beneficence and non-maleficence are in tension in both surgery and drug treatment. In psychiatry, in particular, autonomy and beneficence are in tension in the case of involuntary treatment. And thus an implicit part of the Four Principles approach is to frame ethical judgements which go beyond the resources of the principles alone.

Beauchamp and Childress describe two methods for dealing with such conflicts: specification and balancing. Specification is a way of deriving more concrete guidance from the fairly abstract higher level principles. It is described in outline thus:

> Specification is a process of reducing the indeterminateness of abstract norms and providing them with action guiding content. For example, without further specification, do no harm is an all-too-bare starting point for thinking through problems, such as assisted suicide and euthanasia. It will not adequately guide action when norms conflict. (Beauchamp and Childress, 2001, p. 16)

This looks at first to be a kind of deduction. Much as, once particular assumptions are made, Kepler's laws of planetary motion can be (more or less) derived from Newtonian physics, so a specified rule can be derived from a higher level principle. And just as Kepler's laws are useful in the specific context of planetary systems, so a specified principle – such as that doctors should put their patients' interests first – can be tailored to give concrete guidance to cases of, for example, euthanasia. But although specification is some form of derivation, it cannot strictly be deduction because 'specified' lower level rules have more content, more information, than the principles from which they are drawn.

The second tool for generating an actual duty from apparently conflicting principles is more obviously not a matter of simply unpacking the principles. It is called 'balancing' and complements specification thus:

> Principles, rules and rights require *balancing* no less than *specification*. We need both methods because each addresses a dimension of moral principles and rules: *range and scope*, in the case of specification, and *weight or strength*, in the case of balancing. Specification entails a substantive refinement of the range and scope of norms, whereas balancing consists of deliberation and judgement about the relative weights or strengths of norms. Balancing is especially important for reaching judgements in individual cases. (Beauchamp and Childress, 2001, p. 18)

Thus despite the emphasis on the importance of the four principles, Beauchamp and Childress do still suggest the need for a degree of non-principles-driven judgement explicitly in the case of 'balancing' and implicitly in the case of 'specification'. And thus even on this influential approach to medical ethics, the principles themselves are insufficient to guide practice. (That is why I stressed that there is no higher order principle. The view of which principle should dominate is not determined by the principles themselves but, somehow, from outside them.)

Values-based practice goes further than this, however. Although it concedes that there can be sufficient agreement about some values that they can be codified to provide the basis for ethical codes and guidelines, these remain just a small part of the values that have to be taken account of in guiding medical practice which include individual preferences, desires, wishes, firmly held faith and convictions and so forth. By stressing this multiplicity, it stresses the standing possibility of disagreements and clashes in thinking about particular circumstances.

This contrasts with the way that even where there are well-known clashes in the Four Principles approach, it is tempting to think that there are standard solutions. Thus, for example, the case of the Jehovah's Witness who competently refuses life-saving treatment is taken to exemplify the conflict of beneficence and autonomy and on the standard solution, autonomy is taken rightly to dominate (cf. Beauchamp, 2003; Macklin, 2003). (Things differ in the standard case of his or her young child.) The case is sketched in abstract and ideal terms and becomes, itself, a kind of rule to be applied to further actual cases. Competence in solving standard cases, in applying the principles and giving them standardly approved weight, becomes second nature to medical students keen to pass their ethics course and the element of individual judgement is downplayed.

So VBP makes explicit an idea implicit and often downplayed in conventional thinking about medical ethical practice, that there are diverse values in play and that attempts to codify them in principles are just a small part of the picture. Local context and individual preferences are the norm for VBP. Hence, the downplaying of principles-driven reasoning in the VBP claim:

(8) Ethical reasoning is employed in VBP primarily to explore differences of values, not, as in quasi-legal bioethics, to determine 'what is right' (the 'space of values' principle).

Taken together with the claim that such values are in play in diagnosis as well as treatment, this is already quite a radical view of the place of values in medical care. But there is a third, and yet more radical step, implicit in principle 8 in the rejection of 'what is right'.

Radical liberal VBP

The yet more radical third step is what leads to principles 5 and 9:

(5) In VBP, conflicts of values are resolved primarily, not by reference to a rule prescribing a 'right' outcome, but by processes designed to support a balance of legitimately different perspectives (the 'multi-perspective' principle).

(9) In VBP, communication skills have a substantive rather than (as in quasi-legal ethics) a merely executive role in clinical decision-making (the 'how it's done' principle).

It picks up something that ought to have been a worry about the comments above about the Four Principles approach to ethical judgement. I described it as a *deontological* or *principles*-based approach. But I then went on to suggest that, according to its own methods, the principles themselves are often insufficient for ethical judgement. Both specification and balancing require elements of judgement uncodified by the principles. Values-based practice embraces this feature and suggests that principles only have a limited role, in cases where there is agreement in values. But this should prompt two questions: what governs ethical judgements when they are not constrained by principles? And, why is there ever agreement in values?

Before I address these questions on behalf of radical values-based practice, I will first outline a more modest answer. The more modest approach takes ethical judgements to be more like judgements of facts than they are like arithmetic judgements. Arithmetic can, at least arguably, be formalised in accordance with axioms and thus the correct answer to an arithmetic question can be determined or derived algorithmically from those first principles. This is the picture of moral judgement to which a full blooded principlist account subscribes. Moral judgements are determined by accord with principles. Those are what make such judgements true or false. But the Four Principles account does not seem able to live up to that because extra-principled forms of judgement enter through specification and balancing.

An alternative to principlism is particularism. Moral judgements answer to real moral features of the world: the moral particulars realised in specific cases. And thus one way to interpret the Four Principles approach is on these lines. The principles do not determine the correctness or otherwise of judgements, despite first appearances. Rather, they serve as useful reminders of the sort of things to take into account when thinking through particular cases. Further, when we agree about moral values, this can be because we are correctly responding to real features of the world in the way that agreement about factual matters can be partially explained by those facts themselves impacting upon us.

One might take this to be the way to think about values-based practice: modest particularist VBP (cf. Thornton, 2007, pp. 49–88). If so, it can accommodate Fulford's emphasis on the complexity of particular cases and the necessity to develop skills in responding to conflicting values. But this does not seem to be Fulford's own view which appears to be rather more radical.

The clue to this is the claim that 'conflicts of values are resolved primarily, not by reference to a rule prescribing a "right" outcome, but by processes designed to support a balance of legitimately different perspectives.' Now particularism would also reject the idea of a rule prescribing a right outcome (because it stands opposed to principlism). But this VBP claim seems to go further and to replace the idea of there being a correct outcome, something antecedently good, with a right process (cf. Rubin, 2008). This thought is further reinforced by the claim that 'communication skills have a substantive rather than (as in quasi-legal ethics) a merely executive role in clinical decision-making.' Their role is substantive because the most there is of a 'good outcome' is the use of a right process. It is not that the process is a reliable way to determine the antecedently real moral particulars. Rather, the process is the end itself. So in response to the question 'what makes a value judgement true or false?', the answer seems to be neither accord with a principle or principles, nor accord with the real moral particulars, but rather, nothing further than competing views having been heard. So construed, values-based practice is a radical liberal position.

In a previous paper, I put this point baldly thus: 'Fundamentally, all and any values deserve a hearing. All and any can be valued if they survive the right process' (Thornton, 2011, p. 991). That is to overstate the position. As Fulford pointed out in reply:

> the premise of values-based practice in and of itself sets limits to the values that are 'values-based practice-able'. Thus, racism, and any other form of discrimination, as the NIMHE Values Framework makes clear, is incompatible in principle with 'mutual respect' and hence is by definition beyond the pale of values-based practice. Racism that is to say, is a value that, in Thornton's terms, doesn't even get as far as a hearing within values-based practice; it never gets into the process at all. (Fulford, 2011, p. 978)

This picks up a claim that was already explicit in the 2004 paper 'Ten principles of values-based medicine':

> The shared values which, in VBM, are the proper remit of the rules and regulation of quasi-legal ethics, provide, for a given group, a framework for decision-making; Where values are not shared, VBM starts not from the post modern 'anything goes', but from a principle of *mutual* respect with a range of clear and definite implications for policy and

practice (mutual respect, for example, precludes racism because racism is incompatible with respect for differences. . .) (Fulford, 2004, p. 230)

In other words, Fulford has never claimed that VBP is purely procedural. It has always presupposed a framework of transcendental values, the values without which it would be impossible. But even this framework is deeply contingent. Fulford comments:

> while people's values are highly diverse they are not chaotic. Values-based practice makes use of the (contingent) coherence of people's values to work within frameworks of values shared by the relevant stakeholder group (Fulford, 2013)

If there is sufficient agreement in value judgements then codifications of these judgements – whether ethical or legal or other – can be formulated. But such agreement is not explained as a response to real values 'out there' that command the agreement of right thinking people. The contingency is not merely that such value judgements are true (as empirical judgements can be contingently true) but rather, and more deeply, that there can be such agreement without the judgements answering to an antecedent notion of a good outcome.

This in turn suggests that there are two kinds of value judgements in play: those that are presupposed by the process of VBP and those that are the outcome of it. But neither sort, even including the transcendental values, is objective or independent. Both gain the degree of validity they possess either directly or indirectly from the VBP process. But the fact that without the framework of transcendental values VBP would be impossible is not yet to say that those values are right. To make that claim would require independent purchase on the judgement that VBP is itself good. (Consider an anthropological enquiry of the values that underpin the Beltane fire festival, for example. It is possible that there are some transcendental values for such a practice, without holding which no agent would enact the practice. But identifying them need not commit the anthropologist to endorsing either the festival or the necessary underpinning values.)

This suggests a difficulty with the radical view, however. What is the status of the claim that in VBP, conflicts of values are resolved primarily, not by reference to a rule prescribing a 'right' outcome, but by processes designed to support a balance of legitimately different perspectives? Note first that although it says that conflicts of values are resolved. . . this is in the context of values-based practice. So it should be read as saying: conflicts of values *should* be resolved . . . by processes designed to support a balance of legitimately different perspectives. But now we can ask, why should they? (It may be an analytic truth that they are within values-based practice, but we are invited to adopt this approach.)

The worry, now, is that this seems to be a value of a different order from the values that should be put through the right process of balancing views. It seems to be a higher order value, inconsistent with values-based practice's own approach. This then suggests a dilemma for radical VBP. It can either address the question of why we should value values in the way it suggests, but at the cost of violating its own principles, or it can attempt no such question, in which case it lacks the prescriptive force that would give it teeth.

Authoritarianism

Given this objection to the radical liberal version of VBP, why not adopt the more modest position outlined before which accepts the first two features of VBP but rejects the third in favour of moral particularism? In my earlier paper, I commented on an explanation of agreement in value judgements as answering to independent value judgements that: 'That approach – particularism – perhaps smacks of authoritarianism and, in the context of medicine, recalls the dangers of totalitarian psychiatry' (Thornton, 2011, p. 991).

Fulford agrees that this worry was indeed part of the motivation for rejecting the objectivist leanings of all of his commentators in the *Journal of Evaluation in Clinical Practice*:

> Worse still, there are clear hints of totalitarian leanings (understood as commitment to pre-set 'good outcomes') in all three commentators' positions: Brecher's apparent endorsement of 'moral objectivism' (p. 996) and later denial of patient choice (as 'saddling' the patient with responsibility, p. 997, see above), Hutchinson's advocacy of *Eudemonia* as '*the* Good Life' (p. 1001, emphasis added but Hutchinson's capitalization), and Thornton's moral particularism [2, p. 991], all suggest, as Thornton alone acknowledges, authoritarianism. That may or may not be a 'good thing' in theory. But as Thornton reminds us, when it comes to practice, authoritarianism in the guise of totalitarian psychiatry (involving as it did the imposition of a pre-set view of 'good outcomes') was the basis of some of the worst abuses of medical practice in the twentieth century. (Fulford, 2013)

The phrase 'imposition of a pre-set view of "good outcomes"' might carry either of two meanings, however. It might mean the imposition of a prejudiced view by powerful people. That would fit the label 'authoritarianism'. But it would not justify the rejection of the particularist in favour of the liberal view since the rejection of such a form of authoritarianism is consistent with a particularist picture of values.

Or it might mean that the process of deliberation of VBP answers to, is disciplined by, a, or the, good outcome, antecedent to and independent of the process. But if so, why think that responding to independently existing good outcomes is authoritarian? And can we understand VBP without 'authoritarianism'?

One motivation for thinking that responding to independently existing good outcomes is authoritarian, might be drawn from Rorty's assimilation of a rejection of a religious view of sin and a rejection of the view of empirical judgements or beliefs as picturing or representing the world. Rorty rejects both views as forms of authoritarianism in favour of pragmatism.

> The pragmatists' anti-representationalist account of belief is, among other things, a protest against the idea that human beings must humble themselves before something non-human, whether the Will of God or the Intrinsic Nature of Reality. Seeing anti-representationalism as a version of anti-authoritarianism permits one to appreciate an analogy which was central to John Dewey's thought: the analogy between ceasing to believe in Sin and ceasing to accept the distinction between Reality and Appearance. . . To have a sense of Sin, it is not enough to feel guilty. It is not enough to be appalled by the way human beings treat each other, and by your own capacity for vicious actions. You have to believe that there is a Being before whom we should humble ourselves. (Rorty, 2007, p. 257)

On this view, just as it is a sign of human maturity to reject religious authority in favour, instead, of human agreement, it is also a sign of maturity to reject a picture of judgements as answering to a non-human standard. John McDowell summarises the connection thus:

What Rorty takes to parallel authoritarian religion is the very idea that in everyday and scientific investigation we submit to standards constituted by the things themselves, the reality that is supposed to be the topic of the investigation. Accepting that idea, Rorty suggests, is casting the world in the role of the non-human Other before which we are to humble ourselves. Full human maturity would require us to acknowledge authority only if the acknowledgement does not involve abasing ourselves before something non-human. The only authority that meets this requirement is that of human consensus. If we conceive inquiry and judgment in terms of making ourselves answerable to the world, as opposed to being answerable to our fellows, we are merely postponing the completion of the humanism whose achievement begins with discarding authoritarian religion. (McDowell, 2000, pp. 109–110)

Rorty's view is motivated in part by a general criticism of the idea that empirical judgements and beliefs can represent the world, a criticism which dates back to his attack on the metaphor of the mind as a mirror of nature (Rorty, 1979). In more recent work this has led instead to the emphasis on 'solidarity' rather than objectivity (Rorty, 1991). But even if one did not share his more general anti-representationalism, one might still think that value judgements, in particular, cannot represent a realm of independent values. One reason for that – with echoes of Rorty's work – might be the view that value judgements depend on contingent features of human subjectivity. It is only because of contingent features of our natures and cultures that we are in any position to make the judgements we do. Further, value judgements can be 'hard' in this sense: even having deployed very thorough argument and debate, there seems to be no guarantee of agreement. There are echoes of both of these two views in Fulford's radical version of VBP.

Thus, one way to motivate a rejection of authoritarianism in VBP, construed merely as the idea of being disciplined by some sort of right or good outcome, is to take note of the underlying contingency of value judgements and to conclude from this that the idea of objectivity in this area makes no sense. Such a view would have a precedent in Rorty's more general account of the metaphysics of human thought.

If so, however, there is an alternative to be found in what McDowell goes on to outline. The key idea is that neither the underlying contingency nor the idea that value judgements are hard rules out objectivity.

One aspect of the immaturity that Rorty finds in putting objectivity rather than solidarity at the focus of philosophical discourse is a wishful denial of a certain sort of argumentative or deliberative predicament. On the face of it, certain substantive questions are such that we can be confident of answers to them, on the basis of thinking the matter through with whatever resources we have for dealing with questions of the relevant kind (for instance, ethical questions)... But even after we have done our best at marshalling considerations in favor of an answer to such a question, we have no guarantee that just anyone with whom we can communicate will find our answer compelling. That fact – perhaps brought forcibly home by our failing to persuade someone – can then induce the sideways glance, and undermine the initial confidence. Rorty's suggestion is that the language of objectivity reflects a philosophical attempt to shore up the confidence so threatened, by wishfully denying the predicament. The wishful idea is that in principle reality itself fills in this gap in our persuasive resources. Any rational subject who does not see things aright must be failing to make proper use of humanly universal capacities to be in tune with the world. If we fall into this way of thinking, we are trying to exploit the image of an ideal position in which we are in touch with something greater than ourselves – a secular counterpart to the idea of being at one with the divine – in order to avoid acknowledging the ineliminable hardness of hard questions, or in order to avoid facing up to the sheer contingency that attaches to our being in a historically evolved cultural position that enables us to find compelling just the considerations we do find compelling.

Here too we can make a separation. This wishful conception of attunement with how things really are, as a means of avoiding an uncomfortable acknowledgement of the limitations of reason and the contingency of our capacities to think as we believe we should, can be detached from the very idea of making ourselves answerable to how things are. We can join Rorty in deploring the former without needing to join him in abandoning the very idea of aspiring to get things right… (McDowell, 2000, p. 112)

This suggests two ways of thinking about VBP and authoritarianism. One can reject authoritarianism, construed as a commitment to 'good outcomes' independent of any particular instance of the process of deliberation, and put the emphasis on process or solidarity and motivate it by invoking something like Rorty's rejection of abasement to the 'Other'. One can appeal to this in the case of value judgements in particular because of their connection to the contingencies of human subjectivity and the omnipresence of hard judgements.

But, if so, one will need to shore up that picture against the objection that it does not follow from those motivations alone. That is, one can combine the first two elements of VBP, which I outlined at the start, with a denial of a constitutive role of process and maintain that, even in VBP, value judgements are disciplined by evaluative particulars. This is the second way to think of UBP and authoritarianism. One way to fill this out is to borrow McDowell's own account in which the realm of values is in a transcendental harmony with our subjectivity (McDowell, 1998). That is, only those subjects with a particular kind of mind and life can have their eyes open(ed) to this tract of reality. (Thus the independence of the process or procedure of making value judgements and the values to which it answers is at the level of instances. In each individual case, the process may deliver the wrong judgement but as a whole, the process cannot in general deliver the wrong result.) Such an alternative is at least available to VBP at the cost of adopting, and defending, a particularist metaphysics of values.

Conclusions

I have set out two approaches to values-based practice and authoritarianism with their distinct philosophical costs. But there are reasons to favour the latter.

First, as I argued earlier, proposing or supporting VBP itself presupposes a value which does not seem simply to await the VBP process. (Nor would granting it a transcendental status help, a precondition *if* one wants to practice VBP, since that would still be contingent on that conditional.) Thus the value of VBP itself cannot be accounted for within VBP's resources if they are taken to exclude the idea of a good outcome, independent of a process of deliberation.

Second, as Fulford's fifth principle of values-based practice states: 'In VBP, conflicts of values are resolved primarily, not by reference to a rule prescribing a "right" outcome, but by processes designed to support a balance of legitimately different perspectives (the "multi-perspective" principle).' But surely not just any balance would do? For example, a 'balance' imposed through undue force or influence by powerful parties to a clinical decision would not be a good outcome. So 'balance' is to be understood as something like the right or a good balance, which again seems to presuppose the kind of innocent authoritarianism in question.

Third, as Fulford often stresses, VBP involves the exercise of *skill*. But the clearest way to understand the development of such a skill involves learning how to achieve a good outcome in complex circumstances. This may well resist codification into an algorithm. It may involve sensitivity to context. But that is just to repeat a particularist rejection of principlism about value judgement.

Even if it is possible to position a radical, liberal version of VBP in the broader recent history of western thought, there remain reasons to prefer modest particularist values-based practice.

References

Beauchamp, T. L. (2003) Methods and principles in biomedical ethics. *Journal of Medical Ethics*, **29**, 269–274.

Beauchamp, T. L., and Childress, J. F. (2001) *Principles of Biomedical Ethics*. Oxford: Oxford University Press.

Boorse, C. (1975) On the distinction between disease and illness. *Philosophy and Public Affairs*, **5**, 49–68.

Fulford, K. W. M. (1989) *Moral Theory and Medical Practice*. Cambridge: Cambridge University Press.

Fulford, K. W. M. (2004) Ten principles of values-based medicine. In Radden, J. (editor), *The Philosophy of Psychiatry: A Companion*, pp. 205–234. New York: Oxford University Press.

Fulford, K. W. M. (2011) The value of evidence and evidence of values: bringing together values-based and evidence-based practice in policy and service development in mental health. *Journal of Evaluation in Clinical Practice*, **17**, 976–987.

Fulford, K. W. M. (2013) Values-based practice: Fulford's dangerous idea. *Journal of Evaluation in Clinical Practice*, **19**(3), 537–546.

Hare, R. M. (1952) *The Language of Morals*. Oxford: Oxford University Press.

Kendell, R. E. (1975) The concept of disease and its implications for psychiatry. *British Journal of Psychiatry*, **127**, 305–315.

Macklin, R. (2003) Applying the four principles. *Journal of Medical Ethics*, **29**, 275–280.

McDowell, J. (1998) *Mind Value and Reality*. Cambridge, MA: Harvard University Press.

McDowell, J. (2000) Towards rehabilitating objectivity. In Brandom, R. B. (editor), *Rorty and His Critics*. Oxford: Blackwell.

Rorty, R. (1979) *Philosophy and the Mirror of Nature*. Princeton, NJ: Princeton University Press.

Rorty, R. (1991) Solidarity or objectivity. *Objectivity, Relativism and Truth*. Cambridge: Cambridge University Press.

Rorty, R. (2007) Pragmatism as anti-authoritarianism. In Shook, J. R. and Margolis, J. (editors), *Companion to Pragmatism*. London: Wiley Blackwell.

Rubin, J. (2008) Political liberalism and values-based practice: processes above outcomes or rediscovering the priority of the right over the good. *Philosophy Psychiatry and Psychology*, **15**, 117–123.

Sadler, J. Z. (2004) *Values and Psychiatric Diagnosis*. Oxford: Oxford University Press.

Szasz, T. (1972) *The Myth of Mental Illness*. London: Paladin.

Thornton, T. (2000) Mental illness and reductionism: can functions be naturalized? *Philosophy, Psychiatry and Psychology*, **7**, 67–76.

Thornton, T. (2006) Judgement and the role of the metaphysics of values in medical ethics. *Journal of Medical Ethics*, **32**, 365–370.

Thornton, T. (2007) *Essential Philosophy of Psychiatry*. Oxford: Oxford University Press.

Thornton, T. (2011) Radical liberal values-based practice. *Journal of Evaluation in Clinical Practice*, **17**, 988–991.

Wakefield, J. C. (1999) Mental disorder as a black box essentialist concept. *Journal of Abnormal Psychology*, **108**, 465–472.

Chapter 5

Values-based practice: but which values, and whose?[1]

Bob Brecher

Introduction

Values-based practice (VBP) is founded on a recognition that values play an important part in health care (Fulford, 2013). That is hardly controversial, whatever one's view of what those values should be or what might be their source. Even so, Fulford's advocacy of 'values-based practice' is deeply puzzling; for although it purports to do justice to the full range of whatever values anyone concerned brings to the table, it in fact leaves conflicts between people's values at best unresolved or, worse, simply ignored. The difficulty arises from what seem to be two fundamental shortcomings of the approach. Firstly, it is not even remotely clear what Fulford takes values to be. In particular, how can values be 'based' in skills (Fulford, 2011, p. 976) as though they were something instrumental rather than normative? What, then, does it mean to say that 'Values-based practice is a new skills-based approach to working more effectively with complex and conflicting values' (Fulford, 2011, p. 976)? Until we know how a 'value' might come to be 'based in' a 'skill', we do not even know how to work out what this might mean. Secondly, values are always someone's values; but Fulford glosses over the problem of whose values VBP is supposed to consist in, gesturing vaguely in the direction of liberalism, as if that were something both fairly simply given and normatively uncontroversial. Let us look at these two issues in turn.

---

[1] This chapter is based on Brecher (2011). It develops the material published there and considers Fulford's response to that paper and other criticisms in Fulford (2013).

Debates in Values-Based Practice, ed. Michael Loughlin. Published by Cambridge University Press. © Cambridge University Press 2014.

Values? Which values?

The claim that practice should be 'based on' values is only helpful, or indeed meaningful, to the extent that we have some understanding of the meaning of the term 'values'. So what does Fulford say to help us understand what he means by 'values'? Values, he claims, extend to 'needs, wishes, preferences, indeed to any and all of the many and diverse ways in which people express, directly or indirectly, negative or positive evaluations and value judgments' (Fulford, 2011, p. 976). The final claim here is a tautology – values are whatever is expressed in judgements about value. Apart from that, the 'explanation' seems to equate values with both 'preferences' and 'needs'. But are values, preferences and needs the same thing? Arguably, values, preferences and needs are crucially different.

Some needs – even one's own – are clearly neither values nor the expression of any value; nor are they necessarily the same thing as 'preferences'. Consider needs such as adequate health or human recognition. These are needs we all have, whether or not we know, agree or acknowledge that we do, and thus whether or not we value them. Objectivist views of ethics – such as Len Doyal's and Ian Gough's (1991) classic *A Theory of Human Need* – rest precisely upon the distinction between what people want and what they need. Fulford notes that 'the very term "values" means different things to different people' (Fulford, 2011, p. 976). This is no doubt correct, but it does not tell us anything helpful about what the term designates. He then reports that a survey showed no 'shared meanings' (Fulford, 2011, p. 976). Of course there will be disagreement about what the term designates: but his claim that 'Values are of course not completely individual' (Fulford, 2011, p. 976), shows – albeit without telling us exactly what he takes the term 'value' to mean – that he is talking about something specific. He must be, if his proposal is to have any substantial content. But what is it? Of course 'any attempt to reduce the meaning of the complex concept of values to a definition of the kind for which Brecher calls risks promoting a (Wittgensteinian) illusion' (Fulford, 2013, p. 540); or rather, it would, had I called for it. But I do not. If even something as comparatively simple as a bicycle cannot be defined, but only described, then people's values – unlike, say, a circle – cannot be defined either. What I do call for, and what I do not find anywhere in Fulford's account of what he takes 'value' to mean, is some minimal characterisation of what he has in mind. And that is surely a reasonable request: if we are being asked to subscribe to something calling itself values-based practice then we had better know what it is that we are being asked to sign up to. How can I respond to the question, 'Do you fancy a pint?' if I do not know what a pint is? Nor – of course – would an attempt to define it help, not least because whereas a 'pint' (an imperial measure) can be defined, a pint (as in 'a pint of beer') cannot be.

The puzzle is compounded when Fulford tells us that 'Values-based practice offers a different response ... in being based primarily on learnable clinical skills' and that 'good clinical skills ... are required in coming to balanced judgments' (Fulford, 2011, pp. 976–977). How can values be 'based ... on' 'clinical skills'? If they are based on such skills, then they must have some connection, at least, with them. But what? How *could* clinical skills offer either a basis for values or a basis for making judgements about them? It is as though being a skilled cyclist made one adept at making judgements about whether or not to cycle on the pavement. It does not. Nor do clinical skills, however important, enable one to make ethical decisions about how, when and whether to apply them. What is required in each case is ethical judgement, and this is something quite different from the exercise of a technical skill. Judgements of value may be thought of as requiring a sort of skill (skill in living well or in thinking well, depending on whether we follow Aristotle or Kant); but these are not at all the same *sort* of skills as those in which clinical skills, or cycling skills, consist. If judgements of value can be understood as requiring, let alone consisting in, the exercise of skills at all, this is so in only a metaphorical sense. I have to conclude that what Fulford takes values to be remains mysterious. Granted that definition, being impossible, cannot help. But then, what does?

Certainly not his 'Ten key elements of values-based practice' (Fulford, 2011, p. 979), which are not remotely recognisable as encompassing or exemplifying values. Even if one were to accept that 'values-based practice' can be understood in some (albeit unspecified by Fulford) sense as the exercise of a set of skills (and I admit I have no idea what that sense might be), the 'elements' Fulford outlines are all technical skills: he refers to them as 'learnable clinical skills' (Fulford, 2011, p. 979). They are of course none the worse for that. That said, it remains entirely obscure how the exercise of 'clinical skills' can be what 'values-based practice' consists in – even if one takes a fairly relaxed view of the alleged difference between facts and values. As other contributors to this volume note (see Chapter 3), Fulford's argument that 'values-based practice' is built primarily on 'learnable clinical skills' contradicts his claim that 'values-based practice is derived from philosophical value-theory' (Fulford, 2011, p. 980). For whatever clinical skills he has in mind, they are not any variety of value theory; and whatever he might have in mind in terms of value theory, it cannot be any sort of technical skill.

The view that clinical skills should form the basis of practice constitutes and/or expresses and/or derives from a particular set of values, as does 'evidence-based' practice itself (Gupta, 2011; Hutchinson, 2011). No practice, and no conception of the skills that such a practice requires, is value-free. But that is a different claim from Fulford's apparent claim that they are in some (unexplained) way identical. His own approach is an attempt to instantiate a certain set of values, which is one reason why his vagueness about what values actually are is an important issue for his argument. It may of course be that this is not what he intends, and that I have failed to understand what he is getting at, but thus far his response (Fulford, 2013) to what strike me as the fairly straightforward and fundamental questions I and others raised about his conception of 'values' (Brecher, 2011; Gupta, 2011; Hutchinson, 2011) has failed to enlighten me. If his critics have simply misunderstood him, then he really needs to make it clear exactly how values can be based in skills; and – a different issue – what in turn the values are that underpin such a view of values as thus fundamentally instrumental. In short, Fulford still needs to make explicit, and to justify, his assumptions. They are not self-evident and the responsibility to explain the meaning of his own fundamental claims is surely his.

Some of his assumptions do come to the surface (though are not thereby justified) in Table 5 and the commentary on it (Fulford, 2011, p. 982). What becomes apparent is an insidiously formulaic approach: it is as though all would be well if we could just get the elements of the appropriate code right. This sort of approach will be familiar to many practitioners as it reflects the 'tick-box' approach to ethical practice of many senior NHS (and not just NHS) managers and their political masters. It is as if this particular 'values-based' approach could save clinical practitioners the trouble of exercising their own moral agency and instead enable them simply to check that they had taken account of all the correct 'elements'. Far from promoting more ethical practice, such approaches undermine the critical moral reflection that is the essence of genuine moral deliberation, exemplifying how an increasingly immoral society is dressed in 'ethical' clothes to disguise the fact (Brecher, 2004).

That is presumably not what Fulford intends, though it is what one might expect from an approach that apparently equates making value judgements with learning a technical skill. In the guise of offering 'a new skills-based approach to working more effectively with complex and conflicting values' (Fulford, 2011, p. 976), his proposal replicates neo-liberalism in its acceptance of what 'effectively' is taken to mean and – again – of the moral values underpinning that acceptance.

Whose values?

Whatever his intentions, Fulford's 'new' approach turns out actually to serve today's neo-liberal agenda (see Chapter 6). This impression is unhappily underlined by his proposed 'focus-group approach' to the question of whose values he has in mind. Is it individual clinicians'? Or the Trust's? Or individual patients'? Or the government's? When they clash – as clash they will – whose are to prevail and on what grounds? Merely to observe that ethical 'framework values are often in conflict' (Fulford, 2011, p. 976) is entirely unhelpful, however accurate: the question of how actually to resolve clashes of values remains unaddressed, let alone answered. For example, of course, and as we know all too well, 'respecting autonomy may be in conflict with acting in a patient's best interests' (Fulford, 2011, p. 976) – but that shows merely that the putatively neutral but in reality deeply ideological "Four Principles" approach (Beauchamp and Childress, 2001) at best solves nothing and, more usually, serves simply to invite the clinician, the manager or the Trust to insist on their own way of resolving the conflict. Alternatively, it saddles the patient with responsibility for 'making the choice'; thus at once accepting the ideology of choice, imposing it on the patient and in all likelihood blaming them if that choice turns out to be wrong. Everyone is listened to, everyone's views and values are taken into consideration; and everyone who does not accept the neo-liberal mantra of choice is ignored.

Fulford goes on to claim that 'values-based practice adds . . . a particular focus on the diversity of *individual* values and the need to incorporate this diversity more effectively in clinical decision-making' (Fulford, 2011, p. 977). But this again leaves unrecognised the key practical question of who is going to do what with this 'diversity'. Who is going to 'incorporate' it and how? How – and by whom – are the conflicts that Fulford rightly recognises going to be resolved? It is one thing to observe that different people have different values. Taking it into account – addressing the question of how, precisely, one takes this into account – is something else; and resolving the clashes concerned is another thing again. Fulford notes that 'the approach reflects the diversity of the values of clinicians as well as patients' and that 'it is responsive to the evidence' (Fulford, 2011, p. 977). But these assertions are empty until and unless both the terms 'reflects' and 'is responsive' are cashed out. Unfortunately, Fulford does not do this. Most worryingly, he himself says that his approach 'operates within and is constrained by the framework of shared values incorporated in ethical codes and guidelines' (Fulford, 2011, p. 977). Far from being reassuring, this suggests all too clearly how and by whom the necessary content of the 'framework of shared values' is to be supplied – namely by those in command. Fulford remains silent on the issues of who exactly shares the values in question and how the judgement that this is so might validly be made. In short, he assumes that the 'values' he relies on are in some sense neutral and – whatever their content – shared by all of us.

But they are neither neutral nor shared by all of 'us'. Insofar as the sorts of thing they are supposed to be can be discerned at all, their form is clearly liberal. My objection to that is not that it is a liberal view; but rather that it is an unacknowledgedly liberal view, and thus one quite devoid of the sorts of defence of liberalism that might justify the position. In short, Fulford is asking us to accept a liberal framework of values without being explicit that this is what his 'values-based practice' requires. Furthermore, and more practically, this liberalism masquerading as, it seems, some sort of 'common sense' allows neo-liberals to take advantage of that empty, undefended space by filling it in with a variety of liberalism that would have been anathema to the values espoused by, for instance, John Stuart Mill.[2]

His observation (no doubt accurate) that 'the values likely to be driving' a mental health team's decisions and actions 'were not those of their clients but those of the team' (Fulford, 2011, p. 977) does not help. Is the position that it ought to have been the clients' values that determined what the mental health team did? Fulford implies this. But if so, then, however laudable (or not) that position may be, it does not even begin to address what needs to be addressed. What if a client's values clash with those of the team? Or with dominant political values – such as 'choice'? What if different clients' values clash with each other? Should the NHS institute structures and practices that 'incorporate' *everyone's* values? Again, what would this actually mean?

The problem of conflict between values is ineliminable. In practice it needs to be fairly – perhaps democratically – resolved even if that goes against some parties' values (see Chapter 6). The supposition that conflict can be resolved to the satisfaction of the parties involved, whatever their own values might in fact be, is unrealistic. Either such a supposition is sincere but naïve or (much worse) it is awesomely disingenuous. Either way, the actual outcome is likely to be an imposition of the values of whoever holds effective power. One has only to remember, for example, the use Blair made of 'the evidence base' and of 'values' in his attempted justification of the invasion of Iraq, the corruption of the universities and of course the incipient privatisation of the NHS, to appreciate the point.

The assumption, that liberalism is just obviously right, that underpins Fulford's proposal is all too clear. Here are two illustrations. He maintains that 'values-based practice is entirely consistent with those forms particularly of religious belief (such as the Benedictine tradition of spiritual direction) that are *open and respectful of the beliefs of others*' (Fulford 2013, p. 538, fn.1, my emphasis); that is to say, it is consistent with those forms of religious belief that are compatible with liberalism. Or consider his discussion (Fulford, 2011, pp. 981–982) of the Beauchamp and Childress principles I referred to above: autonomy, beneficence, justice and non-maleficence. He claims that 'the four principles, then, taken together, provide four dimensions for opening up and exploring the *full* values-aspects of a given case' (Fulford, 2011, p. 982 my emphasis). But they do no such thing, however valuable (or otherwise) any one or more of them may be. They reflect *merely one* particular view of what counts as 'the *full* values-aspects' concerned; in this case a liberal view. But liberalism – whether Beauchamp and Childress's or Rawls's (1971) – is neither self-evident nor neutral. Not only might other values be thought

---

[2] For a discussion of the different sorts of liberalism allegedly an influence in Fulford's work on VBP, see Chapters 4 and 6. For Fulford's own thoughts on this issue, see Fulford (2013).

relevant (dependence, patience and equity, for example) but the liberal Holy Quartet might be rejected and/or understood quite differently than from a liberal perspective. So, for example, 'autonomy' might not figure in a person's set of values at all; 'beneficence' and 'non-maleficence' might be understood accordingly; and 'justice' might be interpreted in a radically different way from its liberal instantiation. Perhaps it is his unargued commitment to liberalism that allows him simply to assert that '"dependency, patience and equity" ... are fully compatible with liberalism at least as expressed in values-based practice' (Fulford, 2013, p. 539). But that is either to adopt a view of liberalism, both historically and conceptually, which is to say the least at odds with how liberalism is actually understood (and criticised – see for example MacIntyre's classical analyses (1997, 2009)) or implicitly to insist that liberalism is whatever one wishes it to be. Neither view is remotely tenable.

Fulford's insouciance about whose values his 'values-based' approach reflects allows him to speak of 'Bringing together Values and Evidence' (Fulford, 2011, p. 984) in the way he does. Citing Sackett approvingly, he reports him as saying that

> evidence-based medicine ... involves the integration of three key elements: 1) best research evidence, 2) clinical expertise, and 3) patients' values. There could be no clearer statement of the importance of a twin-track 'evidence plus values' approach to health care decision-making. (Fulford, 2011, p. 984)

This might not seem a particularly startling conclusion. Yet in the context of Fulford's argument it is indeed startling, because his earlier insistence (Fulford, 2011, p. 977) that his approach 'reflects the diversity of the values of clinicians as well as patients' appears by now to have been entirely lost. I am tempted to surmise that, given the likely clashes and contradictions among patients' values alone, to bring in at this stage the clinicians' values earlier claimed to be part of the picture (with the likely clashes and contradictions between those, and the further likely clashes and contradictions between these two already contradictory sets of values) might too easily upset all those neat tables of the elements of 'values-based practice'. If we also bring in the values that managers, Trusts and politicians may care to bring to the table, the disturbance is even greater.

Conclusion

To ask for answers to the question, 'Which values and whose?' is not to ask for definitions. *Of course* it is better if, 'rather than trying to come up with a definition of "value" we look instead at how the term is actually used by those concerned, i.e. by, in the case of values-based practice, those concerned directly or indirectly in a given decision in a given health care context' (Fulford, 2013, p. 540). But it will not do to assume that those people must be committed to liberal values or to liberal conceptions of what values might be. To ask that the liberalism which frames 'values-based practice' be explicitly acknowledged, plausibly characterised and distinguished from the neo-liberalism for which not doing these things makes space is not unreasonable. And the remark that there are 'totalitarian leanings ... in ... Brecher's apparent endorsement of "moral objectivism"' (Fulford, 2013, p. 539) is as uninformed about moral objectivism as it is self-defeating. For Fulford is in fact no less committed to moral objectivism than I am: how else is one to understand his insistence that – to take just one example – 'racism, and any other form of discrimination, as the NIMHE Values Framework makes clear (Fulford, 2011, p. 978, Table 2), is incompatible in principle with "mutual respect" and hence is by definition beyond the pale of values-based practice. Racism, that is to say, is a value that . . . doesn't even get as far as a hearing within values-based practice; it never gets into the process at all' (Fulford, 2011, p. 978)? Either that welcome claim is an instantiation of moral objectivism or it is merely a matter of opinion. If the latter, then it is of no consequence; if the former, then it cannot be squared with moral non-objectivism.

I continue to find it very hard to see how Fulford's proposal might usefully contribute to any genuine resolution to the problem of conflicting values in health care. Indeed, I have to conclude that by reason of its unexamined liberalism it is likely all too easily, and however inadvertently, to contribute to the neo-liberal revolution currently taking place in UK health care.

References

Beauchamp, T. L., and Childress, J. F. (2001) *Principles of Biomedical Ethics*, 5th edition. Oxford: Oxford University Press.

Brecher, R. (2004) Against professional ethics. *Philosophy of Management*, **4**, 3–8.

Brecher, R. (2011) Which values? And whose? A reply to Fulford. *Journal of Evaluation in Clinical Practice*, **17**, 996–998.

Doyal, N. and Gough, I. (1991) *A Theory of Human Need*. Basingstoke: Palgrave Macmillan.

Fulford, K. W. M. (2011) The value of evidence and evidence of values: bringing together values-based and evidence-based practice in policy and service development in mental health. *Journal of Evaluation in Clinical Practice*, **17**, 976–987.

Fulford, K. W. M. (2013) Values-based practice: Fulford's dangerous idea. *Journal of Evaluation in Clinical Practice*, **19**, 537–546.

Gupta, M. (2011) Values-based practice and bioethics. *Journal of Evaluation in Clinical Practice*, **17**, 992–995.

Hutchinson, P. (2011) The philosopher's task: VBP and 'bringing to consciousness'. *Journal of Evaluation in Clinical Practice*, **17**, 999–1001.

MacIntyre, A. (1997) *After Virtue*, new edition. London: Duckworth.

MacIntyre, A. (2009) *Dependent Rational Animals*. London: Duckworth.

Rawls, J. (1971) *A Theory of Justice*. Cambridge, MA: Harvard University Press.

Chapter 6

Reframing health care: philosophy for medicine and human flourishing

Phil Hutchinson and Rupert Read

Introductory comments

An important insight of Fulford's work – which actually precedes his development of 'values-based practice' – is that there is no such thing as 'value-free' diagnosis. To characterise a person as having a particular illness is to make a value-laden claim, whether or not people reflect on what the values are that underlie the diagnosis (Fulford, 1989). We agree with him on this point, but want to ground a view about the role of value judgements in diagnosis in a broader conceptual framework – one which argues that there is no such thing as an approach to health care (including the science of medicine) that is 'philosophy-free'. In what follows we explain and justify this claim before bringing out its significance to Fulford's project and his own underlying assumptions about the relationship between value, philosophy, science and practice.

Medical science (philosophy redundant)

What business does philosophy have in health care? The application of statistical methods will tell us scientifically which medical interventions and diagnostic procedures are most effective. Statistical analysis, in the form of RCTs and their meta-analysis in Cochrane Collaboration-style systematic reviews, has become the benchmark of good scientific practice. Some still hold that a good scientist will insist on finding support for inductive statistical analysis in explanatory work on biochemical causal mechanisms, but wherever one stands, whether one is a positivist who believes that we really only need concern

Debates in Values-Based Practice, ed. Michael Loughlin. Published by Cambridge University Press. © Cambridge University Press 2014.

ourselves with 'Cochrane-style' inductive statistical analysis or whether one thinks it essential to understand the causal mechanisms at work,[1] this is what health care is: evidence-based health care, as it is referred to on the Cochrane Collaboration website. This is why what we here refer to as 'health care' is widely referred to as, and used interchangeably with, 'medical science', and one (valid) reason for this is to differentiate it from quackery, or pseudoscience, such as homeopathy. But does the insistence on seeing health care simply as science, and science of a particular sort, have unfortunate side effects? Is there anything else that can be said, which might qualify as being distinctively medical while falling outside the purview of science?

We ask this because while it has emerged as an assumption of some prominence that philosophy is a sort of proto-science, this is, we submit, a false assumption. Unfortunately, the falsity of the assumption does not seem to impact on its prominence. The assumption might be illustrated by the following narrative presentation: psychology is a relatively new science and as such it is a discipline occupied by and under siege from many folk assumptions and confusions. Philosophers might hold the fort of psychological reason against attacks from the folk beyond the battlements (and quell the internal insurrections), but all we can really expect from the philosophers is that they can hold the fort, not that they might win the battle and establish law and order. For, the idea is, philosophers are simply not equipped to do *that*. One day, the philosophers know, the scientific cavalry will arrive. They will thank the philosophers for keeping the flag of reason flying, but tell them they are no longer needed. The real scientists are here. The neuroscientists are here to win the battle once and for all and establish the neuroscientific laws which will govern the region of psychology from here-on-in. If you are a philosopher who insists on sticking around and questioning the laws, then you must be some kind of anarchist (or libertarian cf. David Colquhoun's *ad hominem* remarks about Michael Loughlin[2]). We can exchange 'psychology' for 'medicine' in this story and the same would apply: on this view, philosophers are redundant following the work of Archie Cochrane and later the emergence of the evidence-based medicine movement in the 1990s. Philosophical hand-wringing about the nature of causality, about whether or not 'evidence' is a concept the content of which is specific to particular domains of enquiry, and philosophical arguments about the problems of Positivism and 'problem of induction' are at best seen as what Taleb (2007) refers to (talking about philosophy in another context) as *weekend problems*[3]: problems that we do not need to bother ourselves with Monday to Friday, when the real important work is being undertaken.

What's wrong with this picture? While such a picture might be operative in the subconscious of many scientists,[4] it will appear to most philosophers to rest on a set of

---

[1] The bio-statistical community is not as one on this. Some seem to be interested only in inductive statistical analysis, others claim that a scientist must be concerned to explain in terms of the underlying causal mechanisms as a part of the overall explanation. See Bausell (2007) for an example of a bio-statistician who holds the latter view. David Colquhoun seems to be an example of someone who holds the former view.

[2] See Colquhoun's remarks about Loughlin, here: http://bit.ly/1ciC4uV.

[3] Taleb's work might in other ways provide support for the line of thought we shall pursue in the present chapter. In future work, we hope to lay out how genuinely precautionary/'via negativa' thinking may undermine EBM and VBP. See also footnote 14 and the final section, below.

[4] See, for example, the recent remarks of Peter Atkins (2011) and Stephen Hawking (2010). See Hutchinson's (2013) discussion of these claims in his 'What Have the Philosophers Ever Done For Us?'

crudely inaccurate assumptions about the discipline of philosophy; for while science by-and-large is about explaining real things and how they interact, philosophy is about explaining or understanding the nature of reality at the most general level. How one meets that question – the nature-of-reality question – determines what sort of philosopher one is (realist, idealist; cognitivist, non-cognitivist; rationalist, empiricist; and so on). So, while the philosopher's domain is not coextensive with that of the scientists, it is the domain which frames the enquiries of the scientist. (The *world* has little concern for academic disciplinary boundaries.) Philosophers do not *seek* to answer the questions of science in lieu of the application of scientific methods to those questions, but rather seek to identify distinctively philosophical questions, questions that cannot be readily reduced to scientific questions (or reduced to mathematical questions, and so on). Philosophers then seek to understand the nature of these questions: for example are they answerable, and if so through the adoption of which methods? Linguistic? Experimental? Or do the questions need reformulating or even dissolving?

Where a medical scientist will want to enquire as to what evidential basis there is for the administration of intervention X to treat illness Y, the philosopher will want to look at that which frames the question: what makes Y an illness in need of treatment?[5] What makes X qualify as something it makes sense to think of as a cure, given the non-curative negative or debilitating effects it has on a person (or society) in addition to its ability to combat the illness? What *counts* as evidence in specific domains of enquiry?

Medical science 'reframed' (some philosophical-ethical aspects of health care)

So far we have talked of philosophers and scientists, as if one can be uniquely one and not the other. However, philosophy is unavoidable, even for scientists: the thought that philosophy can simply be forgone, based in the assumption that it is a proto-science and therefore redundant once we earn the right to drop the 'proto' prefix, is a profound error which contributes to philosophical naïvety and serves to justify philosophical ignorance. The naïvety is to be found in the extent to which one will be missing the distinctively philosophical aspects of one's enquiry; the ignorance will seem justified because in missing those distinctively philosophical aspects one will feel justified in ignoring philosophical suggestions, objections and corrections that might well be pertinent (or dismissing them as being only of interest at the weekend, when the real work has been completed). Rejection of philosophy does not amount to what one might be tempted to assume: it is not to forgo actually doing philosophy, in favour of rigorous science or philosophy-free science; rather it is to commit oneself to doing spontaneous philosophy. Philosophy is unavoidable. Philosophical assumptions frame our investigations, whatever discipline provides the home for those investigations. It is important how our questions are framed. For example, framing certain psychological questions in the same way as one might frame non-psychological medical questions might well result in the misidentification/confusion of symptoms and causes. Philosophy is not an add-on, but always present. It is not what one does when one is still waiting for the frontiers of science to extend to and encompass one's domain. Philosophical assumptions *frame* what one does and, therefore, leaving those assumptions unexamined is simply to accept the frames bestowed by

---

[5] See, for example, Havi Carel's (2008) work.

happenstance. So, to return to the question with which we began: what business does philosophy have in health care?

Beyond the identification of effective medical interventions and effective diagnostic practices (the science part, allegedly) there exist of course concerns about the appropriate ways people might interact, the appropriate ways in which people might be used in drug trials, questions of physician-assisted dying, questions of stem cell research, cloning and so on. One can see these as ethical questions which are separate from the science of health care. So, while one might argue that medical epistemology is the domain of the sciences, beyond that there are questions of an ethical character. Some of those ethical questions are discussed by bio-ethicists, such as questions of stem cell research and cloning; while some are left to professional ethics committees, such as the appropriate ways in which people might be used in trials, for example. But if we leave things at this, we simply accept the frames as they are currently set by medical science. Let us try a little reframing.

Consider the norms governing the physician/surgeon-patient relationship, or more specifically consider the norms in play when a surgeon advises a patient on a particular surgical intervention for preventative reasons: a mastectomy, for example, or a prosta-tectomy. One might be tempted to suggest that the surgeon's judgement here should be guided purely by the balance of probabilities, and in suggesting so one might believe this to be a domain that falls well within the purview of the statistical sciences. The judgement should be evidence based. But in talking of balancing probabilities, what, beyond (or behind) the numbers, is being balanced? Let us assume that there is a statistically high risk of cancer on the one hand; what are we asking our surgeon to balance this against? Does the surgeon need to have empathetic understanding of a life without breasts or a life lived with a high likelihood of erectile dysfunction? Or does the surgeon need only to have consulted the QoLs[6] for those who live a life under the threat of cancer, undergoing regular tests, and then later having to undergo a long debilitating course of chemotherapy in comparison to those who live without the threat, without the tests, and without the chemo, but also have to come to terms with living without their breasts and with massive scars (mastectomy) or with a high likelihood of incontinence and/or impotence (prostatectomy)? Is it unethical of a surgeon to make a recommendation based on their judgement if they have made no attempt to consider the *significance* for the patient, the significance within the culture, of the surgical intervention being proposed? How might one set about answering such a question? This is not a question about what is a right or wrong recommendation, not an ethical question in the standard sense of enquiring after the morally right action or the correct response to a moral dilemma, but rather a question regarding the appropriate 'resources' one believes ought to be drawn upon by the surgeon in arriving at her/his judgement. It is a question about what one should expect from those who make evaluative judgements.

One point we might bring out here is this: we could imagine a response which suggests that the surgeon should merely restrict their advice to the success rate of the intervention, and the possible negative effects (side effects), and others should advise on other things. Here the surgeon avoids the difficult question posed in the previous paragraph by restricting their role to simply providing the data regarding the proposed surgical intervention's success rate, side effects and potential complications. But there are a

---

[6] See Loughlin (2002) for a critique of QoLs, QALYs and the like.

number of reasons for finding such a response unsatisfactory. First, the term 'success' is evaluative and determines what are to *count* as the pertinent data hereabouts. Second, surgical interventions do not take place in a political and economic vacuum. The relative costs of different interventions will be relevant. Moreover, adjudicating between the relative costs of different interventions will involve consideration of the relative outcomes, and appraisal of outcomes goes way beyond the analysis of the data provided by RCTs. It is not merely about a surgeon acting ethically responsibly, it is about the ethical considerations that emerge from the use of finite resources. Whether one likes it or not, it is *political*. Another way of putting this is that good RCTs and systematic reviews of RCTs produce hard data,[7] but as soon as these data are embedded in the context of health care, and judgements are made employing these data, then there are all sorts of evaluative considerations which impact on those making judgements about medical interventions. Finally, simply in virtue of being a surgeon and being prepared to undertake the surgical intervention, the surgeon in and through their actions is expressive of an evaluative stance: what is expressed to the patient is that this authority figure believes in this intervention.

Now, if one were a surgeon and had not thought about this question before in the way we present it here in this judgement scenario, having done so now might lead you to make a more value-literate and ethically informed decision in future. It might lead you to make a more rationally defensible decision, which has a greater chance of being acknowledged as legitimate by one's peers. And this is surely a good thing. Imagine, then, the ability to think about such judgement scenarios in a supported and structured forum with other people, some of whom might be 'stakeholders'. These 'stakeholders' might be people who have had (or indeed have chosen not to have) a mastectomy, had (or chosen not to have) a prostatectomy, or had an extended course of chemotherapy; they might include Macmillan nurses, nurses who have cared for people undergoing chemotherapy, and family members of those who have had a mastectomy, a prostatectomy or an extended course of chemotherapy. Maybe participation in this structured forum would further enhance the rational foundations of the surgeon's judgement and also help patients, family members of patients, and nurses better understand the surgeon's views. The thought that 'stakeholders' engaging in dialogue in a supportive and structured forum will enhance value-literacy and ethical judgement in beneficial ways is the thought that Fulford's (2013) theory of values-based practice (VBP) is built on.

Medicine and deliberation (libertarianism and values-based practice)

Liberal deliberative democracy

Fulford's idea is derived from a particular brand of liberal political theory: liberal deliberative democracy. The idea is proposed in response to a perceived dilemma: while

---

[7] Whether in practice the framing of such 'evidence-based' data can itself really be regarded credibly as apolitical is a question that merits further discussion. Cf. footnote 3, above: arguably that framing ignores deeper questions about the structure of knowledge and the structure of society which substantively condition the meaning, results and importance of RCTs. (See also the opening of the penultimate section, below.)

we are committed to respecting the evaluative beliefs of individuals these often conflict with the evaluative beliefs of other individuals. We want to respect each individual's values but also arrive at collective value judgements on policy issues and the like. Moreover, in arriving at collective value judgements and incorporating those into policy, we want those individuals who might still not share these values to acknowledge the legitimacy of these values-now-made-policy. How might this be achieved? Well, we can identify which are the most robust, best or correct claims. But how do we decide this in a manner which respects the evaluative claims of each individual? What we need to do, so the argument goes, is subject the claims of individuals to a non-prejudicial process whereby the claims can be exposed to the counter-claims and rational scrutiny of others in a supportive forum in the absence of the distorting influence of external forces. In such a forum, the evaluative beliefs will be subject to a process of 'natural' selection' as the weaker give way to the stronger beliefs. Individuals who have submitted themselves and their evaluative beliefs to a deliberative forum will dispense with their weaker, less-defensible, beliefs and emerge with strong – because well-supported and more defensible – beliefs: either those they entered with, now revised, or new ones.

Let us put this another way. Individuals hold evaluative beliefs, which often conflict with those held by other individuals. Societies, being collections of individuals, need to arrive at collective judgements on evaluative beliefs. We need to find a way of arriving at collective judgements, while respecting the beliefs of individual members (resisting authoritarianism) and establishing the legitimacy of the collective judgement, even for those for whom that collective judgement remains in conflict with their own individually held evaluative beliefs.

If we think of liberalism as a spectrum, with libertarians at one end and liberal deliberative democrats at the other, that which determines one's position on the spectrum is the extent of the procedural demands the theorist takes to be justified in imposing on individuals. Libertarians minimise procedural demands because all demands are seen as restrictions on an individual's total freedom, even if those demands are procedural. On the other hand, liberal deliberative democrats make more demands, while still insisting on these being purely procedural (this is taken to be the 'red line', which when crossed leads one to authoritarianism). For libertarians, political institutions should be structured with one goal in mind, which in turn legitimises the authority those institutions enjoy: the maximisation of the freedom of individuals to express their preferences un-coerced. For liberal deliberative democrats, political institutions should serve the same goal, but they can do so in a more indirect manner: an institution can be said to maximise freedom in as much as it promotes reason, social stability and greater legitimacy. A rational, stable society with a legislature that is acknowledged as having legitimate authority – even by those who do not share its values – is freedom enhancing. For liberal deliberative democrats, institutions that involve individuals in processes of deliberation promote reflection and understanding of the values of other individuals, and this promotes social stability and the individual's recognition of the legitimacy of the values that have become incorporated into policy. Where libertarians trust that dialogue, along with the understanding and shared values that might emerge from that, will take place spontaneously through the free association of individuals in civil society, deliberative democrats contend that such dialogue requires (or at least benefits from in important freedom-enhancing ways) promoting and facilitating by the state in structured fora, which form an integral part of the public sphere. Libertarians might charge that liberal deliberative democrats impose unjust freedom-restricting demands on individuals, in demanding that they participate in the structured deliberative fora. In contrast, liberal deliberative democrats might respond that the libertarian's reluctance to promote deliberation through structured fora does not, as the libertarian hopes and claims, result in greater individual freedom but rather subjects the dialogue undertaken in civil society to the distorting, maybe even perverting, influence of dominant socio-economic interests, such as corporate interests. Capitalist societies contain powerful interest groups, and any dialogue that feeds into policy needs to be protected from these. Structured deliberative fora established as an integral part of the public sphere create a space where, so the argument goes, dialogue can be undertaken in a manner that is conducive to free, open and un-prejudiced dialogue because it is free from the distorting influence of powerful interest groups.

Liberal deliberative democracy and health care: values-based practice

It seems to us that the best way to understand the perceived need for VBP is via the thought that right now health care generally operates *de facto* on the libertarian model. This leads to a chaotic cacophony of competing value claims, which in the absence of supportive and structured fora can appear to persist in a state of chaos. In this environment, collective decisions based on evaluative judgements or beliefs transpire to perpetuate the pervading or dominant interests and biases: market interests, managerialist interests, professional interests of the individuals or group with the highest status, gender bias, ethnic/racial bias and so on. Furthermore, in being encoded with these interests and biases the judgements are much less likely to be perceived as legitimate by those who do not share those evaluative beliefs. Fulford, through VBP, wants to implement the ideas of the liberal deliberative democrats and introduce supportive and structured fora where the evaluative claims of individuals (stakeholders) will, through dialogue-induced natural selection free from the distorting influence of prevailing interests and biases, be transformed into rationally defensible beliefs with greater capacity for being perceived as legitimate.

Viewed in this light, Fulford's proposal seems interesting for two reasons:

(1) because it goes beyond the 'bio-ethics' and 'ethics committee' approach, and engages philosophically beyond the usual areas in which medicine has tolerated, and even on occasion invited, philosophical contributions; and

(2) because it serves to expose unacknowledged assumptions to scrutiny – and does so because VBP seems to re-orientate the way one might have hitherto viewed matters.

In this, latter, way it seems to fulfil the task we outlined as that of philosophy at the beginning of our chapter, in contrasting this to the widespread assumption that philosophy is a proto-science. VBP reframes our way of thinking about value: it tells us that both the legitimacy of policy decisions based in collective judgements (evaluative beliefs) and the strength or fitness of those judgements can be enhanced, while retaining a healthy respect for the individual judgements. It finds the middle ground between the poles of on the one hand libertarian anarchy, which actually, somewhat paradoxically, leads to backdoor-authoritarianism owing to the unfettered perverting influence of powerful interest groups, and on the other hand traditional authoritarianism, derived from traditional authorities such as church and state or, in the context of health care, managers and surgeons/physicians.

Medicine and value (the emotivist frame is non-obligatory)

So much for accentuating the positive. We believe there are, unfortunately, stronger grounds for scepticism regarding Fulford's proposal. We want to suggest that despite appearing to reframe the issues at hand, Fulford actually takes on wholesale the framework which is (was) already present. The clue has already been flagged, albeit implicitly, in what we have written in the foregoing. In VBP, Fulford proposes a quasi-deliberative solution to the current libertarian value-anarchy, while all along the problem is to be found in the conception of value which is *shared* by both liberal deliberative democrats and libertarians: *the liberal conception of value*. If we might be forgiven for stretching the frame metaphor, what we are suggesting here is that while it can seem, at first glance, that Fulford has reframed our way of approaching value in the context of health care, it transpires that he has simply remounted the same picture in the same frame. Only the mount has changed. Put less figuratively, we agree that reframing our thinking about value would be beneficial to health care, but note that Fulford has failed to achieve the required reframing because he has remained within the dominant liberal paradigm (see Chapter 5). Liberal political theory is itself unphilosophical in neglecting the frame or assuming there is a possibility of a neutral frame.

There are other ways to think about value. Health care lends itself to teleological analysis, where a *conception of the good* might be useful in guiding deliberations. There might even be (*we* will *here* remain agnostic on this) good reasons for subscribing to a liberal conception of value at the nation state level, but that does not entail that those reasons carry-over into the context of health care. Fulford (2013) writes that 'The point of values-based practice is to support balanced decision making on individual cases where complex and conflicting values are in play within frameworks of values shared by the individuals concerned.' While this has a superficial air of reasonableness about it, one might be forgiven, if one does not share Fulford's liberal assumptions, for finding it a little question-begging. It is question-begging in that internal to it is an assumption that the response to being confronted with a value-conflict should not be simply to identify *the actually stronger claim*. This observation is important to note, because what we would like to bring out is the extent to which Fulford's liberalism is non-obligatory and, ironically, *by his own standards* authoritarian.

What we seek to draw attention to in identifying VBP as liberal is the extent to which liberalism begins by tacitly effecting a decidedly negative valorisation of value claims, in the sense that those value claims are 'translated' into the preferences (or 'interests') of individuals (see Chapters 5 and 8). Liberals treat value claims as little more than *expressions of individual preference(s)*. We suggest that this relegation of value claims to the status of preferences is unjustified; indeed, we would argue that it does violence to the true status/nature of value claims. It does not follow from the observation that individuals often express conflicting values that those values either are of equal status or ought to be considered of equal status (see Chapter 3). Thinking, as Fulford does, that one must treat them from the outset as of equal status, as equally viable expressions of preference, on pain of being authoritarian,[8] is to become confused. It is to fall into a kind of localised relativism. (It is an illicit deduction of a localised relativism from a – not unreasonable – observation of initial pluralism.)

---

[8] Cf. his equation in Fulford (2013) of 'authoritarianism' with a commitment to 'pre-set outcomes'.

The confusion emerges because in attempting to avoid authoritarianism at the level of adjudication between the conflicting claims of individuals one stipulates that each individual's claim must be considered as of equal status (until post-process). If we understand authoritarianism in the way the liberal does – as that which arises from the invocation of non-procedural authority regarding the status accorded to individual value claims – then an appeal to non-procedural authority to stipulate that all value claims must be treated, irrespective of their merits, as of equal status (prior to procedural ratification) is equally authoritarian. So pure-procedural liberals,[9] and therefore Fulford too, enter into an authoritarian regress. This is the way in which modern – more or less Rawlsian – liberalism is constitutively (tacitly) authoritarian. It is authoritarian in its *prima facie* rejection of non-neutrality between values, and in maintaining in practice, as we shall shortly see, a more or less subjectivist view of values. The conclusion of Thornton's (2011) 'Radical liberal values-based practice' remains highly salient. Liberalism somehow seems to think it has a right to help itself to a 'master-value', which Fulford (2013) characterises in the rhetorically appealing language of 'mutual respect'. That really *is* a value, unlike the 'values' that people hold. These 'ordinary' values need respect because individuals need respecting, but they are merely preferences, *even if they are held by those holding them as the most important thing in their lives* (a philosophy or an ethic or such-like) and even if they believe (and are prepared to defend the belief with rational argument) that their values are more important than other values – some of which they may regard as simply *wrong*. Such a belief, it seems, stands in need of 'correction', as their values simply cannot be as important as 'mutual respect', the master-value.[10]

Now a liberal theorist like Fulford might reject this accusation of authoritarianism regarding the status of value claims, and argue that what he/they are seeking is neutrality

---

[9] As will have become evident to a reader versed in recent political philosophy, Fulford's liberalism is of the hegemonic kind: it is broadly Rawlsian, 'pure-proceduralist'. For our objections to Rawlsian liberal political philosophy, see e.g. Read (2011, 2012) and Hutchinson's 'Climate change and the liberal programme' (forthcoming in Makoff and Read's *A Political Philosophy for All Beings*).

[10] What is the status of the claim that: in VBP conflicts of value are resolved primarily, not by reference to a rule prescribing a 'right' outcome, but by processes designed to support a balance of legitimately different perspectives?

> Note first that although it says that conflicts of values *are* resolved . . . this is in the context of VBP. So, it should be read as saying: conflicts of values *should* be resolved . . . by processes designed to support a balance of legitimately different perspectives. But now we can ask, why should they? (It may be an analytic truth that they are within VBP, but we are invited to adopt this approach.) And now the worry is that this seems to be a value of a different order from the values that should be put through the process of balancing views. This seems to be a higher order value, inconsistent with VBP's own approach. This suggests a dilemma for radical VBP. It can either address the question of why we should value values in the way it suggests, at the cost of violating its own principles, or it can attempt no such question, in which case it lacks the prescriptive force that gives it teeth. (Thornton, 2011, p. 991)

> We like to call this dilemma 'the Fulford fork': either liberals have to be (and ought to admit) their authoritarianism (as classical liberals often did, but Rawlsians shy away from doing), or they must give up the claim that pre-set outcomes are distinctively authoritarian. But the latter option opens up just the space we mean to occupy: the space for true rational deliberation, and thus for the development of (say) an Aristotelian alternative to liberalism.

between conflicting value claims. What they are doing is striving for neutrality by attaining a meta-meta-ethical position: liberals are then the alleged champions of plural-ism.[11] However, to give all views equal status is to be committed to one (or more) of the following three claims:

(1) the ontological claim that there exists nothing in the world which can settle or play a decisive role in determining which of a number of conflicting value claims is correct; or

(2) the epistemological claim that we cannot know for certain (or beyond reasonable doubt, or reliably) which of conflicting value claims, if any, are correct/true; or

(3) the substantive moral claim (or psychologically induced stance) that we are resolutely indifferent to which views, if any, are, or can be shown to be, correct/true.

To be committed to the ontological claim entails a rejection of objectivist ethics and of any form of ethical realism (that values might be the sort of things that exist constitutively independent of our thoughts). Commitment to the epistemological claim entails non-cognitivism in practice, because we lack knowledge of the truth or otherwise of a particular moral view or claim. To be committed to option 3, the indifference option, would seem to entail that one was, at the very least tacitly, committed to a form of existential emotivism, whereby one is committed to living and acting as if emotivism (or some form of moral subjectivism) were true. Whichever of these is the view to which Fulford is committed, what is entailed by VBP is that no moral value claim can make a specifically moral demand on any individual without their – alleged and indirect – formal consent in virtue of the claim having been legitimised by having passed through the procedures, as established by VBP.

Put another way, according to VBP, value claims need assent from other individuals, in virtue of having passed through the deliberative process, if they are to be established as being more than mere expression of preference, opinion or interest. What we are concerned with here are the consequences of Fulford's liberal negative valorisation of the value claims for those for whom VBP is being proposed as a solution. VBP professes to avoid authoritarianism and to respect individuals' values but begins by insisting on those values being treated as nothing more than expressions of preference or interests, i.e. not distinctively evaluative *beliefs* at all. Consider: the only thing which can enable an individual's value judgement to achieve the status of more than mere expression of preference, or be formally recognised as politically significant, is it having been legitimised by having passed through institutionalised procedures as prescribed by the theory.

What is the alternative? Well Fulford (2013) would have us believe that the alternative to VBP's negative valorisation of value claims into interests and preferences is the author-itarian ranking of value claims by *fiat*. (Cf. his swift move (Fulford, 2013, p. 539) from

---

[11] We suspect here a *confusion*, among liberals such as Fulford, between process and outcome: just because we *need* to get (plenty of) others to agree, in a democracy, if we are to implement a policy, does not mean that *what* we put forward for agreement should be *defined by* that need so to agree nor reduced to it! To be fair to Fulford, we suspect that this confusion is inherited from Rawls and colleagues – it seems fairly stark, by the time one gets to Rawls's *Political liberalism*, for example in Rawls's notion of the 'proviso'. (For discussion, see Read's article published at www.arsdisputandi. org/publish/articles/000394/article.pdf.)

noting certain philosophers are 'moral objectivists' to discussions of Soviet commissars imprisoning dissidents.) But this is simply not a dichotomy we need accept. Such a dichotomy is, one might say, an artefact of the very negation of substantive values that we are questioning. The dichotomy Fulford sees and tries to overcome is a result of his own failure to overcome genuinely (and then reframe) the way values have been side-lined in the context of health care, especially in the context of EBM. If we reject the negative valorisation, if we resist the liberal's invitation to see all value claims as mere expressions of preference, then we find that we also come to recognise why the dichotomy with which Fulford presents us is a false one, i.e. because value claims are rationally assessable.[12] While expressions of preference about such things as taste (what's your favourite flavour ice-cream?) involve no demand for rational support, value claims do. The category of a value claim is not reducible to an expression of preference, unless one is committed to some form of emotivism as a meta-ethical position (and/or to some substantive moral relativism). It appears to us that the most plausible reading of Fulfordian VBP is that he is so committed. Or at least: that whichever of the three options indicated above one takes, it amounts *in practice* to an accepting of emotivism in the political sphere, or (at least, specifically) in relation to the treatment of value-conflicts in health-related contexts. (Fulford's emotivism should not be a surprise to those familiar with his writings on VBP. He repeatedly reminds his readers of VBP's heritage in the philosophy of R. M. Hare. The observation that Hare's writings are a form of emotivism – a sophisticated form, but still a form thereof – is uncontroversial.)

Medicine reframed (health and the telos of human flourishing)

We have already gestured in the direction of our proposed solution to the problem. The solution is to engage in some genuine reframing; we must reject the subterranean emotivism operative in VBP. Our proposal is what we call *flourishing-oriented medicine* (FOM). Not EBM with a VBP add-on; no negative valorisation, simply the recognition that medical science involves (is in fact saturated by) evaluative concerns, judgements and beliefs (see Chapter 19). Even in the 'strictly epistemological' aspects of medical science such evaluative judgements frame and therefore permeate our investigations (contrary to the dominant self-image, represented in our opening paragraphs). These must be acknowledged and discussed in an attempt to triangulate or evaluate. This is why Fulford starts with the premise of values being in conflict. Our free-floating value judgements can seem to be in interminable and intractable conflict *because* of the liberal-emotivist framework which Fulford simply accepts as unavoidable and seeks to reify institutionally through the processes of VBP. But this framework is non-obligatory. Evaluative concepts in health care have their home in a teleological framework, where to be in good health is to flourish. To be sure, there will be deep discussions and arguments and divisions about what flourishing is. But our value conflicts will seem *less* interminable, less intractable and less inevitable when we see that one of the reasons why our way of seeing the value of a proposed intervention might be at variance is because we had different ideas about what it was to flourish, to live a fulfilling, dignified healthy

---

[12] Note: our understanding of rationality is intended here as a broad one. It will include much that is often illegitimately *dismissed* as 'emotional'. For explication, see Hutchinson (2008).

life. For we can then start to seek together genuinely to reconcile or at least 'triangulate' those ideas.

Why do we speak of 'flourishing-oriented' rather than 'flourishing-*based*' medicine? Because it is about where we are (and want, all things considered, to be) *headed*, rather than about an alleged solid and ethically uninflected evidence-base from which we proceed on the grounds of values that are, regrettably, in practice largely taken for granted and not subject to investigation or rational critique. FOM keeps our eyes collectively on where we are going; it does not deduce everything from an 'evidence-base' and then worry about having to 'add back in' the values that have been left missing from the picture and thus figured spontaneously. VBP is an attempt to bring the 'values' back into the health care picture. But it *mirrors* the assumptions of EBM; it thinks of facts and values as radically different, and complementary. It is an attempt to 'fix' EBM. It fails, as we have shown, to take seriously that values are *more* than just preferences or interests.

FOM would by contrast genuinely integrate fact and value, as part of an indissoluble whole which we actually live. There is an important sense in which, insofar as values and facts actually can be extricated from each other at all, then values come first. In FOM, one would look at the state of health, of flourishing, that could ideally be achieved, and would actually be genuinely desirable (this would be a crucial part of the reconciliation project alluded to above), and at the change needed in a patient(s)/population in order to achieve it, and *backcast* that outcome to determine what therefore needs to be done now: what needs to be considered, what needs to be researched, what options with which to present patients, and so on. It is important to stress here that the goal, the desired outcome, of human flourishing, is an 'open-ended' goal. Keeping clearly aware of that open-endedness would lessen any risk that FOM became 'authoritarian' in a genuinely troubling way, and would suggest instead that much of the requisite goal-setting and backcasting should be framed in terms of a sustainable 'via negativa': much that we take to be health services would be conceived as directed toward their own self-eliminating and the enhancement of people's (collective) autonomy. So: yes to (collective) open-endedness; but FOM would be non-liberal. It would aim with deliberate force at enhancing (certain of) people's capabilities considered over time, indeed over generations, and over a population. Moreover, the word 'deliberate' should be understood in a rich and multiple sense: a *genuine* (i.e. non-liberal) *deliberative* democracy (employing citizens' juries, etc., taking seriously deliberation as a collective rational endeavour) should be what leads this effort at deliberate discussion of and direction toward health. A preference-satisfaction model of values and of value-expression (tacitly based, in effect, in consumer preference, or in individualistic non-deliberation-based voting) is liberal, and is inadequate for the reasons outlined above.

FOM would entail that we look outwards to the political and ecological structure of our society, so as to see how this might (if and when it is wrongly designed or badly operating) conflict with the pursuit of flourishing. And FOM would be *highly* amenable to the idea of deliberative fora, but not on the liberal model. For liberalism empties out these fora of real content, by reducing values to preferences, and rejecting discussion of the frameworks (the conceptions of flourishing) within which those values gain sense. In doing so the space for rational discussion is undermined. FOM would envisage not a totting up of preferences, but a real social engagement, of human beings thinking together about how to decide the issues that structure medicine, and would factor in prevention and precaution (including crucially across a whole population) heavily. Think what it would really be like, to have a National Health Service, rather than what we currently have: a National Illness[-treatment] Service.[13]

The deepest way forward, we would suggest, is a '*via negativa*', a serious emphasis on *precaution* and *prevention*,[14] on the Hippocratic 'First, do no harm.' On doing less, not more. FOM would be a more (explicitly) 'political' medicine – and all the better for it. It would be a collective – a communitarian, or 'societarian' – medicine, not a liberal individualised medicine based on a scientistic fantasy that abstracts from our embodiedness and from our sociality. We are social animals. 'Flourishing' *includes others*. I never flourish as all others decline. Flourishing is ultimately something that a population – a 'herd' – does as a whole. Think of 'herd immunity'. It is far easier to understand this as an ethical goal on the basis of FOM than it would be on the basis of VBP, where its desirability would depend on the happenstance of preference-distribution of individuals. As, in closing, we shall now seek to demonstrate. . .

Flourishing-oriented deliberation

By way of conclusion, let us here suggest a ('hypothetical') judgement scenario and then ask some questions. This time, rather than the mastectomy case we discussed above, we look at a case with yet broader social dimensions.

A deliberative forum has been established by a regional health authority to feed into policy decisions about administering vaccinations to children. The parties – stakeholders – involved in the forum include mothers, fathers, General Practitioners, Nurses, Health Visitors and Health Service managers, some of whom have medical backgrounds and some of whom have no medical background but who do have MBAs. Herd immunity is key, so as to prevent outbreaks of measles in future years or decades,[15] but vaccinations are costly to buy and administer, and parents have a right to protect their children. It should go without saying that there are lots of factors to be considered. However, one matter comes to dominate proceedings and it does so because of an intersection of two popular views held by a number of those participating in the forum. The two views are:

---

[13] Here, we are somewhat encouraged by the following moment, even if it is only a rather brief and isolated one, from p. 128 of the King's Fund Report (2011) on 'Improving the Quality of Care in General Practice: From Treating Illness to Promoting Health'. Therein, 'general practice is regarded as uniquely well placed not just to promote the health and wellbeing of the practice population'. We are however discouraged by the completely trivial account of population health given on the following page: 'The performance of general practices, as providers and commissioners of care, should not only be assessed in terms of whether individuals can access high-quality services. It also needs to be judged on the extent to which it meets the health needs of the wider population, including people experiencing homelessness, veterans, refugees and asylum seekers, people with mental health problems, and those with drug and alcohol problems, who may not actively seek care from general practice.' This name-checking exercise and the repeated use of the word 'people' do not begin to substitute for a serious effort at thinking of the population, 'the herd', as a whole.

[14] In future we hope to demonstrate how FOM, unlike EBM/VBP, can take seriously the precautionary principle, and what positive effects on human flourishing (within the very real limits of knowledge, material resources, ecosystemic limits etc. to which we are subject) this is likely to have. But nothing in our critique of VBP depends upon *that* future critique.

[15] As happened in 2013 in South Wales.

(1) that individuals should have the right to choose (for their children); and

(2) that the MMR vaccine probably causes autism.

In contrast to the vantage point we (the authors of this chapter and our readers) enjoy now, when there are numerous studies and a disciplinary hearing to which one can point which resoundingly undermine the truth of the autism claim, at the time our hypothetical forum occurred there were few such resources. Despite assurances from the health practitioners participating in the forum, the parents were clear they would be betraying their children, and being bad parents, if they condoned the MMR roll-out. The author of the MMR-autism paper that provided the origins for the parents' concerns, while seen as a controversial and a maverick, had not at this stage been struck off and even the health practitioners present at the forum struggled to produce hard data to refute the autism claim. All their talk of herd immunity just felt to the parents like a request to sacrifice their children, or as a smokescreen for cost-reduction strategies (everyone knew that MMR was cheaper than individual measles, mumps and rubella vaccinations). In the absence of a refutation of the autism claim then the individuals should clearly have the right to be cautious and protect their children. This thought was buttressed (principle 1) by a widespread valorisation of a liberal individual 'right to choose'.

The point is that for VBP all participants have interests or preferences that are being expressed here, and it is only the outcome of the forum that can transform some of those into legitimate value claims that can be incorporated into policy. But the truth is that in our scenario the parents were expressing 'self-interest' based in a combination of unreflective individualism and poor knowledge (and that liberal principles made it particularly difficult to resist this combination). Those advocating the vaccination programme were advocating a robust well-thought-through and supported evaluative judgement regarding public health. But: they lost.

While VBP would in this case presumably have supported the potentially disastrous (and actually harmful) witchhunt against the MMR vaccine, and thus ('ironically') would have undermined the result that one might have expected a 'science-based' approach to have given, FOM would not. For, in flourishing-oriented medicine, people are more likely to think carefully of what the precautionary approach would be than to demand 'evidence' (that reducing the MMR vaccine will actually lead to serious harms due to its reduction of herd immunity). Crucially, in FOM, the 'herd' and not just the individual 'stakeholders' will have a *role*. This is how FOM, in emphasising the flourishing of the community as a whole, is superior to the liberal (individualistic) approach of VBP.

How would this work, in FOM? Over time, one would have reason to hope that understanding of the kinds of points we make in sketching out FOM, in the previous section above, would become more general, among medical spheres and also among society more generally. A society that comes to understand itself as directed toward its own flourishing will naturally choose according to the kind of precepts indicated in FOM. But what about in the meantime? In the kind of deliberative forum we envisage – in a deliberative forum structured according to the precepts of FOM rather than of VBP – how would the deliberation and decision-making be approached, and why are we confident that it would be likely to have a different outcome than what actually occurred historically, which would we think merely have been undergirded by a Fulfordian approach?

There are various possibilities here. Briefly, beyond what we have already said, let us make the following two – (we think) decisive – points.

- While VBP is 'purely procedural', *FOM has objectives built into it*. Participants would be *enjoined* to consider these. Herd immunity would not be something that individuals might or might not decide that they valued; it would be structured into the framework of the discussion from the outset. (Fulford might consider this 'authoritarian'; we humbly submit that it is, in fact, merely sane.)
- If one were unconfident of this being enough, one could also introduce additional 'stakeholders' into the deliberative process. One could explicitly create representatives for the community as a whole, and/or for unborn future generations, etc. One could strongly empower such representatives in the deliberative forum: for example, would it not be reasonable to suggest that any proposed outcome that were unacceptable to the voice in the forum representing all those not present, and representing in particular the powerless future people, should be unacceptable in toto?[16] Fulford might think such arrangements for 'proxy representatives' illiberal and undemocratic. We would respond that, while they might be 'illiberal', this would/should not necessarily be judged a *criticism* (for the reasons we have offered above, concerning why a liberal political philosophy can fail to help a society to flourish, etc.); and that our proposals would arguably be *more* democratic than Fulford's. For surely a people is not merely a time-slice; a people – a *demos* – exists over time, and thus should *include* the future ones.[17]

Our MMR 'case study' here undergirds what we have argued. That, rather than 'complement' EBM with VBP, EBM should be sublated. VBP should be dropped, and EBM could morph then into FOM. No longer positivistic and scientistic, and more honestly ethical and political. With deliberative fora that, far from being mere tick-box exercises or amalgamations of individuals' preferences, are actually likely to produce the best and most robust decisions. Decisions that are likely to be compatible with both medical science and human flourishing.

This is how philosophy might be able actually to help enrich medicine and health care. And thus even, dare we say it, to help us all.

References

Atkins, P. (2011) *On Being: A Scientist's Exploration of the Great Questions of Existence*. Oxford: Oxford University Press.

Bausell, R. B. (2007) *Snake Oil Science*. New York: Oxford University Press.

Carel, H. (2008) *Illness*. Oxford: Acumen.

Fulford, K. W. M. (1989) *Moral Theory and Medical Practice*. Cambridge: Cambridge University Press.

Fulford, K. W. M. (2013) Values-based practice: Fulford's dangerous idea. *Journal of Evaluation in Clinical Practice*, **19**, 537–546.

---

[16] Our suggestions here are in part modelled on Read's suggestions in his proposals for deliberative 'guardians for future generations': www.greenhousethinktank.org/files/greenhouse/home/Guardians_inside_final.pdf. We will expand on this parallel, in future work.

[17] See again Read's report on guardians, especially the opening two sections. (In the particular respect under consideration here, we are closer to Burke than to Rousseau. A people is a necessarily asymmetrical 'partnership' between the future, the past, and the present. It is *not* a 'contract' in the liberal – presentist – sense of that word. Being a person who is actually part of a society, and part of a society that is sane, *requires* that we care for the future. Real health care is a key part of this.)

Hawking, S. (2010) *The Grand Design*. Oxford: Oxford University Press.

Hutchinson, P. (2008) *Shame and Philosophy: An Investigation in the Philosophy of Emotions and Ethics*. Basingstoke: Palgrave.

Hutchinson, P. (2013) What Have the Philosophers Ever Done For Us? blog post of a talk given in 2011. Available at: http://viewfromthehutch.blogspot.co.uk/2013/06/what-have-philosophers-ever-done-for-us.html.

King's Fund Report (2011) *Improving the Quality of Care in General Practice: From Treating Illness to Promoting Health*.

Loughlin, M. (2002) *Ethics, Management and Mythology*. Oxford: Radcliffe Press.

Read, R. (2011) Beyond an ungreen-economics-based political philosophy. *International Journal of Green Economics*, 5, 167–183.

Read, R. (2012) On philosophy's (lack of) progress. In Perissinotto, L. and Camara, B. R. (editors), *Wittgenstein and Plato*. Basingstoke: Palgrave MacMillan.

Taleb, N. N. (2007) *The Black Swan*. London: Penguin Books.

Thornton, T. (2011) Radical liberal values-based practice. *Journal of Evaluation of Clinical Practice*, 17, 988–991.

Values-based practice: a new tool or a new package?

Mona Gupta

Positioning values-based practice

Over the last several years, the British psychiatrist and philosopher Bill Fulford has been developing a framework called values-based practice (hereafter VBP) which, in his words, will help 'in coming to balanced judgments in individual cases [where values conflict]' (Fulford, 2011, p. 977). The VBP framework includes ten elements bundled into four thematic areas: (1) practice skills; (2) models of service delivery (which refers to features of services rather than overarching models); (3) some assertions or claims about VBP, evidence-based practice, and values; and (4) the principle of partnership (which refers to a partnership between health care practitioners and patients). The first four of the ten elements are practice skills that reflect competencies practitioners ought to have if they are to make clinical decisions in accordance with the values-based framework; the other six elements are claims or principles advocated by the framework. The practice skills include: (1) awareness of values, (2) reasoning about values, (3) knowledge of values and facts, and (4) communication. The six claims or principles are: (5) that services ought to be user-centred and (6) multidisciplinary; (7) that EBP and VBP work together, (8) that we only notice values when there is a problem; (9) that increasing scientific knowledge increases choices which can demonstrate divergence in values; and (10) that values-based practice involves providers and users making decisions in partnership (Fulford, 2011, p. 981).

Fulford paints a picture of clinical decision-making as operating on a 'twin-track' meaning that both facts and values must be incorporated into decision-making. He argues that in clinical practice, evidence-based medicine (hereafter EBM) offers the facts of medicine, while 'ethical codes and guidelines' offer high-level ethical principles. Fulford

---

Debates in Values-Based Practice, ed. Michael Loughlin. Published by Cambridge University Press. © Cambridge University Press 2014.

implies that while these codes or guidelines can offer a 'framework of shared values', they do not necessarily provide the means to expose and work through conflicts of values. He also suggests that ethical codes have been used to develop rules that do not allow for the necessary reflection required in individual cases. In his view, VBP overcomes both of these problems by providing a practical method for clinical decision-making that can 'work together' with EBM, enabling balanced judgements when values conflict (Fulford, 2011).

Fulford makes several claims about VBP: that it is new, that it is based on learnable, clinical skills, and that it involves 'working more effectively with complex and conflicting values' (Fulford, 2011, p. 976). To describe VBP, he draws on the commonly used metaphor in health care of the 'tool'. On the one hand, he sees VBP as simply an additional tool to add to the clinical decision-making toolbox. On the other, he emphasises its necessity by saying that 'something on the lines of values-based practice will be needed in medicine' (Fulford, 2011, p. 985). It is therefore important to know what VBP will add that does not already exist. In other words, a new tool should have a clear purpose such that its users know exactly when and why to use it, otherwise it could add unnecessary clutter and weight to the toolbox, creating confusion rather than clarity. This is particularly true in the health care environment where new tools are regularly on offer.

In this chapter, I will examine Fulford's positioning of VBP as a practical method for connecting EBM with ethics in clinical decision-making. I will first examine the supposed complementarity between VBP and EBM, exploring whether these two approaches can actually be used concurrently. I will then compare the methods of VBP with various approaches to clinical ethics to expose whether and where the differences lie. Having discussed VBP's role in decision-making, I will then examine an example of VBP in action using a case study written by Fulford (2004). I will argue that as a method for accomplishing its stated goal, to enable balanced judgements where values conflict in clinical practice, VBP does not distinguish itself sufficiently from other approaches with similar aims, particularly those offered by clinical ethics. Specifically, it is unclear that *as a practice* VBP offers something new, that it fosters additional skills beyond what have already been established as important for ethical decision-making, and that it leads to any practical differences in coming to balanced judgements compared to other approaches. At the same time, as a theoretical model, it does hint at 'upstream' values as an important area of moral concern that can be neglected in mainstream ethics discourse. These include values that lie behind frontline care, within policy choices about the social determinants of health, or decisions about which agendas to serve in medical research. VBP may not offer many practical differences to what already exists, but depending on which direction it takes as it evolves, it may be able to play a role in highlighting new areas that deserve moral reflection in health care.

VBM and EBM

Fulford claims that EBM and VBP work together. What is evidence-based practice exactly? What is the role of values within EBM, and where might VBP fit?

EBM is defined as the 'conscientious, explicit, and judicious use of current best evidence in making decisions about the care of individual patients' (Guyatt et al., 2008, p. 783).

According to the authoritative descriptions of evidence-based medicine (Guyatt et al., 2008; Straus et al., 2011), the practice of EBM requires '...the integration of the best research evidence with our clinical expertise and our patient's unique values and circumstances' (Straus *et al.*, 2011, p. 1) or alternatively, the 'integration of individual clinical expertise and patient preferences with the best available external clinical evidence from systematic research and consideration of available resources' (Guyatt *et al.*, 2008, p. 783). With respect to how one integrates patients' values, EBM's developers say only that practitioners must ask themselves the following question: 'What are our patients' values and expectations for both the outcome we are trying to prevent and the treatment we are offering?'(Straus *et al.*, 2011, p. 88). However, once they have identified these values, the authors provide little explanation of how the practitioner actually integrates – in the sense of combining – different forms of knowledge, such as patients' values with research data. Thus, it has fallen to other scholars (Tonelli, 2006; see also Chapters 18 and 19) to try to explain what the concept of integration means and what doing integration actually looks like.

On the other hand, EBM's authors do provide their overall view on decision-making in clinical practice (Guyatt *et al.*, 2008, pp. 643–661). They endorse an approach called 'shared decision-making' in which patients *and* clinicians[1] express what they know about the options, they present their values, they deliberate, and they take a decision together. They recommend various methods that specify values (either those of the individual patient, or those of a general population of patients) and can help with the final decision: practice guidelines, clinical decision analysis (CDA), and the computation of the likelihood of being helped versus being harmed. Practice guidelines typically involve a review of research data about the treatments being considered and their outcomes, as well as the incorporation of values into the recommendations about the 'optimal course of action' (Guyatt *et al.*, 2008, p. 600). Decision analyses express the probabilities of possible outcomes associated with the courses of action for a given clinical scenario as well as the utilities (preferences for those outcomes). They then combine these figures to generate a 'total expected value' for each treatment strategy. For both practice guidelines and decision analyses, the values concerning different treatment outcomes could come from patient representatives and members of the general public from surveys of patients and/or the general public, and/or from published research about preferences expressed by patients. Both guidelines and CDAs can be used in clinical decision-making in the sense that practice guidelines can be applied to the individual case, while an individual decision analysis can be undertaken for an individual patient's decision incorporating his or her own utilities. A third, more complex method which can be used just for a specific patient is to compute the likelihood of being helped compared with the likelihood of being harmed (LHH).[2]

Fulford views the exploration and negotiation of values in clinical practice as operating *in parallel* with EBM and, therefore, with these methods. But it is not clear how this occurs and he does not provide an example. Let us imagine a specific clinical scenario in which there is a clash of values: a patient wants to receive antibiotic treatment for what is almost

---

[1] The values of other parties (institutions, society, families) are not included explicitly in this approach.

[2] The LHH is a ratio of the NNT (number needed to treat) to the NNH (number needed to harm) that can be adjusted to take into account an individual patient's risk factors. The LHH can then be manipulated further to reflect the patient's numerical tradeoff of benefits versus harms of an intervention (e.g. by assigning numerical values to the desirability or undesirability of health outcomes) (Straus *et al.*, 2011, pp. 94–97).

certainly a cold and the practitioner does not wish to prescribe it. Presumably, VBP would involve the doctor and patient each listening to each other's values as well as perhaps exposing societal values (concerns about antibiotic resistance, cost of unnecessary medication to the insurer, cost involved in the patient seeking out other physicians who might be willing to prescribe). Through this discussion, they might negotiate that the patient could have a trial of antibiotics or the doctor might refuse to prescribe the antibiotics, but for either option EBP and VBP are *not* working together since the treatment is not evidence based. Rather, VBP is working in a situation where EBM is not.

If on the other hand, a patient is choosing between two treatment options that are being offered, with one perhaps considered to be more effective according to the rules of EBM than the other, there may be a clash of values in the sense that the clinician wants the patient to choose one option but the patient chooses the alternative. Shared decision-making (as part of EBM) seems to be able to handle the situation without recourse to VBP. The shared decision-making process would allow the patient the opportunity to express his preferences and/or values about matters such as treatment, side effects, inconvenience, cost, while the practitioner has the opportunity to express her preferences or values about, say, the patient's best interests. They will then eventually come to some decision about what to do (e.g. try one of the options and if that does not work try the other, or only accept one option, or only accept the other etc.). Unlike in the previous example, EBM is operating here, but it is not clear how VBP would be deployed and what it would add to this process.

There is another important sense in which VBP and EBP might work together, but do not. Fulford characterises EBM as offering the 'facts' of practice. Yet, several scholars have argued that EBM reflects certain ethical values in spite of its claims that its methods of generating evidence are value-neutral. External values (Gupta, 2009, pp. 32–37) influence what topics get researched and funded and what data get published, while values internal to EBM (Goldenberg, 2006, pp. 2628–2630) reflect the aspects of illness and forms of treatment best captured by its methods and which are, in turn, prioritised by EBM. EBM then, does not reflect merely the 'facts' of medicine, but rather an implicit set of ethical and social values (Borgerson, 2008, pp. 237–244). By portraying EBM as offering the facts of medicine, VBP seems to ignore the values that EBM already brings to the table. This seems at odds with VBP's explicit aim to consider the values of all parties involved in clinical decisions. Why not include consideration of the values that led to the creation of the options under consideration in the first place? VBP is silent on this matter.

Thus, it is not clear that principle 7 is correct, that VBP and EBP actually *do* work together. It does not seem that VBP is intended to be a vehicle to express and debate all values relevant to the clinical encounter for, as I have pointed out, the values inherent to EBM seem to get left out. Nor does it seem that VBP is meant to step in when clinical decisions move beyond the available evidence, as VBP is supposed to work together with EBP, rather than apart or in isolation from it. Perhaps Fulford's intention is that VBP might have something to add to how shared decision-making actually unfolds but this is never explicitly discussed.

Values-based practice and clinical ethics

In this section I want to examine Fulford's broad claims about the practice of VBP: that it is new, that it is based on learnable, clinical skills, and that it involves 'working more effectively with complex and conflicting values' (Fulford, 2011, p. 976). Having chosen the terms 'more effectively', it is fair to ask, 'more effectively compared to what?' I believe this to be an important detail as it is difficult to evaluate the contribution of VBP without knowing to what one is comparing it. We have a hint of the comparators when Fulford states that VBP is only one of a variety of ways of 'working with complex and conflicting values in medicine and health care' including ethics, law, decision analysis, and health economic theory (Fulford, 2011, p. 977). However, he specifically positions VBP as filling a gap between EBM and *ethics* rather than these other approaches (Fulford, 2011, pp. 976 and 985). Furthermore, by characterising ethics as preoccupied with a 'rush to the rule book' in practice (Fulford, 2013), it is clear that he locates the deficiency with ethics, rather than with law, decision analysis or health economic theory to which he does not attribute any specific deficiencies. Fulford also says that the values of VBP are 'wider than ethics' yet at the same time says that VBP operates with the framework of values offered by *ethical* codes and guidelines. The few references he makes to specific examples of clashes of values in clinical practice (autonomy versus best interests) are clashes of *ethical* values. Thus, it is in this context that I will look at VBP as compared to other approaches to dealing with conflicts of ethical values, particularly with respect to VBP's claims of newness, skills-base, and greater effectiveness.

Before going further, it is important to distinguish between various related terms: bioethics, academic bioethics, and clinical ethics. I am not sure what or whom Fulford counts as representative of the kind of ethics he is concerned about as he does not define what he means by ethics exactly. I take bioethics to be the field concerned with moral issues in the health and life sciences, academic bioethics to be the scholarly study of these issues, and clinical ethics (or clinical bioethics) to refer to the practical work involved in defining, analysing and resolving these issues in different types of organisations (e.g. hospitals, research ethics boards, clinical service providers such as home care agencies etc.) and in various contexts such as clinical cases, policy development etc.

Fulford portrays ethics as being primarily about the development of 'ever more detailed ethical codes and regulatory systems' (Fulford, 2011, p. 976). This character-isation ignores the ongoing and lively debate within that field of the many competing values and principles, from a variety of sources including patients and providers that inform clinical practice and how these are to be negotiated (see for example, Wright, 1991; Hoffmaster, 1994; Kopelman, 1994; Thomasma, 1994; Jones, 1999; Gracia, 2003; Adams and Winslade, 2011). Clinical ethics in particular is oriented towards case-based models of decision-making that emphasise the weighing and consideration of a range of values in light of the specific features of a given case. For example, Jonsen *et al.*'s (2010) 'four topics' model explicitly takes into account: (1) medical indications (similar to what Fulford calls the 'facts' of medicine); (2) patient preferences; (3) quality of life; and (4) contextual features (e.g. considerations of the relevant parties and settings). Their method involves assessing the facts of a case of conflicting values in relation to the ethical principles that are relevant to the case in order to identify which principles apply and why. They then recommend the comparison of the case at hand to other cases while keeping in mind the similarities and differences between them. About their overall approach the authors write, 'Ethical issues are embedded in every clinical encounter between patients and caregivers because the care of patients always involves both technical and moral consid-erations.' They also state that, 'Clinical ethics is seldom a matter of deciding between ethical versus unethical, between good and right versus bad and wrong; rather it involves finding the better, most reasonable solutions among the relevant options.' Here Jonsen and colleagues indicate that the aim of their method is not to find and apply a general rule that fits the situation but to negotiate a solution that all parties can live with. The four topics enable the user to identify the facts of the situation and the values held by all concerned parties that will be relevant to finding 'reasonable solutions'. This approach seems consistent with VBP's commitment to exploring the diversity of values held by the various parties involved in all kinds of health care encounters and using this exploration to come to balanced judgements in individual cases.

Phil Hébert's succinct volume, *Doing Right: A Practical Guide to Ethics for Medical Trainees and Physicians*, now in its second edition (Hébert, 2009), is a mainstay in introductory ethics education for Canadian medical students. In this monograph, Hébert offers yet another approach to aid clinicians wrestling with ethical dilemmas in clinical practice. Hébert refers to this approach as an 'ethics decision-making procedure' suggesting that, like VBP, its purpose is to facilitate decision-making in situations where ethical values are divergent (Table 7.1).

Like the four topics, there appears to be substantial overlap between VBP and Hébert's model. The area of greatest correspondence between the two approaches is the four skills of VBP and the seven reflective steps needed prior to clinical decision-making. Indeed it is the skills of VBP, rather than its principles, which seem to be more central to the framework's functioning. For example, a psychiatrist on call alone at night might have to work with a patient in a scenario of conflicting values. Even though the situation might fail to adhere to the principle of multidisciplinary, the four skills of the values-based approach could still apply. Or, there may be clinical scenarios where there is very limited or no evidence. In these cases, the decisions may not be approached using the 'two feet' of EBM and VBP together, but rather by the skills of VBP alone. Hébert's approach seems to be able to cover what VBP's skills can offer. Consequently, it is not clear that in comparison to the objectives and methods of these two approaches, that VBP is new, any more skills-based or necessarily any more effective in working with complex and conflicting values.

Fulford (2013) has pointed out five apparent differences between clinical ethics and VBP. These include: (1) the deeper institutional and service delivery penetration of VBP; (2) the greater sensitivity of values-based practice to the importance of power differentials;

Table 7.1 Ethics decision-making procedure

Step 1 – The case (pertinent facts and circumstances)

Step 2 – What is the dilemma? What decision needs to be made?

Step 3 – What are the alternatives?

Step 4 – How do the key considerations apply? (Autonomy: what are the patient's wishes and values? Beneficence: what can be done for the patient? Justice: is the patient receiving what is fair?)

Step 5 – Consider involving others and consider context (situational factors, others, institutional policies, professional norms, and legal precedents)

Step 6 – Propose a resolution (Weigh these factors for each alternative then make a recommendation)

Step 7 – Consider your choice critically (e.g. when would you be prepared to alter it? Consider opinions of peers, your conscience and emotional reactions. Formulate your choice as a general maxim, suggest cases where it would not apply etc.)

Step 8 – Do the right thing

(Information from Hébert, 2009, p. 23)

(3) the fact that this sensitivity arises from the origins of VBP from psychiatry and mental health; (4) that VBP includes the values of all stakeholders and not just patients; and (5) the extension of VBP to questions of diagnosis as well as treatment.

With respect to the latter four, I see nothing within the approaches to ethical decision-making presented here that prevent them from being sensitive to power differentials, the values of all parties, or to apply to questions of diagnosis, and problems in mental health care. Moreover, the ten elements of VBP do not make specific reference to these points. Further, I am not sure on what grounds Fulford claims that VBP has penetrated institutions and service delivery to a greater extent than clinical ethics in the light of the widespread presence of ethics programmes, committees, and staff in health care institutions (clinical ethics) and universities (academic bioethics) alike.[3] The only examples he cites of are of developments specific to mental health policy and legislation in the UK (Fulford, 2011).

How does VBM actually work?

Comparing VBP to two approaches to clinical ethics has highlighted the ways in which they seem to be very similar. Examining a case example of VBP in action may be able to expose its distinct contribution. In this section, I will examine a case study in which VBP is brought to bear upon the situation (Fulford, 2004). This case features a 64 year old female artist, with a presumed diagnosis of bipolar disorder on the basis of having suffered recurring hypomanic episodes. In the case study, the diagnosis is not at issue. She is referred to a psychiatrist by her GP to discuss the pros and cons of initiating lithium treatment. She makes a decision to start treatment on the basis of research data supporting the efficacy of lithium for the treatment of hypomania, and based on a colleague's successful treatment with this medication. A few months later, she decides to stop taking lithium because she finds it has a side effect (emotional blunting) that disrupts her ability to perceive colour and thus to create art. Her GP refers her back to the psychiatrist to discuss this decision. She and the psychiatrist agree that she will stop lithium but that should she relapse she will receive antipsychotic medication (another option for treating acute mania), if necessary, on an involuntary basis.

Fulford explains that this side effect had been omitted from the original discussion with the patient because it is not important to most people, but that if it had been included, the patient and her physicians would have become aware of the patient's worry about developing it. He claims that the principles of VBP, properly applied, might have led to the disclosure of this side effect and might have influenced the patient's decision to initiate the medication in the first place. Maybe. But it also seems entirely consistent with VBP that a discussion of the values held by all the parties might still not have led to any greater

---

[3] There are, for example, numerous professional societies and meetings such as the Canadian Bioethics Society, the American Society for Bioethics and Humanities, the International Association for Bioethics, and the International Conference on Clinical Ethics and Consultations. There are additionally various educational programmes worldwide offered by university-based centres for bioethics including the Programs in Bioethics, University of Montreal, the Joint Centre for Bioethics University of Toronto, the Centre for Values, Ethics and Law in Australia. Finally, there are organisations that develop bioethics education courses such as the Indian Council of Medical Research and working groups such as the Karachi Bioethics Group that meet to discuss bioethics issues.

awareness of the possibility that the patient might experience a change in her capacity to perceive colour, simply because it might never have occurred to anyone. It is plausible that neither psychiatrist nor patient could even imagine that something like emotional blunting would result in the specific problem of altered perception of colour in this patient at the time that she took the medication. It is rather in retrospect that the patient discovered that she had developed a particular effect and that it had a negative impact on her life. And it seems that the psychiatrist was then able to address the problem in a way that was acceptable to the patient but that also seemed to be consistent with the values of ordinary, clinical practice, for there is nothing within these values that obliges a patient to take a medication that she finds difficult to tolerate.

Fulford goes on to point out that the outcome in this case – the patient's decision to stop lithium – might have been the same whether one uses VBP or whether one uses 'quasi-legal ethics'. He characterises this latter approach as one in which outcomes (like stopping lithium) are prescribed by rules which express right values (like patient autonomy) whereas, '...in VBM stopping lithium is the product of a process aimed at achieving a balance of different, and legitimately different, values' (Fulford, 2004). For Fulford, even if the outcome would have been the same, what VBP contributes differently to this situation is to emphasise process. He goes on to explain that VBP involves a focus on 'how' things should be done rather than 'what' to do (process versus outcome). Now, it is certainly the case, as is evident from the models of ethical decision-making presented earlier, that one element of clinical ethics is coming to some decision about action when clinician and patient find themselves in situations of conflicting values. However, this seems to be inherent in how medicine is practised. Where there is disagreement about the choices to be made in clinical situations, at some point decisions must be taken about the next step. Even no action reflects a decision having been made. The case example illustrates very well the various points at which decisions are made even when VBP is in play.

What about Fulford's emphasis on process? His claim about the importance of process in times of conflicts of values echos the words of Arthur Frank's essay, 'Ethics as process and practice' (Frank, 2004). In this paper, Frank argues that the single, decisional turning point which is the central narrative of many ethical problems is illusory. Instead, we ought to see that situation as itself arising out of many prior situations and continuous in time. The true ethical response is not the pursuit of a certain ethical value, a thing ascribed to a situation (like a 'good' outcome) but rather the constant striving towards a way of being and relating to others that reflects the virtues we consider important. Frank argues that the substance of ethics, namely, choosing certain values as important ones to guide actions and decisions can prevent meaningful exchange about the diversity of individually held values. In his words, 'Ethics-as-process recognizes there can never be a unitary response to the question: "What is at stake for everyone who is involved in this situation?" Ethics that begins with this question is a process of ongoing negotiation, which can only be a respectful, open process if there are no trumps' (Frank, 2004). Yet, even this type of ongoing negotiation – relevant to the communication component and process emphasis of VBP – will involve choices being made, where sometimes the different choice points reflect divergent ethical values. In such moments, certain substantive values will be operating. On the one hand, Fulford acknowledges that VBP is 'constrained by the framework of shared values incorporated in ethical codes and guidelines...' (Fulford, 2011, p. 976) but on the other, he says that 'values-based practice offers no point of values-reference external to the values of those concerned in a given decision' (Fulford, 2013).

VBP does not necessarily advocate that process alone can solve problems of conflicting values but we do not seem any further ahead than where bioethics scholarship and clinical ethics practice has already pointed us: that there are various values that seem to be fundamental to medical practice (e.g. do no harm) and are enshrined in ethical codes, that there is continued debate about what these core values are; that the interpretation of these values in specific situations is person and context dependent; that sometimes these interpretations or even the values upon which they are based will conflict; that a careful and empathic exploration of the values of all parties may help to illuminate areas of convergence and divergence; and that sometimes decisions must be taken even when there is continued divergence, and/or distress about the divergence.

What *could* VBP offer that is distinct?

There is an ambivalence that runs throughout Fulford's discussion of VBP. On the one hand, he describes it as a tool that is intended to *support* balanced decision-making in individual cases, implying that it is a process or method that leads the parties towards decision-making but does not itself contribute to the content of those decisions. On the other hand he denies that VBP strives towards a value-neutral procedure because the basic premise of VBP itself is a value, that of mutual respect (Fulford, 2013).

As a method, VBP does not seem to occupy a position that is distinct from what is offered by various other methods of clinical, ethical decision-making. Thus, I do not see VBP as a new or complementary tool for clinicians. Since VBP already endorses at least one value – mutual respect – it seems more promising for VBP to acknowledge and make explicit its own underlying values, including the framework values that constrain it, rather than to claim to be a value-neutral tool. Such an acknowledgement would clarify what VBP is and how it could influence clinical practice for the better, in ways that existing models cannot. For VBP to say something new, it needs to say something substantive about values, otherwise it seems to be largely replicating existing techniques for approaching conflicts of values (see Chapter 3). In other words, rather than being a new tool, it seems to be more like a new package for the tools that we already have.

If Fulford could resolve this ambivalence, VBP has the potential to offer something stronger than what is currently offered by clinical ethics. Fulford writes that VBP adds a particular focus on the diversity of *individual* values and that it includes the values of all individuals involved in situations where values conflict such as patients, clinicians, carers, managers, and policy-makers (Fulford, 2013). Fulford's use of the word 'individual' is important here. In what sense are all of these individuals' values relevant? While specific people are involved in any given clinical situation, the reason to include their values is *not* as specific people *per se*, but because those values represent the values of the profession or the institution that person represents. Indeed, the point of professional values is exactly to constrain individual values. We do not want a physician's personal values about which services are important to influence where they refer patients or what treatments they provide. We want their reasoning about these things to be influenced by what the profession as a whole has determined to meet the standard of care. Therefore, these individuals' values are important to include inasmuch as they represent the values of a larger entity: such as an institution or a profession.

If we take seriously VBP's commitment to acknowledging *all* values involved in health care, then this would seem to include a whole host of values such as those operating in the background conditions (e.g. in social policy) that contribute to clashes of values arising in frontline care. Why include the values of the medical profession or the individual patient but ignore the values of the society? Discussions about whether a person should be involuntarily hospitalised might be enriched by examining the social policy decisions that make it difficult for that person to live in the community including, for example, the paucity of safe, affordable, supported housing. In its current form, VBP (and clinical ethics) focuses largely on 'downstream' values, evident at the point of clinical decision-making. This emphasis comes at the expense of 'upstream' values – those that give rise to the social and economic conditions that create health problems, those that focus our attention on certain health problems and not others, and those that shape and constrain the options we are willing to provide to address health problems. If VBP were oriented towards the inclusion of upstream values, it would have the potential to offer a perspective that was both distinct and more radical than what is currently offered by mainstream clinical ethics. It would be distinct because background conditions are often accepted as given in clinical ethics while the particulars of the situation at hand are (understandably) given priority. It would be radical because once it is clear that values are part of every aspect of health care, including the 'facts' of medicine, it might transform providers and recipients of care into participants in the political and economic debates about which values are at play in health care and on what grounds. As VBP evolves, it will be worth following closely how it specifies itself practically, and what vision of ethical health care it stakes out.

Conclusions

In this chapter, I have examined the positioning of VBP as a practical method that fills the gap between EBM and ethics in clinical decision-making by offering a method for identifying and exploring the values of all parties concerned. I have argued that the description of the model lacks detail about how it works, which makes it difficult to compare it to the approaches it criticises, namely those offered by clinical ethics. Further, VBP does not live up to its assertion of working together with EBM nor does it substantiate its claim of working more effectively with conflicting values compared with other approaches which might attempt the same. As a method for accomplishing its stated goal, to enable balanced judgements where values conflict in clinical practice, VBP does not distinguish itself sufficiently from clinical ethics. However, if VBP acknowledged its normative position, it has the potential to draw attention to important areas of moral concern that can be neglected in mainstream ethics discourse. These include 'upstream' values that lie behind conflicts of value frontline care, whether these relate to political, economic, or social policy choices. VBP may not offer many practical differences to what already exists, but depending on which direction it takes as it evolves, it may serve an important role in highlighting new areas that deserve moral reflection in health care.

References

Adams, D. M. and Winslade, W. J. (2011) Consensus, clinical decision making, and unsettled cases. *Journal of Clinical Ethics*, **22**, 310–327.

Borgerson, K. (2008) *Valuing and Evaluating Evidence in Medicine*, Doctoral Thesis, University of Toronto (unpublished). Available at:

www.academia.edu/902043/Valuing_
and_evaluating_evidence_in_medicine,
accessed 8 May 2013.

Frank, A. (2004) Ethics as process and practice.
Internal Medicine Journal, **34**(6), 355–357.

Fulford, K. W. M. (2004) Ten principles of
values-based medicine, www.wpanet.org/
detail.php?section_id=11&content_id=519,
accessed 3 May 2013.

Fulford, K. W. M. (2011) The value of evidence
and evidence of values: bringing together
values-based and evidence-based practice in
policy and service development in mental
health. *Journal of Evaluation in Clinical
Practice*, **17**, 976–987.

Fulford, K. W. M. (2013) Values-based practice:
Fulford's dangerous idea. *Journal of
Evaluation in Clinical Practice*, **19**(3),
537–546.

Goldenberg, M. J. (2006) On evidence and
evidence-based medicine: lessons from the
philosophy of science, *Social Science &
Medicine*, **62**, 2621–2632.

Gracia, D. (2003) Ethical case deliberation and
decision making. *Medicine, Health Care and
Philosophy*, **6**, 227–233.

Gupta, M. (2009). *Is Evidence-Based Psychiatric
Practice, Ethical Practice?*, Doctoral Thesis,
University of Toronto (unpublished).
Available at: https://tspace.library.utoronto.
ca/handle/1807/19274.

Guyatt, G., Rennie, D., Meade, M. O. and
Cook, D. J. (editors) (2008) *Users' Guides to
the Medical Literature*, 2nd edition. McGraw
Hill Medical.

Hébert, P. (2009) *Doing Right: A Practical
Guide to Ethics for Medical Trainees and
Physicians*, 2nd edition. Oxford University
Press.

Hoffmaster, B. (1994) The forms and limits of
medical ethics. *Social Science & Medicine*, **39**,
1155–1164.

Jones, A. H. (1999) Narrative based medicine:
narrative in medical ethics. *British Medical
Journal*, **318**, 253–256.

Jonsen, A. R., Siegler, M. and Winslade, W. J.
(2010) *Clinical Ethics: a practical approach to
ethical decisions in clinical medicine*.
Electronic book, available through
University of Ottawa Library, accessed
2 May 2013.

Kopelman, L. M. (1994) Case method and
casuistry: the problem of bias. *Theoretical
Medicine*, **15**, 21–37.

Straus, S. E., Glasziou, P., Richardson, W. S. and
Haynes, R. B. (editors) (2011) *Evidence-based
Medicine: How to Practice and Teach EBM*,
4th edition. Edinburgh: Churchill
Livingstone.

Thomasma, D. C. (1994) Clinical ethics as
medical hermeneutics. *Theoretical Medicine*,
15, 93–111.

Tonelli, M. R. (2006) Integrating evidence into
clinical practice: an alternative to evidence-
based approaches. *Journal of Evaluation in
Clinical Practice*, **12**, 248–256.

Wright, R. A. (1991) Clinical judgment
and bioethics: the decision making link.
Journal of Medicine and Philosophy, **16**,
71–91.

Values or virtues?

Richard Hamilton

If we know anything about values, it is that there a lot of them around and that they are terribly important. Debates rage about whether children should learn Biblical stories or instead be offered 'values education'. Australia's economy revolves around digging up lumps of metal, which are then transported to China where 'value' is added by turning them into cheap (and often toxic) children's toys. Upon entering my local supermarket, I find myself magically transformed into a 'valued customer' whom it is the store's sole mission to delight. Politicians and other low rent types are encouraged to embrace a clearer commitment to values. In medicine too, the jargon of values has spread like a *staph*. infection in a badly cleaned ward. Patients have them, doctors too, and we should do our best to respect them in anything and everything we do.

F. W. M. Fulford's values-based medicine (VBM) takes values seriously. It has been self-consciously developed (and skilfully marketed) as the 'values' counterpart to evidence-based medicine. In his contribution to this volume (Chapter 10), Harry Lesser contrasts the team-based approach advocated by Fulford with various competitors. The first of these is paternalism, in which doctor knows best and browbeats the patient into accepting his decisions. Since this model is officially disfavoured, a much greater danger is the approach Lesser refers to as 'consumerism'. In a consumerist model, under the guise of respect for autonomy, the patient (usually sick and often distressed) is given a range of options and is then left to her own devices to peruse them, bereft of expert guidance. Fulford also counsels against bioethical imperialism, in which a philosophical expert derives a solution from *a priori* postulates which all must accept on pain of irrationality.

Since much of what follows will be critical of VBM, I want to stress that I endorse neither paternalism nor consumerism, and although the dangers of bioethical imperialism

Debates in Values-Based Practice, ed. Michael Loughlin. Published by Cambridge University Press. © Cambridge University Press 2014.

are somewhat overstated, good reasons exist to be suspicious of much mainstream bioethics. Certainly, no ethical decision should ever be settled by appeals to authority, be that medical or philosophical. I have written at length elsewhere against the fiction of value neutrality that often underpins such appeals, so I am also in profound sympathy with this aspect of VBM (Hamilton, 2010, 2013). Values are ubiquitous in health care and no decision which neglects them will do.

Does Fulford's VBM provide the best support for a team-based model of decision-making? I suggest not. We should respect the seriousness with which most parties approach clinical deliberation but we cannot do so with the faulty value theory Fulford endorses. Indeed, the jargon of 'values' is best left to grocers. The best way to take values seriously is to stop talking about values. Or so I shall argue.

In what follows, I defend an alternative Aristotelian model of collaborative medical decision-making without Fulford's unfortunate meta-ethical baggage. At its core is the conception of *phronesis* (practical reasonableness) as personified by the figure of the *phronimos* (the virtuous person). The *phronimos* need not be an individual and, in our context, it is best to see her as the personification of the deliberative process itself when conducted by persons of good faith with sufficient knowledge of the particulars of the situation and a sense of which virtues it summons. This is a strenuous ideal but so it should be when people's lives are at stake.

I

Selina, a 35 year old professional in a long term stable relationship, had been trying to conceive for over a year and was about to start IVF when she became pregnant. She is in good general health, a non-smoker and a moderate drinker. She has avoided alcohol in the last year and is taking folate supplements. Aside from the difficulties of conceiving and occasional minor menstrual issues, her reproductive health is good with no family history of birth difficulties. She strongly favours a homebirth and has found a supportive midwife. Her GP is adamantly opposed. Although she works in the CBD she lives in a semi-rural suburb many kilometres away from the nearest maternity unit.

Planned home births are a hot topic in contemporary Australian health care. The AMA is adamantly opposed while the Royal Colleges of Midwives and Obstetricians jointly support the option for low-risk pregnancies. Both cite competing data sets but a Cochrane Review is inconclusive. While it is possible to profile risk, it is not possible to predict difficulties accurately in an individual case. Equally, one cannot predict accurately a fatigued obstetrician or a badly cleaned ward.

In a sometimes acrimonious debate, the AMA and its supporters question the competence of midwives to detect complications, while midwifery groups imply questionable pecuniary motives behind the AMA's support for medical intervention in unproblematic pregnancies. Australia has one of the most medicalised birth regimes in the world and women who opt for home births sometimes complain of undue medical pressure. If, nevertheless, we adopt a charitable interpretation of the motives of all parties involved, then this issue seems to fit perfectly with what Fulford has in mind when he talks about legitimate disagreement.

The central ethical question here concerns risk, as it does in most questions surrounding patient autonomy. At one extreme, the paternalist assesses risk on the patient's behalf and attempts to mitigate it, even if this means overriding her wishes. The libertarian at the other pole asserts the patient's sovereignty, even in the face of lethal danger, which seems an untenable position when it is not solely the mother's life that is in peril. Our options are thus paternalism, consumerism, mainstream bioethics and a VBM approach.

The AMA position adopts an aggressively paternalist stance. Consequently, many women who would like to opt for a home birth feel bullied. Australia's highly medicalised birth regimes put us at odds with comparable health care systems where home births are routine. While geography affects matters, it is hard to see how Australia differs that radically from Canada. So, the AMA's stance is problematic.

Let us consider consumerism. On this model, mothers considered as customers choose birth options, as if perusing a menu. Thus starkly stated, the problems are obvious. The interests of the child, who is not a consumer, go unacknowledged. Furthermore, Selina is not simply asking to make her choice unmolested. She is asking for her choice to be facilitated. In a health care system where a significant proportion of any ensuing costs is borne by the public purse, it is unclear who the customer is. Moreover, proper decision-making requires more than information. Minimally, it involves presenting the mother with the risks in an intelligible manner. This requires a conducive emotional atmosphere, which is yet another reason to reject the AMA's bullish approach. A woman's ability to exercise autonomy requires an array of social, political and psychological factors to be in place, which make the consumerist model inappropriate.

Perhaps, we might consult the bioethicists. Mainstream bioethics is dominated by what Fulford refers to as a 'quasi-legal' approach, typified by Beauchamp and Childress' Four Principles. Although these have become a mantra in medical education, with many students believing they have 'done' ethics if they can list them off, they generate some notorious problems. Perhaps the greatest problem is how to resolve conflicts between the principles. One might say that the principlist approach does better at outlining the contours of an ethical problem than actually solving it.

Raanan Gillon suggests a way out of the impasse (Gillon, 2003). He believes that a principlist approach encompasses all of the factors that a morally serious person should consider. Conflicts between the principles can be resolved by treating 'respect for autonomy' as the core principle from which the other principles derive. For instance, beneficence facilitates autonomy while justice concerns itself with the equitable distribution of opportunities to exercise autonomy.

Gillon's solution has all the merits of vacuousness. Both Selina and her GP could present themselves as upholding respect for autonomy. For Selina, this is expressed in her right to choose a home birth. Her GP sees himself as protecting Selina's future autonomy and that of her child. One might prioritise current autonomy over potential autonomy but it is not obvious that this is anything more than a fiat. Further problems arise. As Onora O'Neill (2007) suggests, we need to know whether, in respecting autonomy, we are respecting mere choice, in which case it is unclear that all choices merit respect, or whether we respect the reasoning upon which such choices are based. The fact that we routinely disregard the choices of infants and the insane implies that we respect reasoning not mere choice.

Indeed, I would go further than O'Neill and argue that autonomy, as it is typically understood, is not a medical value at all. It is rather a structural feature of the political and legal context in which health care operates. Viewed thus, many ethical problems in medicine are not problems within medicine but rather a conflict between the practice of medicine and its institutional setting. Autonomy's passing resemblance to some genuine medical virtues, such as respect for human dignity, may obscure this. I will develop this point below. For now, I want to emphasise that the veneration with which the four principles are treated notwithstanding, they offer little practical guidance and there is indeed a danger of them lapsing into the type of arbitrary stipulations against which Fulford warns.

Consequentialism is the competing tradition within mainstream bioethics. It would approach Selina's situation by assessing the most likely outcomes and attempting to analyse the decision retrospectively in their light. The problems besetting consequentialism are as grave as those that confront principlism. Simply put, the ethical problems arise precisely because we do not know the most likely outcome. Consequentialists proceed as if we did. Moreover, consequentialism misses what is really significant morally speaking about decisions involving risk. Selina could follow the advice of her GP and the AMA, play safe and still have a catastrophic event. If the focus of the evaluation is on the outcome, as for a consequentialist it surely must be, then this is no different from a case in which a woman was reckless in respect to risk and suffered a catastrophe.

Of course, there are various 'sophisticated' forms of consequentialism which would attempt to avoid these problems by vacuously expanding the concept of an outcome. Many defenders of consequentialism see this ability of the theory to absorb objections and difficult cases as a strength; I am inclined to see it as a weakness. It was one which was introduced by J. S. Mill when he responded to obvious problems with Bentham's hedonic calculus by distinguishing between 'higher' and 'lower' pleasures, despite the fact that nothing in the principle of utility permits an honest philosopher to do this. Clearly the subject of moral evaluation in most cases of risk cannot be the outcome, over which the risk taker has little control, but the attitude towards the risk that she takes.

Once again, I will develop these points below. I presume that most readers who sympathise with VBM are familiar with the problems with mainstream bioethics, so I will not dwell on them. To sum up, the first stage in resolving Selina's predicament is neither to browbeat her into submission, nor to leave her to her own devices, nor to invoke some lofty bioethical consideration, be it principlist or consequential. It is rather for all the parties involved to sit down together and deliberate in a spirit of openness and humility.

II

Selina's midwife manages to get a case conference convened involving Selina and her partner, her GP and a supportive obstetrician. In the course of the meeting, Selina makes clear her reasons for preferring a home birth. The GP lays out his reservations and does his best to convince her of the risks. The professionals in the meeting have received training in the communication skills associated with VBP, notably 'patient-perspective' and 'multi-perspective' skills. At the end of the meeting, although he still has strong reservations, the GP reluctantly supports Selina's decision with certain provisos. If any routine tests detect abnormalities or if there are complications during labour Selina will abandon the home birth.

Unusually for health care, decisions about birth often involve a relatively lengthy timeframe. Nevertheless, as Fulford (2013) rightly notes, a decision cannot be left hanging in the air. This speaks to a broader observation: ethics is about decisions and actions, not primarily belief. In the jargon of twentieth-century analytic philosophy, ethical propositions are action guiding. It is this feature of ethical utterances which struck R. M. Hare (1952, 1977) from whose meta-ethics Fulford draws inspiration.[1]

A vegetarian declares that eating meat is abhorrent. Superficially this has the appearance of a factual statement. But, of course, this appearance is misleading, for it is, *inter alia*, an expression of the speaker's attitude. In this respect, it has affinities with my preference for Wagyu steaks. My preference, however, is only a recommendation to other steak lovers. The vegetarian's utterance has a more categorical character. She is enjoining all who hear her to refrain from eating meat. If she fails to persuade, her utterance has misfired. If we discover her in a steakhouse, we would figure that she is a hypocrite or else that she did not understand the language that she uses.

Hare intends to draw our attention to two features of moral utterances: they are universal in their scope and they override other considerations, such as those of aesthetic taste or convenience. The vegetarian expects all, and should be expected herself, to refrain from eating meat, even at the loss of the pleasures and convenience of meat eating. Hare's view is a refinement of the earlier emotivist meta-ethics associated with the logical positivists. Ethics presented a troublesome case for their semantic theory since by rights it ought to be consigned to the category of nonsense. This hardly accorded with the serious practical roles that ethical talk plays. The emotivist solution was to stress the expressive and persuasive function of moral talk. Ethical statements state neither empirical nor logical facts; they express emotions and attempt to persuade.

Although Hare adopted the basic elements of this view, he realised that classical emotivism cannot do justice to the gravity of ethical talk. Our ethical judgements seem subject to certain kinds of rational constraints which other evaluative judgements do not. If my friend is considering a holiday and I suggest tropical North Queensland, I am not thereby obliged to accompany him. Yet, my suggestion both expresses my pro-attitude towards wintering in tropical North Queensland and attempts to persuade my friend to share that attitude. Unlike moral statements, it lacks universalisability.

Hare's analysis superficially resembles Kant's famous Categorical Imperative. However, on Hare's account, the universality and seriousness are features of the speaker's utterance. Any overriding judgement that demands universal assent would qualify as a moral judgement. For Kant, by contrast, one judges the moral worthiness of a motive by how well it stands up against objective criteria. Whatever quibbles one might have with Kant, Hare's position deprives ethics of objectivity altogether. The seriousness with which we treat someone's moral claims is, at best, a mark of respect towards the person advancing them, though subjectivism is necessarily silent on why we should treat others with respect.

Hare was keen to emphasise the importance of tolerance and mutual respect for conflicting opinions. Fulford too shares this emphasis. His version of VBM is a form of radical liberalism (see Chapter 4). He expresses his distrust of mainstream bioethics as follows:

> In quasi-legal ethics, the assumption of 'right' values, and its consequent proliferation of rules and regulatory authorities, inevitably leads to a model of the ethicist as an expert. And ethicists, like scientists, may indeed bring a range of relevant expertise to policy, practice,

---

[1] It is worth noting that Hare himself eventually adopted a much more robust form of utilitarianism, perhaps in recognition of some of the problems that his meta-ethical position generates.

education and research in healthcare. As we saw earlier, however, where legitimately different values are in play, the particular value prescribed by a quasi-legal ethical rule, however enlightened, will necessarily conflict with the very different values of many of those to whom the rule is intended to apply. (Fulford, 2004)

The worry here is that the ethicist will arrogate to herself the paternalistic authority which doctors have traditionally claimed. Fulford's guarantee against this danger is to adopt a form of non-cognitivism in which there is no danger of either clinician or bioethicist knowing best because the concept of knowledge is inapplicable in a moral setting. Outside the very minimal constraints of formal consistency and factual accuracy, there is no way of saying one set of values is better than another.

Fulford's central message is that we should respect legitimate disagreements about values and the decision-making process should facilitate this. When stated thus, the message seems innocuous: who would dispute that we should respect legitimate disagreement? What this obscures, however, is the distinction between disagreement that is genuine in the sense that there are real differences of opinion at stake, and the smaller subset of such disagreements in which the values of all sides must be given equal weight. For instance, as a good liberal, Fulford would surely wish to give less weight to some particularly intolerant religious fundamentalist's views than to those of a fellow liberal who believes in promoting autonomy and patient choice.

The trouble here is that the question of which values are legitimate and worthy of respect is itself a moral question and one which Fulford provides us with no tools to address. To illustrate this, suppose that a patient refused to be treated by a physician of a different race for no other reason than racial prejudice. Contrast this with an indigenous patient who requests that an indigenous health care worker be present during his treatment, believing that he will be more likely to receive culturally sensitive care. Most serious folk would agree that the hospital is under a *prima facie* obligation to consider the latter request and would not be morally culpable if they disregarded the first.

Circumstances obviously matter. It might be inordinately difficult to provide an indigenous health care worker and the patient's life may be in imminent danger. The patient may know this full well and be using the request to buy time. In such a circumstance, the right thing to do may well be to disregard the patient's request and explore his reasons for asking. Similarly, the hospital might accede to the racist's request out of a desire to protect the wellbeing of its staff. Any answer must take account of fine-grained situational details and that is why the 'solutions' proposed by mainstream bioethics often seem so wildly implausible. Fulford appears to vacillate between this reasonable position and a rejection of right answers *per se*. This ultimately undermines all the positive aims that VBM promotes. It trivialises the seriousness of the deliberative process and it risks opening the door to old style paternalism, albeit covered with a figleaf of consultation.

A common phrase which occurs whenever Fulford discusses bioethics is 'quasi-legal'. He is rightly concerned with the legislative pretensions of many bioethicists who would seek to circumvent the hard work of *in situ* deliberation. In rejecting this parallel with the law, Fulford appears blind to another, namely, adjudication. In complex legal cases, a judge or jury must weigh up a range of facts and values and reach an outcome in a timely manner. It need not follow that the solution arrived at transfers seamlessly to other cases, and part of the business of legal interpretation involves working out appropriate comparisons. Nevertheless, legal reasoning when it works well (for instance, where a decision is reached which cannot be successfully appealed) is able to reach a decision even in morally contested cases. There is an obvious parallel here with Ronald Dworkin's 'right answer thesis'.[2] By way of contrast, I will call Fulford's position the 'no right answer thesis'. While we should not circumvent the deliberative process by assuming that any party has that right answer at the outset, without the goal of a right answer, deliberation risks degenerating into a 1960s style encounter session with participants sitting in comfy chairs emoting. At worst, however, there is a danger that medical decisions will simply become exercises of power (see Chapters 5 and 6).

Like law, ethics is an attempt to hold power to account, and nowhere is this more vital than in medicine. Philippa Foot, who begins her book *Natural Goodness* (Foot, 2000) with a critical discussion of Hare, concludes with a discussion of Nietzsche. There might seem to be a world of difference between the poetic ravings of the wild-eyed German immoralist and the genteel musings of the urbane Anglo-Irishman. However, both writers express the predicament of a culture which has lost the traditional source of moral authority.

One source of Foot's rejection of Hare's subjectivism is her belief that it offered an inadequate response to the horrors of Nazism. If ethics is ultimately a matter of attitude and persuasion, then the field goes to he who shouts loudest or carries the biggest stick. To his credit, Hare tackled the obvious objection of the consistent Nazi who upon learning that he is in fact Jewish commits suicide. Hare evades this problem (to his own satisfaction but to no one else's) by arguing that a fanatic can never be properly informed (Hare, 1977). Yet Foot finds equally unsatisfactory the Kantian project of vindicating morality from a standpoint external to the everyday affairs of men and women. She follows MacIntyre (1984) and Anscombe (1958) in urging a recovery of the Greek ethical tradition which pre-dated the rise of modern theism and thus feels no need to vindicate ethics in an external locus of authority and is thus unperturbed by its absence. I hope to show how such an approach can provide a stronger foundation for a collaborative approach to medical decision-making.

III

Aristotle opens his *Nicomachean Ethics* by remarking that 'it is a mark of an educated person to look in each area for only that degree of accuracy that the nature of the subject permits' (Aristotle, 2004, I: iii 1094b). This should also be our starting point. He stresses the practical nature of ethics; that it involves a set of skills with deep analogies to activities such as playing a musical instrument, acquired first by the training and only later by theoretical reflection. He also discusses the limitations this places on our ability to generalise about people, whether individually or collectively, and argues that 'we should be content' with generalisations that are 'for the most part true (*hos epi to pulo*)' (Aristotle, 2004, I: iii 1094b). Although we must generalise, our generalisations can never have the precision of those of mathematics and it would be folly to attempt to make them more precise.

Aristotle here captures both the centrality of practical reason to ethics and the peculiar features of practical reason. *Phronesis*, the master virtue of practical reasonableness, is the ability to discern what the situation demands and act upon it. We learn to act ethically by a

---

[2] Cf. Ronald Dworkin (1978) but we should be mindful of the important differences between ethics and law such as the lack of a substantive mechanism for adjudicating disputes.

combination of emulation, trial and error, and reflection, and the only test of whether we have mastered the skill is whether we can proceed unsupervised. Virtue thus requires an exquisite sensitivity to context combined with a sense of the big picture. The virtuous are able to grasp the rational principle (*orthos logos*) at stake in any given situation. They characteristically get things right and can thereby act as role models for others. Indeed it is better to see phronesis not as a 'monolithic virtue' but rather as a suite of practical skills including comprehension (*sunesis*), sense (*gnome*) and more general intelligence (*nous*) (Russell, 2009, pp. 18–19).

Virtue ethics shares a suspicion towards the sorts of all-purpose solutions in which much mainstream bioethics trades (Hursthouse, 1999). There can be no substitute for the process of communal deliberation by epistemically and morally virtuous agents. Perhaps an Aristotelian should be sympathetic to VBM. There is, however, a world of difference between insisting that the right answer to any moral problem is occasion sensitive and only available to the practically wise, and Fulford's 'no right answer thesis'. Fulford shares with both paternalism and mainstream bioethics, a conception of what a right answer must look like; he has simply lost hope that one can be found.

The predicament is illustrated by H. L. Mencken (1949) in 'A good man gone wrong' which discusses an adulterous couple who conspired together to murder the woman's husband. Mencken argues that the murder occurred because of, and not despite, the man's fundamentalist Christianity. Once the initial sin of adultery was committed the man decided that he was doomed anyway. Thus in 'his eyes the step from adultery to murder was as natural and inevitable as the step from the cocktail shaker to the gutter in the eyes of a Methodist bishop' (Mencken, 1949). Beneath Mencken's characteristic cynicism is a profound point. It is the plight that confronts all rigorist moral theories when they encounter the real world in all its complexity.

The real danger of absolutist ethics is not that anyone will actually live by them, nor even the sheer difficulty of doing so. It is that by rigidly sticking to some code the person fails to develop the necessary skills to negotiate moral complexity and ambiguity without sliding into defeatism and moral recusal. That ability to maintain a relatively even keel in the face of ambiguity is the mark of virtue. It is to this we now turn.

IV

Several months later, having decided upon a home birth, Selina goes into labour two weeks early. The midwife in attendance phones Selina's GP who upon examining Selina and the baby advises an immediate hospital admission. Selina is reluctant and wishes to proceed with her original plan.

The central ethical question throughout Selina's case has been that of risk: risk to the mother and child. There are also secondary risks to the health professionals involved, especially in an increasingly litigious environment. As our scenario has developed, the risk profile has clearly altered: what began as a routine unproblematic pregnancy has now become complicated. While many might have initially sympathised with Selina's wish to have a home birth, our evaluation of her may change if she doggedly sticks to this plan in the light of the increasing risk. Aside from anything else she has made a promise to her GP.

As mentioned above, the dominant thinking about risk has been consequentialist. Consequentialist approaches fare badly in such a situation. Notwithstanding the considerable technical ingenuity consequentialists deploy, in the final analysis it is this unpredictability that creates the ethical problems. Even with a mathematically rigorous risk profile, human beings are complex biological systems and like all such systems we embody elements of unpredictability and randomness. It is worth also noting a theme in much recent psychology: human beings, even those with some degree of mathematical training, are notoriously bad at dealing with probabilities. Some of the finest mathematical minds in the world were working in the financial sector. They could neither predict nor prevent the Global Financial Crisis of 2008, even if in retrospect we see that it was inevitable.

Risk resembles luck but it also differs in significant ways. As Athanassoulis and Ross point out, 'risk is not something that happens to us, but something that we choose to become involved in' (Athanassoulis and Ross, 2012, p. 3). Crucially from a moral point of view, risk involves, or at least should involve, deliberation. It is the quality of that deliberation that determines whether a decision to take a risk expresses courage or foolhardiness. It is a central Aristotelian thought that we reveal our character through our decisions as much as through our actions. Deliberation, decision and action form a triad through which our virtues come to be known.

Making reasonable decisions about risks 'requires good character, which, in turn, involves wisdom and well-regulated feelings and desires' (Athanassoulis and Ross, 2012, p. 3). It might seem that virtue requires a person to stick doggedly to her decisions in the face of adversity. The stereotypical virtuous figure is one who does not allow herself to be led astray by temptation or inconvenience. Such a picture fails to do justice to the occasion sensitive quality of practical reasonableness. Stubbornness can as often be a vice as it is a virtue.

Suppose that, as the obvious dangers affecting her pregnancy become manifest, Selina continues to demand a home birth. Perhaps, she has read Hare and realises that moral statements must be consistent and she insists that she (and anyone else who found herself in the same position) ought to stand by the principle that she had adopted and that moreover this principle was so serious that she was prepared to risk her life for it. In other words, it would satisfy the criteria of universalisability and overridingness. Genuine moral agreement seems possible. Selina's autonomy looms large. But does it override other considerations, such as the risks to her child, the GP's genuine concern for her health and wellbeing and no doubt equally genuine fear of being sued should something go wrong? This is less clear. Would the appropriate solution be then to accept that there is no right answer?

We could, following Gillon's advice, treat respect for autonomy as first among equals and (regretfully perhaps) accept Selina's plan. If the only option was legal intervention, then this might be the wisest course. Certainly it would be dangerous to invoke some legal mechanism to prevent her from having a home birth. However, there remains the pressing danger to the infant, either direct or indirect in the form of losing its mother in childbirth. Moreover, unless Selina decides to have the child in complete privacy, then her decision makes a call upon others. To say that she has a right to a home birth (unless interpreted very narrowly to mean the state should not prevent her) is to claim rights against other people, in this case primarily the midwife. Should the midwife assist at her birth she faces the very real prospect of de-registration. If she does not and Selina or the infant dies, she would face other consequences.

Dealing with this issue in terms of rights, duties and obligations is crass. This is partly why the four principles seldom help in guiding us through real moral problems. The worryingly legalistic tone of concepts like autonomy is not accidental. As I suggested above, the concept of autonomy is not properly speaking a medical concept at all but is rather a feature of the institutional setting in which medicine operates. It is quite possible to imagine a health care system that functioned without a concept of autonomy. If we believe the standard Whiggish story, such was our own health care system before the heroic rise of modern bioethics.

But there are other possibilities. We could have a medical system in which the over-riding consideration was concern for human dignity when people are at their most vulnerable. No elderly patient would ever be left alone and dehydrated because a nurse was worried about violating their autonomy and the patient was too deaf to hear the offer of a cup of tea. Health care staff would attempt to involve patients in the decision-making process as the best way to honour their dignity. Clinicians would sometimes make decisions on the patient's behalf, if such consultation was difficult or impossible, with the nurse acting as the proxy defender of the patient's interests.

Someone might reasonably interject that this is precisely what contemporary health care aspires to being. They would be right. Much of what is glossed under the quasi-legal concept of respect for autonomy is better seen in the medical setting in terms of dignity. The understandable outrage of patients when their interests are disregarded more often than not expresses a visceral recognition that they have been humiliated rather than an appeal to an abstract principle. Most reasonable patients recognise that there are occasions where time pressures or imminent danger mean that full consultation is not an option.

Many feminists have noted that our paradigm example of the autonomous person is that of an adult (typically male) in a situation where he has power and a wide range of choices, not a vulnerable and often frightened or anxious person who may well have some degree of cognitive impairment being forced to choose between a small range of unpalatable options in a very short time period.

It seems clear therefore that there can be vicious and virtuous ways of respecting patient autonomy. What makes paternalism offensive is less that it disregards hallowed political principles drawn from the Magna Carta than that it is just plain rude. There is however a similar rudeness in the consumerist model which would refuse to give patients guidance when they are in most dire need. It is safe to assume, however, that neither paternalism nor 'respect for autonomy', whether in its lofty principlist variety or more tawdry consumerist version, captures how the best medical professionals regard themselves. It is more fruitful to see medical practice as embodying, or aspiring to embody, a set of epistemic and moral virtues.

What the obsession with autonomy misses is that choice *per se* is not obviously worthy of respect. Some choices are neutral, such as a firm decision to avoid walking on cracks in the pavement, and others are despicable such as the decision to spread a particularly cruel piece of gossip. From a virtue perspective, what we admire are those choices which reveal a person's moral and intellectual character. In the first case, what the choice reveals is perhaps a certain immaturity, while the second choice reveals malice. Restricting someone's ability to exercise choice can restrict her ability to express her character. It also restricts her ability to develop her character through making mistakes which she subsequently regrets.

Suppose then, rather than leaving Selina to her own devices, which is clearly not an option, or imposing a solution upon her against her will, which is equally unpalatable, all those involved deliberated virtuously. I have suggested that such a process has the best chance of arriving at the right answer. It may not be one that generalised, even to other similar cases. It would not and could not be the sole decision of any party, no matter how knowledgeable or well intentioned. In the course of a deliberative process the crucial ethical question will be clarified, namely, the extent to which Selina is acting reasonably in respect to the risks of her situation. There is no way of knowing this from a position external to her situation, one further reason why consequentialism fails. The clinicians involved bring a technical understanding of risk which Selina does not have. At the same time, Selina brings her understanding of her reasons for wanting her home birth. It is for these reasons also that neither the blanket paternalistic opposition to home birth nor the equally unreflective advocacy of mother's rights adopted by some home birth advocates can be defended.

Obviously such a deliberative process takes time. By the time Selina's pregnancy has reached this stage, it may be too late for extended discussion. But the picture being defended here is one in which all parties have already acquired the virtue of practical reasonableness which is only gained through practice and subsequent reflection on one's own mistakes and others', and of our respective successes. Through this we refine our understanding of what the situation calls for. The acquisition of practical wisdom is necessary precisely in order to make decisions when one is called upon. The key feature of ethical decision-making which is lost in one-size-fits-all theories of ethics is its timeliness. Aristotle defined practical reasonableness as the capacity to make correct decisions, *pros ton kairon*, or as the occasion demands. The *phronimos* or virtuous person is just the one who is able to know what any given situation demands and act decisively.

I suggested earlier that we need not see the *phronimos* as an individual. Indeed, the broader context of Aristotle's thought stresses that we only ever acquire practical reason in an appropriate communal setting and moreover Aristotle's self is radically different from contemporary liberal ones in that it is constitutively social. It is therefore fitting to see the *phronimos*, in our context at least, as the personification of the deliberative process itself when conducted in good faith by persons of at least moderate epistemic and moral virtue and with sufficient knowledge of the relevant features of the situation. Actual deliberative processes may fall short of this ideal but at least it gives us a benchmark by which they can be evaluated and an ideal to which they can aspire. And it does so without the unfortunate baggage, inherited from scientistic twentieth-century moral philosophy.

Conclusion

Observant readers will realise that I have not offered a solution to Selina's problem, but that is entirely in keeping with an approach that emphasises process over product. Where I have differed from Fulford is that I am confident that the right answer is what will emerge when such a process is properly conducted. It might seem that I am advocating an alternative to Fulford's values-based medicine which could perhaps be described as virtues-based medicine but that would be wrong. I do believe that the jargon of value is unhelpful and is probably best left on the stock market trading floor. If anything, it would make far more sense to talk about practice-based values (better, virtues) than the converse. I have also raised grave concerns about Fulford's meta-ethical stance. But I hope that it is also clear that I regard most of what Fulford proposes in a positive light and that the commitment to a mistaken meta-ethics hampers the very positive contribution that the team-based model of decision-making hopes to bring to medicine and the profound and complex moral problems that it generates (see Chapter 3).

References

Anscombe, G. E. M. (1958) Modern moral philosophy. *Philosophy*, **33**(124), 1–19.

Aristotle (2004) *Nicomachean Ethics*, translated and edited by Roger Crisp. Cambridge: Cambridge University Press.

Athanassoulis, N. and Ross, A. (2012) Luck and risk in medicine, with A. Ross. In Cowley, C. (editor), *Reconceiving Medical Ethics: An Anthology*. London: Continuum Press.

Dworkin, R. (1978) *Taking Rights Seriously*. Cambridge, MA: Harvard University Press.

Foot, P. (2000) *Natural Goodness*. Oxford: Oxford University Press.

Fulford, K. W. M. (2004) Ten principles of values-based medicine. In Radden, J. (editor), *The Philosophy of Psychiatry: A Companion*, Chapter 14. New York: Oxford University Press.

Fulford, K. W. M. (2013). Values-based practice: Fulford's dangerous idea. *Journal of Evaluation in Clinical Practice*, **19**(3), 537–546.

Gillon, R. (2003) Ethics needs principles – four can encompass the rest – and respect for autonomy should be 'first among equals'. *Journal of Medical Ethics*, **29**(5), 307–312.

Hamilton, R. P. (2010) The concept of health: beyond naturalism and normativism. *Journal of Evaluation in Clinical Practice*, **16**(2), 323–329.

Hamilton, R. P (2013) The frustrations of virtue: the myth of moral neutrality in psychotherapy. *Journal of Evaluation in Clinical Practice*, **19**(3), 485–492.

Hare, R. M. (1952) *The Language of Morals*. Oxford: Clarendon Press.

Hare, R. M. (1977) *Freedom and Reason*. Oxford: Clarendon Press.

Hursthouse, R. (1999) *On Virtue Ethics*. Oxford: Oxford University Press.

MacIntyre, A. (1984) *After Virtue: A Study In Moral Theory*, 2nd edition. Notre Dame, IN: University of Notre Dame Press.

Mencken, H. L. (1949) A good man gone wrong. *A Mencken Chrestomathy*. New York: Vintage Books.

O'Neill, O. (2007) *Re-Thinking Informed Consent In Bioethics*. Cambridge: Cambridge University Press.

Russell, D. (2009) *Practical Intelligence and the Virtues*. Oxford: Oxford University Press.

Values-based practice, competence and expertise[1]

Gideon Calder

In any profession, standards of practice matter – and one way of gauging such standards is by way of concepts such as 'competence' and 'expertise'. Such terms help mark out stages of graduation between the states of complete novicehood and being a seasoned professional. Any such process will have an ethical dimension. To progress along it, practitioners will need to show not only that they know appropriate facts or have good enough skills, but that they have due awareness of how to treat others. But is ethics something that people – for example, practitioners or of this or that profession – might be *expert* at practising? Do we know what *competence* means, in ethical practice? These two questions seem pressing insofar as professional standards include at their core an ethical component, and those standards need gauging – for example so that people might qualify as a practitioner in the field in question, or progress within it. And they matter together, insofar as expertise and competence are placed on a continuum, and in part mutually defining: the former an advanced status, towards which the latter is a necessary step on the way. Yet the questions are slippery. To many, tying up terms such as competence and expertise with the normative dimensions of practice will strike odd notes or (more than

[1] This chapter builds on work presented firstly at a research seminar at the School of Social Policy, Sociology and Social Research at the University of Kent, then at the University of Brighton Philosophy Society, and lastly at the Contemporary Aristotelian Studies Group panel at the spring 2013 Political Studies Association annual conference in Cardiff. I am grateful to all concerned for feedback gained in those settings, and also to Gillian Smith, whose research at the University of South Wales has influenced my own take on issues broached here.

Debates in Values-Based Practice, ed. Michael Loughlin. Published by Cambridge University Press. © Cambridge University Press 2014. **108**

that) be flatly problematic. In a general way, it is not self-evident that values are something people can be good at.

In this chapter, these issues will be explored in connection with values-based practice (VBP). While 'values' under VBP are 'wider than just ethics' (Fulford *et al.*, 2012, p. 7) questions about how we gauge competence in handling them seem especially pressing for a framework which places such stress on the evaluative. A salient feature of VBP is the insistence that neither facts nor rules should serve as sole or final arbiter in cases where value conflicts arise in clinical practice. This case is convincingly made. It also suggests that insofar as VBP itself seeks to offer ways of assessing practice – through elements such as 'awareness of values', 'partnership in decision-making' and so on (Fulford *et al.*, 2012, pp. 208–210) – then questions of competence and expertise are clearly relevant to how we understand it as a framework. These elements are, *prima facie*, things at which individuals may be better or worse. The same goes for the general task of resolving conflicts between values, in complex professional scenarios – a task for which, presumably, some will have far more developed knowledge and skills than others. Under VBP – and again, the supporting case is forceful – good practice involves not just applying rules, or knowing facts, but practical engagement with scenarios which may be negotiated in better or worse ways.

This in itself does not give us a fleshed-out sense of what expertise or competence might look like, or assess how compatible with VBP this or that understanding of either term might be. In fact, I shall argue that subscribing to VBP leaves little space for the promotion of something like ethical *expertise* – which, as the idea of ethical expertise is questionable in any case, by no means necessarily counts against it as a framework. On the other hand, it does seem to require recourse to a robust sense of ethical *competence*. In the next section I highlight certain key relevant points about VBP, and in the following two sections I consider how it might relate to the very idea of ethical expertise. I then draw conclusions about why, rather than expertise, VBP seems both to need, but make difficult, a viable model of competence in resolving conflicts between values. Some of its own core claims – particularly as regards the nature of values – seem to get in the way of achieving, on its own terms, a coherent sense of the competencies on which VBP must rely.

Facts, rules, and 'good enough' values-based practice

Like most theoretical positions, VBP partly sets itself apart and defines itself in terms of what it is not. And a key part of what VBP is not lies in the line it takes on resolving conflicts of values. I shall assume for the purposes of this chapter that such value conflicts are a given. Of course, any such assumption will rest on an intricate background apparatus of contestable claims in both moral and social theory. Here we are going to set aside those claims, and those contestations. We are instead going to make a fairly innocent existential point about professional practice. Namely: it involves conflicts between different princi-ples and priorities, all of which are applicable to situations we find ourselves in – but which, as we might say, 'pull us in contrary directions' (Fulford *et al.*, 2012, p. 13). Being a decision-making practitioner is, in part, characterised by this experience of conflict. Being a *good* decision-maker requires finding a way of negotiating the conflict in an effective and justified way. So, given that decisions need to be made, and that even non-decisions are a kind of decision, practitioners need to find a way of dealing with this conflict – of emerging from the dissonance with (if not a neat or complete resolution of it) at least a decision that is defensible in 'values' terms.

What resources should we call on, in negotiating a way through this? At this point, VBP, in staking out what it is not, steers us away from two familiar ports of call. One is 'the facts'. The other is 'the rules'. It is not that VBP entails a rank disregard for 'the facts' or 'the rules' when it comes to making judgements in a practice setting. Rather, it counsels against exclusive or ultimate reliance on either, and instead makes appeal to the authority of practitioners in the negotiation of value conflicts. This is key to what Neil Gascoigne has helpfully labelled VBP's 'anti-authoritarian *ethos*' (Gascoigne, 2008, p. 87). So on the one hand, '*all* decisions, whether overtly value-laden or not, are based on the two feet of values and evidence' (Fulford *et al.*, 2012, p. 31). When we 'think evidence,' we need to 'think values too' (Fulford *et al.*, 2012, p. 32). Thus decisions – even in clinical diagnosis – about factual matters are always 'valuey', and never purely factual. And resolving a value conflict *solely* by recourse to an appeal to 'the facts' will always be warping and one-sided: no real resolution at all. And on the other hand, conflicts between values will not be resolved by a rule – a relevant principle, or element of a code of practice – prescribing 'the right outcome'. Work needs to be done in relating those principles to the particular situation one has found oneself in. Principles are several, and will apply in complex ways. And the application itself is carried out by the decision-maker, not by the principles themselves: 'There is always, in any given case, *an element of individual judgement* involved in deciding what in those particular circumstances the appropriate balance of principles should be' (Fulford *et al.*, 2012, p. 15, emphasis in original).

Both of these points seem to me vitally important. Neither is by any means 'owned' exclusively by VBP: both have been doing the rounds since Aristotle, in different versions and registers. Yet this does not distract from their current resonance, particularly in the clinical context. Their impact is especially important in those fields of professional practice most prone to assumptions that scientific facts resolve dilemmas, or that the right outcome is determined by 'the rules'. It is vital for those seeking to engage critically with the practice of ethical decision-making, and to enhance it, that conflicts of values are not taken as a kind of temporary inconvenience to be neutralised by the intervention of whichever of 'the facts' or 'the rules' – off-the-shelf 'conflict resolvers', we might say – is deemed to trump the other and serve as the ultimate arbiter.

This general message is particularly crucial in the pedagogic sphere, wherever ethics takes a central place in the 'training' of practitioners (see Calder, 2007). Here, the temptation to invoke and promote ready-made 'conflict-resolvers' is especially strong. They come in especially useful when considering what counts as competence within the practice in question. The competent practitioner must be 'good enough' at carrying out the core aspects of the role. On qualifying, a professional will expect to feel entitled to say 'I know how to negotiate conflicts of values in an appropriate way, within my field of practice'; and others will expect this of that professional. It is tempting, for students, teachers, and relevant professional bodies to define this exclusively by reference to appropriate following of rules, or handling of evidence. The 'expert' practitioner will be further up the scale: exceptional at these core aspects of the role, or at a greater range – so will know more facts, or find a following of the rules more wired-in to their every decision. But this creates tensions. For reasons to which we will return in the following two sections, terms such as 'competence' and 'expertise' can produce a jarring effect when used in connection with values and ethics. Unlike microbiology, statistics or piloting a fighter jet, values may seem an unlikely backdrop for talk of degrees of proficiency. This is partly because – as is acknowledged in the framing of VBP – the terrain here is conflictual. Values are disputed, open to interpretation, reflexive, and enacted through practice. So it is not clear that competence in the handling of values is the same kind of thing as competence in handling evidence, or in following rules. And yet, if they are a core part of practice, then it seems there must be standards in their handling.

So, *is* VBP something one might be competent or expert at? Bill Fulford writes:

> just as we need evidence-based medicine because of the increasing complexity of the *evidence* underpinning medical decision-making, so, increasingly, do we need values-based medicine because of the increasing complexity of the *values* underpinning medical decision-making. (Fulford, 2008, p. 12)

While we may be more readily attuned to notions of 'competence' and 'expertise' being applied to the handling of evidence and the following of rules, the clear corollary of Fulford's claim here is that what goes for facts must go for values too. If the need for values-based medicine is this pressing, and on a par with the need for evidence-based medicine, it follows that we require standards of 'competence' and 'expertise' in negotiating the 'increasing complexity' of values. But is this tenable?

To answer this, it is helpful to consider further the very idea of ethical expertise – why it may jar, and in what terms it might be important. In the next section I offer three 'takes' on the very idea, as a way of teasing it out.

The very idea of ethical expertise

So, neither 'competence' nor 'expertise' sits next to the term 'ethical' in an unproblematic or comfortable way. Perhaps this is a signal that neither should sit there, and that there is a fundamental tension in designating someone an 'ethical expert'. Yet there are two reasons to resist this quick conclusion. One is that the tensions of ordinary language are not necessarily signposts to fundamental conceptual no-go areas. Just because a phrase jars in the context of everyday parlance need not entail that it is radically incoherent. The other reason is that ethical expertise *is* indeed invoked as a notion in everyday parlance. It does some work in contemporary society. By the same token, this does not carry with it a guarantee of conceptual robustness. All sorts of notions are invoked without apparently hanging together at the conceptual level. Still, that they are invoked and wield influence itself makes them worthy of interrogation.

How are they invoked? Both explicitly and implicitly. On the explicit side, take university websites. Here we find directories of staff expertise, where research interests are listed next to suitably posed photos of their owners, looking pensive or approachable, in ways presumably designed to make the institution in question look like a cutting-edge hotbed of valuable knowledge purveyed by members of an intellectual elite. One such area of research will often be ethics. It will be slotted into the template without a hiccup. So here, nominally, we have experts in professional ethics. (Name: Professor Joanne Smith. Areas of research expertise: applied ethics, especially euthanasia and organ donation.) One reason they will be billed as such is that the news media place such store by expertise. I expect that most who have been introduced on a radio discussion programme as an 'ethics expert' find it a disconcerting experience – though even as the description is coming through one's headphones, one can see how the rationale goes. 'If he's *not* an expert, this guy – like, if he doesn't know things about right and wrong which laypeople don't know – then who is he to advise the rest of us on the pressing moral issues of the day?' The credentials for punditry include being a card-carrying expert. To be sure, it may be that the term is intended to attribute knowledge of the academic field – concepts debates, traditions of thought – rather than (say) being expert at *actual*, real-life ethical decision-making at work, or at home, or when witness to an aggressive argument between a couple in a pub, or wondering whether or not to buy *The Big Issue*. But the subject matter of ethics is such that it faces both ways. While experience says that Joanne's advanced critical endorsement of Kant is in no way a guarantee of her reliably honouring the categorical imperative in every detail of her everyday life, Joanne being designated an expert in *ethics* points beyond her purely textual knowledge in ways which are difficult to disambiguate. Meanwhile universities' habits of self-promotion and the media's positioning of pundits may say more about the cultural and political place of 'expertise' in contemporary societies than they do about the particular textures of ethics itself. Discourses of 'expertise' are closely aligned to power, control and authority, in ways which one need not be a paid-up disciple of Foucault (see e.g. Foucault, 1984) to accept as obvious. Along with being classified as a purveyor of 'expert knowledge' comes the privilege to speak and act with authority, as arbiter and judge. Perhaps the fact that the figure of the 'ethical expert' carries what purchase it does can be largely explained as a side effect of a culture where knowledge must be couched in terms of expertise in order to be taken seriously, and wield influence.

The implicit appeal to ethical expertise is significant too, partly in ways already noted. Because standards of proficiency are part and parcel of the assessment of suitability for practice on professional educational programmes, standards of exceptional performance will need to be in some way measurable too. Here too, ethics may seem to sit oddly in relation to other elements of the curriculum, just because it concerns values as well as other more routinely measurable forms of academic knowledge and skill. But standards are appealed to even so – as they are in wider civil society when those who spend a lot of time thinking about or researching ethical issues are consulted for their 'wisdom' on matters moral. When the vicar or the imam, or indeed the leader of a module on professional ethics, is assumed to have a headstart in grappling with moral complexities, we know what people mean. It is part of the *jobs* of these people to think about ethics. If *they* are not expert at it, who is?

But again, that the notion of ethical expertise is appealed to in contemporary social life, is not by itself any guarantee of its coherence. Among the general lines of response to the very idea, we might single out three. These are non-exclusive, but still distinct.

(1) The term 'ethical expertise' is a fundamental oxymoron.
(2) Use of the term 'ethical expertise' reinforces the dominance of 'scientistic' versions of wisdom.
(3) The term 'ethical expertise' can make sense, but only if we frame very carefully what we mean by 'expertise'.

It is worth saying something briefly about these general positions, before considering them more specifically in relation to VBP. Taking (1) first: there are various directions from which such a claim might come. It may reflect assumptions in line with *emotivism*, developed by Ayer (1936) and Stevenson (1944), but summed up helpfully by Alasdair MacIntyre: 'the doctrine that all evaluative judgements and more specifically all moral judgements are nothing but expressions of preference, expressions of attitude or feeling, insofar as they are moral in character' (MacIntyre, 1985, pp. 11–12). Viewed this way, ethics, being a matter of personal preferences, is not something in which one may be expert insofar as preferences themselves are not rankable according to some putatively 'objective' public standard. Neither, on emotivist terms, can preferences be wide of the mark, or improved upon through intensive research or years of practical experience: they are not true or false. Ethical expertise is no more self-coherent as a notion than expertise in having a favourite colour.

Point (2) comes from a different angle: the objection here is not to the sense of the term 'ethical expertise', but to the social implications of its being deployed. Again, there are different ways of making this point – but here is an example. The idea that some may feel the need for ethics to be 'legitimated' as a field of enquiry and practice through the claim that it is a site of 'expertise' tells us more about the cultural power of 'expert discourse' than it does about ethics. In other words, it is as if knowing about and practising ethics has to be 'like' a natural science – must deal in 'hard facts' – in order to be taken seriously. This in turn reinforces the ways in which appeals to scientific knowledge are used as forms of social control: invoking expertise is on these terms an exercise of power.

Proponents of (3) strike a different note again. Here, the idea is that there is nothing *inherently* problematic about the notion of 'ethical expertise', either as a pairing of concepts or in relation to current social trends and structures. If the term jars, this is for contingent reasons – some of which may reflect concerns raised under (1) and (2). The term sounds odd because of the dominance of a certain model of expertise – facts-based and rules-based, and more or less scientistic. Takers of this stance may bring in the 'Dreyfus and Dreyfus' account of expertise, which finds its roots in the phenomenology of Heidegger and Merleau-Ponty.[2] From this angle, human understanding is fundamentally orientation-based rather than fact-based or rule-based: a matter of knowing *how* rather than knowing *that*. Dreyfus and Dreyfus outline five stages of skill acquisition, from the status of 'novice' to 'expert' (on which more later). Expertise on this account is not characterised by an accumulation of factual knowledge, or by sharpened powers of reasoning, or in other intellectualised terms. Rather, it is a kind of non-deliberative, spontaneous knowing what to do: 'rapid, fluid, involved' and quite distinct from 'the slow, detached reasoning of the problem-solving process' (Dreyfus and Dreyfus, 1986, p. 27). 'Principles,' they argue, 'play no role in mature, practiced decision-making', for which rationalisation amounts to 'the invention of reasons', post hoc, as a (necessarily misrepresentative) way of accounting for a process which has been fundamentally intuitive (Dreyfus and Dreyfus, 1986, p. 35). Bicycle riding, car driving and airline piloting are the usual examples used of cases where advanced knowledge is not, for this model, accountable for in terms of propositions. Viewed thus, the expert at ethics will not be someone who invokes the correct rules in the right way, or is steeped in case

---

[2] There are other kindred versions of the model, for example in Patricia Benner's much-cited work on nursing (2000). Dreyfus and Dreyfus's model is taken here as emblematic of this general stance, rather than exhaustive or definitive of it.

studies and comparative analysis of competing traditions in normative ethics. Or rather, these are not sufficient for expertise. The mark of expertise will be the resolving of problems in a more or less spontaneous, non-deliberative way. The expert is not beset by dilemmas, and does not wrestle with them: it is as if they already know what to do. In these terms, for Benner (2000), for example, ethical expertise is not oxymoronic, precisely because 'expertise' has been redefined away from the scientist model. It is the state of practising well ('exquisitely', to use Benner's phrase) *without* principles, rules or guidelines.

Ethical expertise and values-based practice

How, then, do positions (1), (2) and (3) relate to VBP? In each case, for different reasons, it seems difficult to conceive how VBP might be compatible with notions of ethical expertise.

Firstly, we look at position (1). Is the very idea of 'ethical expertise' oxymoronic, from the point of view of VBP? And relatedly, is VBP emotivist, in MacIntyre's sense? At the core of the model developed by Fulford is R. M. Hare's version of prescriptivism, according to which values are action guiding – this being crucial to the claim that 'values as well as evidence underpin *all* decisions' (Fulford, 2008, p. 11). Now for some (Hare among them, it should be stressed) there is a clear wedge between Hare's position and simple emotivism, in that Hare seeks to couch moral thinking as a form of rational argumentation, by stressing the sense in which moral utterances express universal (rather than just subjective) prescriptions subject to logical constraints (Hare, 1952). So our judgements are not self-legitimating, or legitimated purely by appeal to our subjective preferences. Rather, they are what Hare calls 'covertly universal' (1952, p. 154). In seeking to justify a particular judgement, we will invoke a universal rule from which it may be logically derived. That rule in turn must be justified with reference to some more general rule or principle. But on Hare's model the chain here cannot be infinite – and it stops not with some ultimate rational ground, but at an individual preference. Here is MacIntyre, on this point:

> the terminus of justification is thus always, on this view, a not further to be justified choice, a choice unguided by criteria. Each individual implicitly or explicitly has to adopt his or her own first principles on the basis of such a choice. The utterance of any universal principle is in the end an expression of the preferences of an individual will and for that will its principles have and can only have such authority as it chooses to confer upon them by adopting them. (MacIntyre, 1985, pp. 20–21)

So for MacIntyre, Hare ends up tracking back towards emotivism.

And it does seem that VBP takes us to a similar place. For rather than seeking to ground judgements in facts or rules as a last resort, VBP commends a 'radical liberalism' (echoing what Gascoigne calls its anti-authoritarianism) two dimensions of which are, in this respect, key. One is the claim that 'values are wider than just ethics, extending to needs, wishes, preferences and so forth' (Fulford *et al.*, 2012, p. 7). It makes little sense to suggest that all of these might be covertly universal, precisely because the net has been cast in such a way that it includes (for example) entirely self-regarding choices and preferences – 'what makes me tick,' in the words of one trainee doctor focus group member cited in an account of the diversity of what VBP will count as a value. The second key dimension of VBP's radical liberalism is its emphasis on process and 'values democracy':

like political democracy, the values democracy of values-based practice supports decision-making through good process rather than prescribing pre-set right outcomes. (Fulford *et al.*, 2012, p. 34)

As Tim Thornton glosses this claim:

in response to the question: what makes a value judgement true or false, the answer seems to neither accord with a principle or principles nor accord with the real moral particulars or values, but rather nothing further than competing views having been heard. . . . Fundamentally, all and any values deserve a hearing. All and any can be valued if they survive the right process. (Thornton, 2011, p. 991)

VBP's ultra-tolerant stance vis-à-vis values –in terms of both (i) what constitutes a value, and (ii) what corroborates it or confirms its applicability – locates it close to full-on emotivism. For (i) is sufficiently vague and elastic as to include potentially what MacIntyre calls 'any preferences of an individual will'. And with regard to (ii), the process itself – rather than the value having any relation to an independent moral reality, or separately established principles – is what does the work. Values are less constrained by logic even than on Hare's terms, in which (as we have seen) the constraints bite less than at first it may seem.

So – back to position (1). Is ethical expertise oxymoronic, from the point of view of VBP? If not, what would an expert in VBP be expert *at*? They would not be an expert on values, or indeed on decision-making. Any presumption that this or that individual might have an expert 'take' on which values are paramount, or how they should inform a decision would run right against the logic of democratic process. There being no pre-set right outcomes, the expert values-based practitioner could only be someone exquisitely attuned to the process – and the competent practitioner someone well enough attuned to it. Strikingly, this suggests that there *is* an overriding operative value: the value of process itself (see Chapter 6). But appreciation of this value – in so far as the whole of VBP depends on it, and VBP is not, quite pointedly, the province of experts – seems more readily associated with a standard of competence, rather than expertise. We will return to this point later.

Relating position (2) to VBP offers a more straightforward box to tick. The very genesis of VBP in opposition to facts-based resolutions of value conflicts, and the whole tenor of the position, are very much in sync with the critique of scientistic expertise. From the point of view of VBP, over-reliance on the scientific model is problematic epistemically (it obscures the 'valuey' dimension of e.g. clinical diagnosis), ethically (it thwarts or gives no airing to values at odds with facts-based decision-making) and prudentially (it makes, because of the previous two points, for poor decisions). VBP does not come packaged up with wider social-theoretical critique of the workings of power through regimes of knowledge. It is not explicitly Foucauldian. But there is nothing in the core claims and motivations of VBP which might be deemed radically at odds with such a line of analysis – and much which overlaps with it. In a sense, a critique of the tyranny of 'facts' and 'rules' – and by implication, the notion that expertise consists in mastery of these – is precisely what VBP takes its cue from, in proposing its own alternative.

Does that then point to a consonance between VBP and position (3)? The Dreyfus and Dreyfus account of expertise is developed in opposition to (as they see it) more orthodox, facts-based and rules-based models. In this respect there are some areas of consonance between VBP and Dreyfus-style accounts of ethical expertise – such as Benner's, in the nursing context – which root themselves in creating space for intuition, and in developing capacities, such as 'attentiveness' and 'responsiveness' (Benner and Wrubel, 1989), in tune with a model of 'best practice' centred on orientation and 'knowing how'. But the Dreyfus model can seem mystical in its account of expert attributes, and elitist in its implications. Both of these put it at a distance from the democratic, anti-authoritarian tenor of VBP. On the one hand, Dreyfus-style expertise consists in an ineffable-seeming capacity to know the right answer, without pausing to deliberate. This does not seem an asset on VBP terms, in which so much is staked on the value of process in pursuit of balanced decision-making. In this way, VBP involves a necessarily temporal element. It must unfold through time: issues must emerge, and be considered, in more or less transparent ways in order for decisions to be reached. Spontaneity is not a virtue, under this framework; indeed, it is a kind of abnegation of the requirements of the process. Appeals to the ineffable offer nothing in the context of 'balanced decision-making based on dissensus' (Fulford *et al.*, 2012, p. 112), precisely because the idea that best practice consists in operating in ways opaque to others obstructs, rather than facilitates, the negotiation of conflicting values. And on the other hand, Dreyfus's model of expertise seems affirmatively elitist in so far as it locates idealised knowledge in the intuitions of the exceptional, rather than (say) propositions which are accessible to most (on this, see Luntley, 2011). VBP has no space for the notion that certain values, or certain 'takes' on a situation, might occupy a space of automatic privilege in the decision-making process. The Dreyfus-style expert could not claim a superior intuitive orientation towards the values conflicts at stake in any given situation.

So, in sum: VBP seems, overall, hostile to notions of ethical expertise, even if there are some affinities between it and the Dreyfus model of the expert. Whatever 'best practice' is, on VBP terms, substantiating it seems not to require (nor, indeed, to be positively threatened by) either an appeal to notions of expertise, or the interventions of expert individuals. However, it does seem necessarily to avail itself of notions of competence, for reasons expanded on in the next section.

Competence and novicehood

On the basis of a simple scale with novicehood at the 'entry level', competence at the qualifying stage, and 'expertise' at the most advanced end of professional practice, then VBP seems a framework set up to work without the need for input at the expert level – the theoretical basis for which is in some ways antipathetic to the idea of expertise in values. This is largely because of its anti-authoritarian, radically liberal character. But what about competence? Can we speak of 'good enough' values-based practice?

It seems to me that we have to be able to, for VBP to be coherent and viable. For reasons already noted, this point might seem banal, or circular. *Any* framework for practice must, within its own lexicon, define what counts, or does not, as practice befitting the framework – and define competence as what counts as 'good enough' in this respect. Yet VBP's anti-authoritarianism and radical liberalism give this task a particular, potentially problematic aspect. The framework must be set up so that it is accessible and inclusive with regard to people arriving with different kinds of 'baggage' in terms of their own values. But there is a tension between this priority, and the requirement to establish the values on which VBP itself depends. It is a tension between process and substance.

It is worth stressing that this tension is not inherent in the very idea that practice should be values-based. The force of the case for VBP rests to a large extent on the claim that the priority of values is too readily neglected in discussions of clinical practice – even in the professional ethics literature. For a sense of why specifically *values-based* competence is vital to address, consider this passage in an overview of 'The professional responsibilities of medicine':

> To be trustworthy the doctor must, of course, be knowledgeable and skilled, be fully informed of the most recent clinical studies, and be able to assess their strengths, weaknesses, and implications. Without professional competence, the physician is not deserving of trust. Competence, therefore, is more than a matter of competitive pride, personal curiosity, ambition, or prudence. Being knowledgeable and skilled is essential to trustworthiness and, hence, a moral obligation of physicians. (Rhodes, 2007, p. 78)

This passage reads like a gift to proponents of VBP; it makes their point for them. It is written as if the value of competence (specifically, in handling evidence accessed via the 'most recent clinical studies') lies in its instrumental contribution to the inculcation of trust. Trust is what is substantively valuable, and professional competence serves as a conduit to realising this value. From this angle, competence in one's orientation towards values themselves does not intrude on the picture. There seems no room for the sense that having an appreciation of the value of trust is what might make one knowledgeable and skilled. Against this, VBP gains a vital part of its own impetus from the insistence that what is crucial is not just the value of competence, but competence about values – and that these are as integral to practice as the capability to assess the 'strengths, weaknesses and implications' of clinical studies. Indeed, values will *inform* such assessments.

It seems vital to give VBP its due in this respect, and to recognise the distinctiveness of its contribution in a climate where evidence is often fetishised in ways which either squeeze competence out, or reduce its scope to evidence-handling. I mentioned earlier the temptation – on the part of both curriculum designers and students – to appeal to facts and rules, as if demonstrable knowledge of appropriate amounts of both is sufficient evidence of competence in this regard. This suggests that competence involves 'knowing the right answer', with 'the right answer' being defined in terms of relevant already-in-place facts and rules. But this is a reductive and incomplete picture of the competent practitioner. To be sure, knowledge of facts and rules is *necessary* to their work. But it is not sufficient. 'Competence', being an attribute of an individual, involves skills and orientations, as well as awareness of evidence and procedures. It sits separately from the latter. Rule-following does not by itself a competent practitioner make. It is readily compatible with incompetence. Competence also implies the capacity to orientate oneself with the specifics of a context, weigh up different relevant factors (for example, when 'the facts' and 'the rules' pull in different directions), and to 'own' one's decision, rather than presenting it as simply derived from rules or facts. Joan Tronto extends this point:

> Professional ethics should be about more than teaching professionals that it is wrong to lie, to cheat and to steal. The guiding thought that ethical questions occur in a context should centrally inform professional ethics. . . . [W]e should not permit individuals to escape from responsibility for their incompetence by claiming to adhere to a code of professional ethics. (Tronto, 1993, p. 134)

And to extend the point further: neither should we permit individuals to escape from responsibility for their incompetence by claiming to have acted on the available evidence.

So again, it is not in the notion of values-based competence itself that the tensions lie, for VBP. Rather, it is in the architecture of the framework itself, and the conception of values operative within it. In the exposition of the framework we find consistent reference to the transition from novicehood to competence. At points, it seems as if the beginner is likely to be nearly there already:

> Don't forget you already possess many, if not most, of the skills, and if some are new to you . . . you will find them relatively easy to adopt. (Fulford *et al.*, 2012, p. 204)

On the one hand this is a passing remark – a word of encouragement for trainee practitioners. Yet it also speaks of something problematic about the relationship between process and substance in VBP. For it seems as if, for all its inclusiveness and tolerance on the question of values, VBP relies on an appeal to prior substantive value commitments (see Chapter 6). This is a familiar feature of process-driven accounts of value,[3] in which (as Thornton puts it) 'the idea of right process replaces right outcome' (Thornton, 2011, p. 911). On the one hand, we find the wish to remain maximally open as to the possibility of what emerges from the process, coupled with a denial that we might know in advance what value consists in. The value of the process lies not in its capacity to deliver some 'right' result identifiable before it kicks in – as some kind of royal road to good practice – but in the process itself happening in the right way. It is the process *itself* which is good practice (see Chapters 3 and 4). On the other hand, on closer inspection of the requirements for the process to run its course, we find the need for prior commitments. It is not an accident that trainees must 'already possess' much of the orientation which VBP promotes. It is a requirement of it.

This presents what is a fairly standard kind of paradox of liberalism, or of stances of toleration towards conflicting values. At some point, this toleration has to stop. There are values about which liberals cannot be liberal. VBP's anti-authoritarianism leads it to frame values in a maximally inclusive and generous way. Expressed as a dress code, it might seem to be 'come as you are'. Or to switch metaphors: you are invited to bring to your practice your own ingredients – your own preferences and sense of priorities – to be fed into the mixer along with those of others, and the contextual particularities of different professional situations to be encountered in your field of practice. Expertise is not required; in fact any appeal to it will be anathema to a process set up as fundamentally democratic and without presumption about prior authority or the ordering of values. But then it turns out that there was a dress code, and that actually the ingredients matter – and that things were not as super-tolerant as they seemed at the outset (see Chapters 3, 8 and 10).

In VBP it matters precisely because in Tronto's terms, we cannot rely on the procedures themselves – the rules, the framework – to produce good practice. Certain attributes and capabilities on the part of the practitioner are also a prerequisite. These competencies include value commitments – an openness towards outcomes, a sensitivity to context, a willingness to engage in certain ways with practice situations and to enter into professional relationships in a certain spirit. These are things about which VBP cannot be super-tolerant. On these, it must lay down the law, impose

---

[3] For further discussion (albeit in a rather different context) of this feature of process-driven accounts of value, see Calder and Ceva (2009), which features a kind of critical dialogue between process-based (or procedural) and substantive accounts of the negotiation of conflicting values.

restrictions, and be clear about what is inadmissible (see Chapters 4, 5 and 6). It seems to me that this is not a problem with substantive value-commitments, or the notion that these will sit prior to any process doing its work, in order for it to be a process of the desired kind, and for the process itself to have prescriptive 'shoving power'. Rather, the problem is with defining values in a 'come as you are' way, and presenting the process as if it, by itself, is what is constitutive of good practice. All practice invokes standards of competence. In values-based practice, competence includes the handling of values – and signing up to the process requires prior values commitments which are not neutral, or revisable in the light of the flux and unpredictable course of the process, but substantive, and enduring.

Conclusion

I have argued that VBP's anti-authoritarianism, and its proximity (if not equivalence) to emotivism, make it inhospitable to notions of ethical expertise, and certainly to any recommendation that the views of experts take special priority in the processes of values-based practice. But this cannot be stretched as far as scepticism about competence. VBP requires standards of competence insofar as it seeks to offer an assessable model of practice. These standards include prerequisite orientations, attitudes and preferences – all included in the broad definition of 'values' with which VBP operates. This suggests that VBP is not, as advertised, a framework in which 'good practice' is determined by right process, but is also constrained, informed and dependent on prior, substantive value commitments. There is a tension between this feature of VBP and its anti-authoritarianism. If, as I have argued, an appeal to such substantive, operative value commitments is *inevitable* in any such process, this suggests that it is on the side of VBP's anti-authoritarianism, or radical liberalism, that something has to give.

References

Ayer, A. J. (1936) *Language, Truth and Logic.* London: Victor Gollancz.

Benner, P. (2000) *From Novice to Expert: Excellence and Power in Clinical Nursing Practice*, commemorative edition. Englewood Cliffs, NJ: Prentice Hall.

Benner, P. and Wrubel, J. (1989) *The Primacy of Caring: Stress and Coping in Health and Illness.* Englewood Cliffs, NJ: Prentice Hall.

Calder, G. (2007) Theory, practice and 'teaching' professional ethics. In Smith, S. R. (editor), *Applying Theory to Policy and Practice: Issues for Critical Reflection.* Aldershot: Ashgate.

Calder, G. and Ceva, E. (2009) Values, diversity and the justification of EU institutions. *Political Studies*, 57(4), 828–845.

Dreyfus, H. L. and Dreyfus, S. E. (1986) *Mind Over Machine: The Power of Human Intuition and Expertise in the Era of the Computer.* New York: Free Press.

Foucault, M. (1984) *The Foucault Reader*, edited by Rabinow, P. Harmondsworth: Penguin Books.

Fulford, K. W. M. (2008) Values-based practice: a new partner to evidence-based practice and a first for psychiatry? *Mens Sana Monographs*, 6, 10–21.

Fulford, K. W. M., Peile, E. and Carroll, H. (2012) *Essential Values-Based Practice: Clinical Stories Linking Science with People.* Cambridge: Cambridge University Press.

Gascoigne, N. (2008) The value of 'value'. *Philosophy, Psychiatry and Psychology*, 15(2), 87–96.

Hare, R. M. (1952) *The Language of Morals.* Oxford: Clarendon Press.

Luntley, M. (2011) Expertise – initiation into learning, not knowing. In Bondi, L., Carr, D., Clark, C. and Clegg, C. (editors), *Towards Professional Wisdom: Practical Deliberation in the People Professions.* Farnham: Ashgate.

MacIntyre, A. (1985) *After Virtue: A Study in Moral Theory*, 2nd edition. London: Duckworth.

Rhodes, R. (2007) The professional responsibilities of medicine. In Rhodes, R., Francis, L. P. and Silvers, A. (editors), *The Blackwell Guide to Medical Ethics.* Oxford: Blackwell.

Stevenson, C. L. (1944) *Ethics and Language.* New Haven, CT: Yale University Press.

Thornton, T. (2011) Radical liberal values-based practice. *Journal of Evaluation in Clinical Practice*, **17**, 988–991.

Tronto, J. (1993) *Moral Boundaries: A Political Argument for an Ethic of Care.* New York: Routledge.

Wishing to remain ill: an unacceptable value?

Harry Lesser

The contributors to this volume would probably all agree that the appropriate model of the relationship between medical staff, of all kinds, and their patients or clients is the 'team' model, in which the client is herself or himself part of the cooperating group actively working to produce a cure or an improvement, and whenever possible is consulted as a member of that team. This has obvious advantages over the 'paternalist' model (of the past, but not yet dead) in which the patient takes one free decision, to consult the doctor or other medical practitioner, and then is expected to do what they are told, despite being the person most affected by the choice of treatment and despite the denial of autonomy. It also has advantages over the later 'consumer' model, in which the patient or client is simply presented with the options and left to choose between them, and so is not getting the full benefit of the medical expertise available and is not encouraged to contribute as much as possible to their recovery.

The adoption of the team model has the consequence that questions of what to do medically cannot be settled by appealing simply to one set of values, such as the doctor's assessment of what is in the patient's best medical interest, or the patient's assessment of what they most want. Rather, there is a wide range of values, whether in the form of wants and desires or of moral opinions, which may have to be taken into account, and a range of people – the patient or client, the medical staff, the patient's family – whose values may be relevant. Much of this volume is about how the taking into account of these values should be carried out. The question then arises as to whether there can be desires or moral beliefs which are held by patients or other members of the team, but which are so much at variance with working towards cure or improvement that they should not be taken into account at all. This chapter argues that there are indeed such values and tries to give some account of what they are: the wish to remain ill is a key instance, but not the only one. The practical problem is not simply to be aware of these values, whether in oneself or others, or to refuse to act on them, but, since they are obstacles to the restoration of health, to get rid of them. The problem is made worse because they are values which are often held unconsciously. But recognising their existence is a start.

It is important to note that this issue arises not only on the individual level, but also with regard to medicine's political and social context. The amount of money, and therefore resources, available, the types of treatment available, and decisions as to which classes of patient should be given priority, all of which involve assuming certain values as being more important than others, may all be imposed on the medical team, whether as intended or unintended consequences of political or economic activity. As facts, these may have to be simply accepted, at least in the short term. But the values behind them do not have to be accepted, even if altering them is much harder than altering the desires of individuals. So the issue has to be discussed on both the individual and the social level.

On the individual level, the most important 'unacceptable' value is the patient's wish to remain ill. This, though, needs to be carefully defined. First of all, it can be entirely rational to reject a form of treatment on the ground that, though its chances of success are high, the cost, whether in terms of pain, discomfort, disfigurement or conceivably mutilation, is too high to make it worthwhile. Equally rational would be a decision to reject treatment because it would lengthen a person's life but leave their quality of life greatly worsened. Even when the price to pay is low, and the feeling of the medical staff is that the patient is being irrational, and rejecting a considerable benefit because of fears of a relatively small cost, this is still something at least to be taken into account. Again, there can be valid non-medical reasons for wanting to postpone treatment, even though this increases the risk of its being unsuccessful: deciding to postpone an operation in order to finish a piece of work would be an example.

But there is a type of wish to remain ill, very often unconscious, which works against the patient's conscious wish to get well (as may be shown by the fact that they have sought medical treatment), even under circumstances in which they and those around them would be considerably happier if they were well and cured. This often arises from the advantages to be derived from being ill, or of being 'on the sick list'. Illness is an excusing condition, which enables children to escape rebuke or punishment, and adults in addition to escape responsibilities and hard work. It also creates an obligation on other people to be 'nice' to the person who is ill, and to look after them. There are 'minuses' as well – having what one says not being taken seriously, and being required to be properly grateful and cooperative. But for some people the advantages outweigh the disadvantages, sometimes in the short term, sometimes in the longer term. Freud (1910) summed this up with regard to mental illness by saying 'A number of people who find life's problems too difficult to solve have taken flight into neurosis and in this way won an unmistakable, although in the end too costly, advantage through illness' (Freud, 1963, p. 85).

That there are sometimes advantages in being ill is clear. They are of various sorts: as indicated above, they can be either positive, negative, or both, because there can be the positive benefit of being looked after, and the benefit of being excused from various tasks and responsibilities. They can also be either general or particular: one might wish to escape from responsibility in general or from some specific onerous or dangerous task.

Again, one might wish to obtain sympathy in general, or sympathy from a specific person. It is clear that some people seek these advantages, either by malingering, i.e. pretending to be ill and/or faking the symptoms, or by hypochondria, i.e. exaggerating the importance of relatively minor symptoms. (There can of course be other motives for, or causes of, hypochondria.) What requires evidence is the claim that the cure of a genuine illness can also be delayed or even prevented because of what is being gained by being ill. A good source for this evidence is the work of Freud; but in order to see why what he says is good evidence one must take what he says in stages which he himself did not always distinguish.

Freud (1938) gives a host of examples of involuntary actions and conditions, including forgetting names and words with unpleasant associations, slips of the tongue and pen, 'bungled' actions and errors in general, which, though genuinely involuntary, appear nevertheless to be motivated, because of the way they fit in with a person's conscious desires or aims. Thus the President of the Lower House of the Austrian Parliament opened a sitting, from which he privately expected little good, with the words 'I declare this sitting closed' (Freud, 1938, p. 101). Other examples have to do with a person's moral values, rather than their wants, but again quite conscious values. An example is the lady who said that her son in the army was with the 'Forty-second Murderers' (Freud, 1938, p. 115). Another is a person I once heard speaking of someone pushed into the Catholic priesthood without a vocation, and saying that his mother sent him to the 'cemetery' (instead of 'seminary').

If this occurs so often when the desire or moral assessment that fits with the involuntary action is conscious, it is reasonable to suspect that at least sometimes there is an unconscious desire, and to regard mistakes as evidence, though not conclusive evidence, of unconscious or unadmitted desires. This suspicion may be confirmed by the subsequent awareness of the person who has acted in error. A chilling example, from the time of the First World War, is of a man in Europe, estranged from his wife, still in America, but wanting (or so he thought) a reconciliation, who meant to write to her 'It would be fine if you could come on the *Mauretania*', but wrote instead '*Lusitania*': not surprisingly, he wrote the whole letter out again (Freud, 1938, p. 170). A pleasant example comes from Freud's friend Lou Andreas-Salome, who describes how she repeatedly let milk boil over and spill on the floor, at a time when it was scarce and expensive, and only after this had stopped happening realised that she had been doing it to enable her dog to lick up the spoilt milk, and had stopped doing it when the dog died: 'I was even more fond of him than I was aware' (Freud, 1938, p. 222).

This, though, shows only that involuntary actions and words can fit in with wants and values. We could add dreams: one does not have to agree with Freud that all dreams are wish-fulfilments, but one could accept that many are, and that our values are involved in what we dream and in how we react to it, whether in the dream or on waking. Freud himself (1925) wrote a section of a paper on our moral responsibility for the content of dreams, in which he says 'Obviously one must hold oneself responsible for the evil impulses of one's dreams. In what other way can one deal with them?' (Freud, 1963, p. 225). But what is the evidence that one can apply this to illness?

Freud provides evidence for this of various kinds and in various places. In the first of the three papers 'Further recommendations in the technique of psychoanalysis' (Freud, 1913), which deals with 'beginning the treatment' and 'the dynamics of the cure', Freud discusses his experience, over ten years, of giving gratuitous treatment, and his conclusion that the effect of not charging is to make it that much harder to effect a cure. 'The absence of the corrective influence in payment of the professional fee is felt as a serious handicap;

the whole relationship recedes into an unreal world; and the patient is deprived of a useful incentive to exert himself to bring the cure to an end' (Freud, 1963, p. 145). This involves the effect of the absence of an advantage in being cured, rather than the presence of a benefit in being ill, but the point is the same. It should be noted that Freud, unlike some Freudians, did not hold that the fee had to be a high one, but merely that the results of not charging at all were unsatisfactory.

A little further on in the same paper Freud discusses neurosis in poor people, and says:

> Perhaps there is some truth in the widespread belief that those who are forced by necessity to a life of heavy labour succumb less easily to neurosis. But at all events experience shows, without a doubt, that in this class a neurosis once acquired is only with very great difficulty eradicated. It renders the sufferer too good service in the struggle for existence...The pity which the world has refused to his material distress the sufferer now claims by right of his neurosis and absolves himself from the obligation of combating his poverty by work.
> (Freud, 1913, p. 146)

Freud makes it clear further on that there are exceptions to this, and that some people still get well even under these conditions. But he still thinks that his experience justifies the assertion that, even though illness is an involuntary condition, and these people are genuinely ill and not malingering, nevertheless, if a person is deriving much benefit from being ill effecting a cure becomes harder and sometimes proves impossible. Freud is speaking, of course, of mental illness. But many of his patients had physical problems, even if their cause was psychosomatic. So it is reasonable to regard what he says as general evidence for the existence in many people of a wish to remain ill, whether or not this is admitted. The evidence is, in one sentence, the numbers of people who remain ill as long as there is an advantage to be gained from illness.

In 'Analysis terminable and interminable', Freud (1937) gives another kind of example, of a patient who 'found his present situation quite comfortable and did not intend to take any step which would bring him nearer to the end of the treatment.' He was finally cured, though in the event only temporarily, by Freud's fixing a date for the end of the treatment, 'no matter what progress he made or failed to make' (Freud, 1963, p. 235). Despite this partial success, Freud was normally very reluctant to set such limits. But his 'maverick' follower Stekel did it as a matter of course, setting a limit of four months treatment for all his patients. 'Whoever cannot be cured in four months', he claimed, 'cannot be helped (according to my experience), because he does not want to be helped' (Stekel, 1949, p. 622). Stekel also found that the limit concentrated the patient's mind, and that from around the twelfth week there were often notable advances towards a cure.

In this work Stekel gives us two other pieces of evidence that the great obstacle is often the patient's wish to be ill. He says 'As long as the patients see that they can tyrannise their family and their environment, they will never give up their compulsions' (Stekel, 1949, p. 353). One may compare this with Freud's remark that sometimes an illness is directed at a particular person, and is cured when that person goes away. And he sums up the situation, still in the context of limiting the period of treatment, by saying 'If [the physician] recognises the patient's resistance and its sources, if he shows him repeatedly that he does not want to get well, if he fights his "will to illness", he will obtain the same results in a shorter period of time' (Stekel, 1949, p. 622). This will obviously be less often true when the illness is definitely physical; but some (of course by no means all) physical illnesses may well have a mental component which is delaying recovery.

So Freud and Stekel between them produce a large body of evidence that in mental illness, and in physical illness which is in part psychosomatic, a common key factor is the patient's wish to be ill, which can end either if she or he recognises this wish and refuses to act on it any longer or if the situation changes (or is changed) so that there are no longer advantages in being ill. Another kind of evidence, important but harder to assess, comes from fiction and biography. There are many accounts, from both fact and fiction, of people using illness to control others or to get what they want. The fact that these carry conviction, whether as stories or as interpretations of the behaviour of real people, is evidence (though not proof) that many of us have at least a vague awareness that these things do happen, even if not in as 'tidy' a way as they do in fiction.

A real example of this would be Florence Nightingale herself, whose ill health, after she returned from the Crimea, enabled her to organise the whole nursing profession, because she could stay at home and devote herself to the research and 'brain work' while sending others out to put the results of this into practice (Woodham-Smith, 1964). A fictional example would be Maugham's Louise, in his story of that name. Louise's heart condition enables her to be beautifully looked after by two husbands (in succession) and a daughter, Iris, and to do nothing she does not want to do, while still doing everything she does like doing. This ends only when Iris falls in love and Louise is persuaded not to stand in the way of her getting married. On the morning of the wedding, Louise has a heart attack and dies, 'gently forgiving Iris for having killed her' (Maugham, 1951, volume 1, pp. 438–443).

Neat endings are part of fiction's stock in trade; but the way Louise operates is drawn from life. We should note also that maintaining the illness is not necessarily an aim simply of the patient or client. It can be imposed by the family or the medical staff, or can be something in which they all collude. This, though, may well be not as common as it once was, for at least four reasons. One is the abandonment of the idea that all deviance from the norms of one's society is a sign of mental illness – the idea that caused political 'rebels' in the Soviet Union (see, e.g. Bloch and Reddaway, 1984) and unmarried mothers in the UK and USA to be hospitalised for long periods. Another is the pressure to get patients out of hospital as quickly as possible, in order to treat those waiting in the queue. A third is the fact that lengthy bed rest is no longer used as a treatment, and the aim is to get patients up and about as soon as practicable. Finally, we may note that there is evidence that the 'scapegoating' described by Laing and Esterson (1964), in which a family might deal, unconsciously, with its problems by having a troublesome member declared mentally ill and consigned to hospital, was, even in those days, a very rare phenomenon, fighting tooth and nail to keep a family member out of a mental hospital being much more common. Nevertheless, although as a society we have moved, over the years, from a situation in which there was a problem of people who were not ill being treated as if they were, and people who were ill having their 'illness' needlessly prolonged, to a situation in which the main problem is one in which people who are ill cannot obtain treatment as quickly as they should or even cannot obtain it at all, we should not regard the old problem as being extinct.

The question remains of what should be done about this possibility of the patient or client wishing to remain ill and the further possibility that the family and/or the medical staff may collaborate with them. First, the mere awareness that these are possibilities may sometimes be enough to prevent their becoming actualities. Second, the members of the team, and of the family, while treating the patient with sympathy and doing their best to ease any suffering, can still also do their best to make sure that there is no advantage in continuing to be ill. Third – but this relates only to the kinds of neurosis and psychosomatic illness with which Stekel was dealing – the patient can be told, occasionally or repeatedly, that it is their own wish to be ill which is hindering recovery. But this, though appropriate in some cases of mental or psychosomatic illness, is obviously going to be worse than useless for other patients, including many of those for whom it is true. Freud once observed that the remarks made by ignorant and insensitive people, for example that a person unable to move properly would leap up if the house were on fire, were in one way quite true, but that did not mean that they could simply cure themselves and leap up. Moreover, it would be disastrous if medical teams got into the habit of telling patients that it was all their own fault and they should simply decide to get well!

Indeed, it may be that the most important way of dealing with this 'unacceptable value' is a combination of using the team model, which encourages the patient to contribute to their recovery, and trying to make sure that being 'ill' is not more advantageous for them than being well. This last has two sides to it. One is avoiding indulging people who are ill, as opposed to treating them with respect and sympathy. The other, which is often the responsibility of society rather than the medical team, is to try to ensure that the life to which they have to return when they get well is, at the very least, tolerable, and if possible better than tolerable. (See Freud's remark above about neurosis in poor people.) But, although often little can be done by medical staff in this respect, it may be that if the team model is being used, so that what happens after 'recovery' can be discussed with the patient or client, and it is recognised that being cured of this particular condition is not the end of their problems, at least more can be done than has previously been the case.

All this assumes a relatively uncomplicated situation, in which the advantages of being ill are fairly clear and easy to understand. There is a puzzle as to how something involuntary, such as an illness, can be motivated and have its cure delayed or prevented as a result of the motivation. (One would be inclined to regard this as self-contradictory, if there were not so much evidence that it happens.) But the motivation itself is intelligible: the advantages are genuine, and worth having – the patient's 'mistake' is to choose these benefits rather than the benefits of a cure.

There are two ways in which things may be more complex. First, one may be dealing not with a desire but with a moral feeling, though an irrational one – a feeling that one ought to be ill or has no right to be well: this may be one element in some cases of anorexia nervosa. Stekel, again in contrast to Freud, thought that as well as desires being repressed (i.e. not consciously acknowledged) there could also be a repression of moral or religious ideas (see Dabrowski, 2010). Key factors in dealing with this might be bringing the ideas into full consciousness, which is likely to result in their rejection, and trying to adjust the patient's self-esteem. 'Adjust' seems the appropriate word, because it would seem that these ideas can arise either from a sense of worthlessness, or from an 'arrogant' wish to have an exceptionally sensitive and self-punishing conscience, or perhaps from a combination of these feelings, which, though opposed, could act as responses to each other and as mutual reinforcers.

But illness, it seems, can have even more complex aims. This has, though indirectly and unintentionally, been argued by the late Thomas Szasz, particularly in his conversation on television with Jonathan Miller (Miller, 1983). Szasz, as is well known, held that the phenomena classed as mental illnesses were either physical illnesses or not illnesses at all. Those that are not illnesses should be viewed from a moral and political standpoint; and we will then find, Szasz says, that they have motives which are complex and unusual, and whose existence we are reluctant to admit. His example is anorexia nervosa in adolescent girls: anorexia in boys or adults would require a different explanation. What he suggests is that it is a protest against becoming normal adult women and accepting the role that society allots to women. 'Can you blame them?' he asks at one point. So their failure to eat is as politically motivated as the protest of a hunger striker; but the nature of the motivation is a lot harder to understand.

Now, in one respect the evidence is against Szasz. The evidence is that the political hunger striker is in control in a way that the anorexic is not (for example, the anorexic often has no accurate assessment of the state of her body, or of the way her life is at risk). The anorexic is genuinely ill, and in need of help. But if what we have argued above is correct, this does not exclude the possibility that her illness is motivated and even may have a political dimension, whether or not the one suggested by Szasz. Moreover, if we reject Szasz's dichotomy between illness and motivated behaviour, there is a further consequence. On the one hand, we may say that the anorexic is ill, even though her behaviour is motivated; on the other, we may want to say that sometimes people who are physically ill have a motive for their illness. And this motive may be a complex political or personal motive, rather than a mere wish to avoid responsibility and be looked after.

How often this happens is uncertain: one would expect it to be infrequent but not unknown. Once again, the team model may create a 'political' environment in which it is unlikely to occur, though not impossible. This is so for two reasons: the aim of cure is made very specific, as one of the strongest values to be maintained, so that the introduction of values opposed to this is not easy; and the way in which values from different people and different sources are considered makes it harder for any one person, even the patient or client, to impose their programme on the team.

Nevertheless, the team has to guard against 'unacceptable' values. The wish of the patient to remain ill is one of the most important of these, but it is not the only one. What also has to be considered is the wish of a member, or even several members, of the team to punish the patient or keep them under control, rather than to help them recover or reduce their suffering. There is a long history of this in the treatment of mental illness, from the days when flogging was used as a treatment, to beating up patients in order to control them, to the punitive use of ECT. Things have greatly improved, but even now there are accounts of the excessive use of control and restraint. And nurses and doctors are in general, whether dealing with mental or physical illness, well placed to get away with punishment under the guise of treatment or, in the case of mental patients, of necessary control.

As with the patient's desire to remain ill, there are fewer problems when these desires are conscious. The nurse who takes the opportunity, when off-duty, to admit and express her or his anger ('I'd like to tie him up and torture him, the way he's tortured me' was once said to me by a mental nurse on a Medical Ethics MA course) is probably very unlikely to act on it; it is the unadmitted fear or anger or contempt that can be dangerous. Once again, the team model may be useful. The paternalistic model encourages the conscious idea that patients should be controlled and sometimes the unconscious one that they need to be punished. The consumer model leaves the patients in control but can foster resentments. The team model, as well as giving the patient or client more control may also enable the medical staff to interact with the patient in ways that may check inappropriate behaviour without implying that the patient is in some way subordinate.

Paradoxically, one factor that may contribute to a dangerous situation is the refusal to be judgemental. The evidence for this is admittedly anecdotal, but worth giving, since it consists of the observations of someone who had been a nurse at a leading children's hospital. What she observed was that because the children were ill they were never punished or told off when they were naughty. The effect on some of them was to make them feel that they were in a place with no limits and to become very frightened, and sometimes as a result to behave still worse. One might also suspect that resentments among the nurses were being stored up. This is not to suggest that they should have been punished; but setting limits on their behaviour and being prepared to be appropriately verbally judgemental might have produced a better situation – provided, of course, that this was not overdone or done too harshly. Analogously, making polite suggestions to adult patients that they should modify their behaviour might prevent the building up of resentments. This, again, though not easy to do, is somewhat easier if the team model is being used.

So, patients, clients and medical staff can all develop values which need to be rejected (or even better, 'strangled at birth') rather than being taken into account. It is important to stress the exceptional nature of these values. Respect for the patient requires that there be a presumption that their values, whatever they are, should be taken seriously, and that this kind of rejection is not normally appropriate. Thus we may contrast the unconscious wish to remain ill with the holding of religious or moral values which do not prevent cures but do mean that the most efficient method of treatment is unacceptable. This can arise both with patients themselves and with parents whose children need treatment. It would seem that here the right course is to try to find ways of accommodating both sets of values: Jones (2003) has a very interesting discussion of how this can be done, using as an example the ultra-orthodox Jewish community of north London. But one should note that there can be cultural practices (usually, perhaps always, ones not in fact required by any religion, such as female genital mutilation) which should be rejected and not accommodated, given the harm that they do. Hence, as well as singling out the desire to remain ill as a value that should not be accommodated, we should note that patients and clients can have other values that similarly should not be accepted, even though these are very much the exception.

With regard to the values of the medical staff, the situation is a little more complicated. Again, there needs to be a presumption that their values be respected, unless they are based on a wish to punish or to control, rather than a wish to cure or alleviate. But there is always the possibility that the wish to cure may nevertheless result in the wrong treatment being given, or at any rate the wrong treatment for that patient; and sometimes, though it is hard to define when, the patient knows best. A good fictional example, based on actual events, is Gilman's *The Yellow Wallpaper* (1899). This story has sometimes been misinterpreted: it is not a ghost story, nor a feminist tract, but an account of a woman with post-natal depression which as a result of being given the wrong treatment turns into psychosis. Gilman later explained (Gilman, 1913) that she wrote the story because this is what, she believed, would have happened to her had she not broken off the treatment: she wrote it 'to save people from going mad'. She sent the story to the doctor who had recommended the treatment: he did not acknowledge it, but she found out later that he did change his treatment methods. She also mentions at least one person who was encouraged by the story to save her sanity by breaking off the treatment. It is of course very hard to say when the patient should persevere with the doctor's recommendation and when they should trust what their own mind and body seem to be telling them: and mistakes in both directions can do much harm. So there is a kind of symmetry: with both the patient's values and the medical staff's values there is one kind of desire which needs to be rejected from the start, because it conflicts with the whole purpose of treatment, and there can be other values, which, even though they do not radically conflict with the aims of medicine, need, either in this particular case or in general, to be rejected, because of the harm involved in acting on them.

Finally, we need to consider the social and political values that may be imposed on patients and medical staff, whether indirectly or directly. The overall fixing of resources, and the allocation of resources for different kinds of treatment and different groups of patients, necessarily involves political and moral value judgements, whether or not this is admitted; and these judgements are thus indirectly imposed on the people who have to work within these resources. In addition, there may be instructions or recommendations as to what kinds of treatment may be given and to whom. Both of these have in one sense to be 'respected' more than the values of members of the team and in another sense less. On the one hand, they may simply have to be complied with, there being no choice in the matter. On the other, there is no presumption that they have to be respected in the normal sense of the word. This is not a purely psychological point: it means also that a person is not obliged to come to terms with them, in the way that they often (though as we have seen not always) have an obligation to come to terms with the values of other members of the team. Thus a patient, or a member of the medical staff, or a whole team, might decide that, though one must accept these values, or their consequences, for the time being, one should work politically to change them. Or they might decide that acceptance should be minimal – as much as the rules absolutely require but no more. In an extreme case they might decide to ignore them altogether, or to subvert them, if this were possible. For example, euthanasia is sometimes carried out, even though it is illegal: there are those who speak of us having 'back street euthanasia', analogous to the back street abortion of the past.

But one question here is whether at this level there are values which everyone involved in medicine would agree were unacceptable, as opposed to those which are disputed. There certainly could be, even if this is not the case at the moment: it is not impossible that racism or sexist values might be incorporated, or the level of resources be unacceptably low – as many, though not all, would say it is already. And the crucial difference from the values of team members remains: that, even if it is a personal opinion that certain values are unacceptable, on the political level it can still be a person's right, and sometimes their duty, to act on this opinion and resist them in whatever way is practicable and does not offend against other values. On the personal level this should be very much the exception, but there are values which need to be rejected: this chapter is an attempt to say what the most crucial ones are, and how they can be resisted.

References

Bloch, S. and Reddaway, P. (1984) *Soviet Psychiatric Abuse: Shadow over World Psychiatry*. London: Gollancz.

Dabrowski, K. (2010) Remarks on Wilhelm Stekel's active psychoanalysis. *Heksis*, **2**, available online.

Freud, S. (1910) The future prospects of psychoanalytic therapy. Reprinted in *Therapy and Technique*. New York: Collier, 1963.

Freud, S. (1913) Further recommendations in the technique of psychoanalysis. Reprinted in *Therapy and Technique*. New York: Collier, 1963.

Freud, S. (1925) Some additional notes on dream-interpretation as a whole. Reprinted in *Therapy and Technique*. New York: Collier, 1963.

Freud, S. (1937) Analysis terminable and interminable. Reprinted in *Therapy and Technique*. New York: Collier, 1963.

Freud, S. (1938) *The Psychopathology of Everyday Life*. Harmondsworth: Penguin Books.

Freud, S. (1963) *Therapy and Technique*. New York: Collier.

Gilman, C. P. (1899) *The Yellow Wallpaper*. Boston, MA: Small and Maynard.

Gilman, C. P. (1913) Why I wrote *The Yellow Wallpaper*. *The Forerunner*, available online.

Jones, B. (2003) *Childhood Disability in a Multicultural Society*. Oxford: Radcliffe Medical Press.

Laing, R. D. and Esterson, A. (1964) *Sanity, Madness and the Family*. London: Penguin Books.

Maugham, S. (1951) *Collected Short Stories*, volume 1. London: Heinemann.

Miller, J. (1983) *States of Mind: Conversations with Psychological Investigators*. London: BBC Publications.

Stekel, W. (1949) *Compulsion and Doubt*. Cambridge: Liveright.

Woodham-Smith, C. (1964) *Florence Nightingale*. London: Collins Fontana Books.

Values-based practice and global health

Sridhar Venkatapuram

Introduction

This chapter examines VBP in relation to global health. Given that both topics are large in scope and complex, the discussion focuses on three aspects framed as three questions. First, where does VBP stand in relation to the still evolving global health movement? Indeed, the global health movement is multifaceted and inclusive of such aspects as conceptual analysis, programmatic proposals, national security, international relations, science, development, international trade, ethics and so forth. The focus here is on VBP's relation to an aspect that cuts across many of these dimensions, namely, global governance for health. The discussion explores the link between VBP's framework for the governance of the 'clinical encounter' and discussions of global governance for health. There are interesting parallels between the call for better and more governance at the global level in the pursuit of health, and VBP's aim to produce better outcomes through better governance of the patient-health care provider engagement that integrates science and values.

Second, how does VBP relate to the growing understanding that in all human societies most of the 'action' regarding health outcomes happens outside the clinic/health care domain? VBP aims to be the complement to evidence-based practice ('science') in health care by highlighting and managing the values involved in the clinical encounter. In doing so, it gives much consideration to and takes as given that the sources of values are, in fact, coming from outside of the clinical encounter. However, producing a site of exemplary deliberation and value management could be quite difficult if the surrounding environment is amoral or where values are deeply in conflict and contested. In contrast, evidence-based practice (EBP) is thought not to have this problem as the state-of-the-art evidence or

Debates in Values-Based Practice, ed. Michael Loughlin. Published by Cambridge University Press. © Cambridge University Press 2014.

science is typically believed to be generalisable across all human beings and societies. For VBP, holding the surrounding environment constant while focusing on the interrelations between patient and health care provider may help clarify reasoning, but it may also exclude important moral/value dimensions. Furthermore, the causal pathway between the environment of social values and the experience of health is direct and robust. There is now an established and growing evidence-base on the social causes of disease and their distribution patterns, as well as the effectiveness and efficiency of interventions addressing the social determinants of health at the population level (World Health Organization and Commission on Social Determinants of Health, 2008). And it is well understood in social epidemiology as well as other disciplines such as social medicine, health promotion and economics that social arrangements affecting health are profoundly shaped by social values and choices. So, in order to serve as a complement to what EBP may identify as the best scientific response – a component part of which includes the clinician's response in the clinical encounter – we need to see where VBP stands in relation to the important role of social values and social determinants of health. This concern about the surrounding social values that shape the clinical encounter is valid anywhere VBP is applied. But it comes to the forefront in the context of global health because it is much easier to recognise in a developing country context that social values and choices are directly related to health outcomes.

Third, applying VBP is argued to be better for producing more successful clinical encounters than bioethics principles, human rights, legal regulations and professional guidelines (Fulford *et al.*, 2012, pp. 11–23). This is a bold claim that requires further scrutiny. Fulford and colleagues have gone some way to show how VBP can help resolve value conflicts through a set of case studies (Fulford *et al.*, 2012). Nevertheless, there are reasonable disagreements on how to prioritise a number of competing ethical claims or value conflicts in health justice discussions. For instance, when health care resources are finite, which they are in every society and particularly in developing countries, difficult decisions have to be made about how to allocate these resources, often with life or death consequences. A dominant view within societies with highly organised health care systems as well as international development organisations is that resources should be allocated in a rational way, understood as being cost-effective – maximising health outcomes in a population given finite health care resources. However, such cost-effective rationale is rarely adhered to completely as other competing values such as rule of rescue, rights, or equity are also realised. Furthermore, at the clinical level it is very unlikely that anywhere in the world is the concern for what is best for the patient the primary and only concern in the clinical encounter. An individual clinician or committee of individuals implicitly or explicitly prioritise actions across competing and divergent action-guiding dimensions of health such as need, urgency, numbers, persistence through generations, causes, consequences, differential experience, and so forth (Venkatapuram, 2011). In eschewing the extant action-guiding ethical and legal frameworks in health care, does VBP provide sufficient conceptual tools to indeed produce 'balanced decisions' across these distinct and incommensurable value dimensions of health?

Health (including longevity) is one of the most important and daily concerns of every human being and has been argued to be a special moral good, as it is both intrinsically and instrumentally valuable to human beings (Venkatapuram, 2011). Good health is a component of wellbeing which is of intrinsic value. Good health also allows people to pursue their life projects, or determines their equality of opportunity to pursue life plans, and so has important instrumental value (Anand, 2002; Sen, 2002; Daniels, 2008). Thus, VBP as a framework to govern the patient-health care provider engagement has to be evaluated in relation to the special moral and value-laden nature of health. In so far as VBP aims to inform individual behaviour, we can see it as being a moral framework. If it intends to govern how individuals act together in relation to health then it is an approach to health justice. And so, rather than being a simple analytical or heuristic aid, VBP can be seen as having both a procedural and substantive account of health morality/justice. VBP identifies various principles for the procedure of determining health outcomes. It is also a substantive account of health morality/justice as it asserts some starting values such as mutual respect. And it forbids other values such as racism from entering the deliberation or influencing actions.

The three questions regarding the relation of VBP to global health and global justice are meant to both explore the global applicability of VBP as well as to confront the procedural and substantive moral/justice aspects of VBP. One approach to test a particular moral argument is to confront it with alternative approaches or real world data. I do not aim to reconcile VBP and these issues fully or to make definitive conclusions about its coherence. Rather, my aim is to extend the discussion about VBP into areas that seem underexplored.

Global health

Global health as a conceptual term has achieved remarkable salience since the turn of the millennium. Eschewing the term 'international health' – which was largely a euphemism for developing country health issues – universities, governments, think-tanks, international organisations, philanthro-capitalists, academics and journalists among others have rapidly adopted the term 'global health'. The term is thought better to reflect the reality of globalisation where the actors that do and can impact the health of people across borders are now more diverse than nation-states. The term is also seen better to reflect the growing interdependence of societies, particularly the shared risks and vulnerabilities to disease and premature mortality. The diversity of transnational actors affecting health as well as the increased health interdependence are understood to form a new global layer of activity and analysis supervenient to domestic health actors and issues. Nevertheless, some use global health as a synonym for international health or tropical medicine – to mean health elsewhere, or in poor countries. For example, the discussions on 'global mental health' are largely about mental health of individuals and groups living in developing societies (Editors, *Lancet*, 2011). In any case, following on from the rapid diffusion of the concept of global health, and drawing on the discipline of international relations, there is now increasing rhetoric regarding global governance for health, or global health governance. In fact, current discussions about global health almost invariably include references to governance. Any analyses of how things are currently occurring or *should be* with respect to global health invariably draw in the concept of governance (Pang *et al.*, 2010; Frenk and Moon, 2013).

All health is global

Values-based practice (VBP) can be seen as a prescription for the good governance of the clinical encounter. And though it may appear that the targets of discussions about global governance for health are at a different level in contrast to VBP's focus on the governance of the health care provider-patient engagement, they are clearly linked in numerous ways.

Consider three links. First, there is the notion that everyone's health is now global. Whether one lives in Jakarta, London, or Kansas City, factors that impact our health, whether good or bad, have extra-national dimensions. A virus isolated in Jakarta can lead to a flu vaccine available in Kansas City. Or the actions of a company based in Kansas City can impact pathways to disease in New Delhi. Thus, the clinical encounter, whether in Jakarta or London, is significantly shaped by the governance or lack thereof of global actors and processes. And what happens in the clinical encounter, such as whether and which antibiotics to prescribe or whether to quarantine a patient with MDR TB, could have global implications. So the prescription to use VBP in the clinical encounter implicitly has global dimensions to it in the background. And the state of global governance for health shapes to varying degrees the governance of the clinical encounter.

One aspect of this has already been identified in the VBP literature related to the differences in cultural values of patients and health care providers due to immigrant backgrounds of both participants. But the global factors influencing the clinical encounter go far beyond the personal value differences of individuals due to different global origins or religions. Whether or not there will be a clinical consultation in the first place could be significantly determined by the type of health issues that are supported in a country by international actors. The health care in developing countries is most often organised around single disease, vertical health programmes. Someone with malaria, TB or HIV/AIDS may get access to a clinical consultation, while someone with cancer may not. Or it could simply be that in some places most health care providers have emigrated to other countries so the clinics lie empty. The occurrence of a consultation between the patient and provider, and the scope of that encounter, are both profoundly determined by the external social, economic, and political environmental aspects occurring from the local to the global level. The governance of the clinical encounter is linked very clearly to the global governance of institutions and process.

The global health movement

Second, there is an interest in taking VBP global – to advocate for and apply VBP outside the UK, where it originated, to other countries, particularly to developing countries. The possibility and practicality of transporting VBP across national borders is directly connected to the current state of global institutions and processes. The exporting of VBP and application in other countries makes VBP a part of the global health movement. Of course, contributing to the protection and promotion of health of people throughout the world, particularly those who are worst off, is a good thing. However, the present global health movement has within it a diverse range of actors, with a variety of motivations, propounding various kinds of politics and ideologies, using various kinds of evidence, and having diverse levels of accountability. There is a palpable atmosphere of a gold rush as there are indeed millions of dollars up for grabs (Mccoy et al., 2009; Ravishankar et al., 2009). As in the California gold rush, there is a veritable stampede towards newly discovered terrain in the belief of opportunity and advantage. One philosopher has described global health as a 'growth industry' (Wolff, 2012). Academic programmes are being rebranded as global health programmes; mega-research projects are being funded on promises of solving the endemic problems of the global poor; new degrees are being created; trans-national partnerships, particularly with institutions in developing countries, are being actively pursued, and various claims or stakes are being pounded into the ground through definitions, frameworks, and policy prescriptions. And such claims are being furiously disseminated through academic publications, lectures and social media. Moreover, in case it needs to be pointed out, all of this action is mostly going one way – from developed countries to the rest of the world. There are very few if any global health experts or centres in developing countries. Joining the global health movement means that despite holding the intention of improving the health of people who are worst off in the world, VBP advocates enter a terrain of unequal global distribution of power, knowledge, resources and agency. While any new actor wanting to join the global health movement must reconcile themselves with good and bad aspects of the movement, VBP advocates have a pressing reason to do so. That is, VBP is said to have a concern for ethics as well as the broader concern for values. Thus, advocates of VBP have the intimidating task of reconciling VBP with the global health movement which has a complicated mix of values such as charity, self-interest, national-interest, scientific knowledge, justice, economic interests and so forth.

Global health governance

The third link between VBP and global health governance has to do with the similarities in both discussions about purpose and challenges. In a recent article titled, 'Governance challenges in global health', Frenk and Moon (2013) begin with identifying incomplete health agendas, new and resurgent threats to health as well as a rapidly changing landscape of actors and norms affecting health. They write, 'A robust response to this complex picture requires improved governance of health systems – certainly at the national level but also at a worldwide level in what could be thought of as the "global health system."' In a similar vein, advocates of VBP start with asserting the growing complexity of the health and health care systems, and that alongside organised efforts to find the best scientific evidence through EBP, what is needed is better governance of the patient-health care provider engagement.

Frenk and Moon proceed to identify three challenges to global governance for health including the sovereignty challenge, the sectoral challenge, and the accountability challenge. While VBP advocates do not explicitly identify these three challenges to governance at the clinical level they are, nevertheless, there. For example, for Frenk and Moon, the sovereignty challenge entails two problems. On the one hand, states are no longer the dominant actor when it comes to containing and controlling health risks and implementing interventions. In the era of rapid globalisation, nation-states have become less able to control the flow of people, goods and capital as well as health threats across borders. On the other hand, states still have much power in being able to act domestically and in concert with trans-national efforts at protecting health. But they function in a context of unequal global distribution of threats, resources and power as well as conflicting interests of different states and other non-state actors. Such a description of the challenge of sovereignty is not dissimilar to the issue of autonomy and personal responsibility of the patient. A patient has always had differing levels of agency to determine their own health or manage their impairment. At the same time, individuals still have much agency in determining their own behaviour. And many policies are geared towards holding people responsible for the consequences of their actions. Where to draw the line between personal versus social responsibility for health is unclear and does not seem answerable by scientific research. VBP may offer a procedural account for how to draw the line in different contexts. But why should it abstain from taking a substantive position on responsibility when it does not abstain on other aspects, such as racism? (See also Chapters 3, 6 and 7.)

By sectoral challenge, Frenk and Moon mean the problem that health is determined by policy-making in multiple sectors, and not just in health care. They consider it a challenge as it is difficult to ensure that other sectors will take the concern for health seriously. This challenge is present at the individual level as well. The health of a patient is determined by a range of factors, and not just by access to health care. But it is unclear how a clinician can influence these other determinants despite recognising that some of them have a profound negative impact on health. Safe and affordable housing, freedom from physical violence, employment, and education can have direct bearing on the health of a patient. But clinicians, particularly in private health care systems, hardly engage with these other domains, even when they know that they are directly impacting their patients' health. The VBP framework does recognise that multiple actors and disciplines must be involved in the care of the patient. The component of 'partnerships' attempts to recognise the importance of different expertise and values of a variety of actors involved. But the involvement of 'social care' actors in VBP reflects the way health and social care are linked in the UK. In other countries, particularly developing countries, beyond the clinical management of a particular disease, it is unclear what guidance VBP would offer clinicians about going beyond the clinic, or how to convince actors, if they exist, to contribute to producing better health outcomes for a patient.

Frenk and Moon's final challenge refers to the problems of legitimacy and account-ability of the growing diversity of actors at the international level aside from nation states. They identify as problems the limited accountability of inter-governmental organisations to governments rather than the people directly affected. This is a problem especially where the people see their own governments as illegitimate. And then there is the lack of any accountability for non-state actors such as foundations, corporations, experts and journal-ists that influence governance across countries. Such accountability challenges are also present in the clinical encounter, particularly in developing countries. A variety of actors are often involved in determining whether there will be a clinical encounter and its scope. And where there is a consultation, it is unclear who is accountable to whom. In fact, the acute inequalities in knowledge and power between the patient and provider, particularly when the patient is impaired and/or poorly educated, would make it hard to maintain that there is mutual accountability, or that the provider is accountable to the patient. There are also the invisible actors who determine both the economic underpinnings of such an encounter, and the scientific and medical protocol to follow. VBP recognises that there are various actors involved in the clinical encounter aside from the patient and provider. But VBP takes no position on who is a legitimate actor in the encounter or who is accountable to whom and why (see Chapter 5).

While it is undeniable that novel health issues have emerged as part of increased globalisation, exuberance for the global health movement and for various visions of global health governance could benefit from more critical scrutiny and informed reasoning. Many public health practitioners, and now by extension global health practitioners, implicitly value health as a valuable good or ultimate goal. And this may also be the case for VBP. What is striking about the article by Frenk and Moon is that in no other discipline or discussion would national sovereignty be problematised as a challenge or hurdle in the path towards a worthy goal. The erosion of sovereignty may be identified as a problem, but national sovereignty itself would hardly be considered a problem. The presumption of health as being a special moral good that trumps all goods and values is often taken for granted in medicine and public health. However, much more careful analysis needs to be done before framing national sovereignty as a good to be traded for the sake of health. The ease with which public health professionals advocate many paternalistic or liberty restricting policies will likely meet significant resistance at the international level. Nevertheless, the comparison between discussions on global governance for health versus the governance of the clinical encounter may prove to be fruitful, if only to help VBP advocates recognise the link between the two levels and the presence of similar issues though with different units of analysis in both spheres.

Health and basic social arrangements

The second question posed in the present discussion is how does VBP relate to the growing understanding that in all human societies most of the 'action' regarding health outcomes happens outside the clinic/health care domain? This question is not something that is uniquely being applied to VBP. It is something that is confronting health care as well as the related ethical and legal frameworks. The understanding that preventative and curative health care is only one component of the multi-factoral causal pie of an individual's health challenges any scientific or moral framework that focuses exclusively on health care. The distinction between the concern for health versus health care is much more recognisable in developing countries where it is easier to see that the social, physical, economic and political environments directly impact health and longevity. If VBP is to be applied in developing countries, one of the pressing issues that needs to be addressed is whether VBP aims to produce better health care outcomes, or health outcomes.

Over the last four decades, epidemiologists have produced compelling evidence that health outcomes (e.g. life expectancy, mortality rates, obesity and cognitive development) are distributed along a social gradient; each socio-economic class – defined by income, occupational grade or educational attainment – has worse health outcomes than the one above it (Macintyre, 1997; Marmot et al., 1997; Kawachi et al., 2002). There is a health/illness gradient from top to bottom of the social hierarchy within societies. Research also shows that the steeper the socio-economic gradient (i.e. more social inequality), the lower is the overall health and wellbeing of the entire population; everyone in that society is worse off in the domain of health and many other domains than they would be otherwise (Deaton, 2003; Wilkinson and Pickett, 2009).

The remarkable findings on the social distribution patterns of ill health have motivated numerous research studies on the underlying causal determinants. The important thing to note here is that unlike studies which try to identify what causes a disease in one individual rather than another, these studies aim to identify what causes disease in certain individuals and in differing amounts in different social groups. The main hypothesis is that the causal factors are in the social conditions, the factors affecting social groups differently in different places on the social hierarchy. Where one stands on the social gradient determines the types and levels of harmful exposures and protective factors in pathways to ill health and mortality.

The research has so far illuminated a whole range of social determinants (discrete things and pathways) to ill health over the entire life cycle, starting from the social conditions surrounding the mother while still in utero to quality of social relationships in old age. To be clear, while availability of health care is crucial, other more influential causal determinants include such things as early infant care and stimulation, safe and secure employment, housing conditions, discrimination, self-respect, personal relationships, community cohesion and income inequality (Marmot and Wilkinson, 1999; Berkman and Kawachi, 2000). What is relevant to the reasoning about the scope of social justice is that these determinants operate at levels ranging from the micro, such as material deprivations and individual level psychosocial mechanisms, to the macro, such as community cultures, national political regimes and global processes affecting trade and respect for human rights. The possibility that extra-national, global determinants may have significant impact on the health and longevity of some individuals and social groups requires that the causal analysis as well as the ethical analysis has to start with a global scope.

Such social epidemiological research challenges both the prevailing individual level explanatory paradigm in epidemiology as well as the social inaction regarding harmful social or 'structural' conditions domestically as well as globally. While the level of expenditures and quality of health care, individual behaviours, and genetic risk factors clearly have a causal role, it is the social conditions that are most correlated with prevalence of preventable ill health and mortality in a society. Such findings overwhelmingly motivate the understanding that mitigating preventable ill health and premature mortality in individuals as well as their unequal social distribution (i.e. inequalities) requires substantial changes to basic social institutions, processes, policies and values (Krieger and Birn, 1998; Marmot, 2006; Commission on Social Determinants of Health, 2008).

The empirical research in social epidemiology thus extends the moral scope of the concern for health and health inequalities much wider than health care or even public health, deep into the basic structures of domestic and, indeed, global society. Many extant approaches to social justice are simply ill equipped to evaluate the ethics of such a broad relationship between social and global arrangements and ill health/health inequalities (Venkatapuram, 2011). The assumptions and theoretical structures erase much of the health injustices or push these concerns outside the scope of justice. To wit, the discipline of bioethics is transforming at present as bioethicists have only just discovered that much of health is determined outside the clinic and by values of those aside from the patient and doctor/researcher. Bioethics principles, informed by moral philosophy, aimed to govern the behaviours of individuals in relation to health related issues. However, in the light of the research on social determinants of health, principlism and the bioethics principles are having to give way to reasoning that situates the clinical or research encounter within a broader theory of good social arrangements ('social justice') informed by both social and political philosophy as well as the social sciences.

Competing value claims in health governance

It is interesting, therefore, that advocates of VBP question the usefulness of the bioethics principles as well as many of the familiar ethical and legal frameworks supposed to guide action such as human rights, legal regulations and professional guidelines. Of course, they do it for different reasons. Advocates of VBP assert that where VBP is implemented sufficiently, the health outcomes will likely be better and more fair or just. Producing 'balanced decision-making within a shared framework of values' could also be interpreted as another way of saying the outcomes will be fair, or will satisfy all the parties involved. However, such balanced decision-making is not brought about through a reasoned prioritisation of competing values, or even through consensus. To recall, the third question I posed was: what resources does VBP offer to navigate competing or conflicting values? Aside from the procedural and substantive aspects of the framework which goes some way towards organising different values, Fulford and colleagues argue for something called dissensus. They write, 'Dissensus differs from consensus in that differences of values instead of being ironed out (as in consensus) remain in play to be balanced according to the particular circumstances of a given decision within a framework of shared values' (Fulford *et al.*, 2012, p. 191). This novel approach to resolving value conflicts requires much more scrutiny than can be given at present. However, perhaps the foremost concern regarding dissensus is that while it foregoes consensus, it does not rank whether one pattern of dissensus is better than another, even for the same clinical encounter. A variety of value settlements are possible and equally as good. Such resolution to managing value conflicts may appear to be unsatisfactory, especially to practitioners who hope to find immediate guidance from VBP as well as philosophers who seek to rank clearly competing health related moral claims or values.

The tentativeness or incompleteness in the formulation of dissensus as a way to manage value conflict is similar to how value conflicts are being discussed in other related areas. In the face of reasonable disagreements about which values to pursue in public policy, there has been much philosophical consideration of value pluralism and means to achieve partial agreements (Sunstein, 1995). Such reasoning about how to achieve levels of agreement or incomplete orderings has also drawn on social choice theory in economics (Sen, 2009, pp. 107–108). And, in turn, these efforts to show how there is a possibility to move forward in the face of deep value conflict, or when there are multiple dimensions to consider, have also been applied to health care and health equity issues (Ruger, 2007). Whether dissensus is the same or analogous to incomplete orderings may need to be further explored, if only to see whether the analytical framework offered in the former discussions could be of help to VBP. At present VBP places 'clinical judgement' as something in between science and values which has to reconcile multiple factors to achieve dissensus.

Conclusion

An individual clinician or group of health care providers may in the first instance express their value as doing what is in the best interests of the patient. However, they implicitly or explicitly prioritise actions across competing and divergent action-guiding dimensions of health such as need, urgency, numbers, persistence through generations, causes, consequences, differential experience, and so forth. Even if the commitments to various implicit and explicit values of VBP are justified, there is still much uncertainty as to whether VBP has the requisite tools to produce balanced decisions in relation to health, and whether it will be able to produce a shared framework of values. Given the current state of global affairs, there will be little difficulty in VBP being taken up and applied in other countries, particularly developing countries. Rather than feasibility being the barrier, this discussion has posed three questions in relation to the conceptual coherence of applying VBP in a global context. First, what is the relation of VBP to global health? Second, what is the relation of VBP to an understanding of the broader social and global determinants of health? Third, what resources does VBP offer to navigate the longstanding value conflicts in health decision-making?

In exploring these questions, I have attempted to confront the procedural and substantive aspects of VBP which I understand to be a framework for health morality/justice. Indeed, it is a minimal account as it largely focuses on the site of the clinical encounter, and identifies a few starting values as well as excludes certain other values. I would argue that VBP, when it is applied in different parts of the world, will have to take a position on a number of other values. These include such things as discrimination based on gender, sexuality, tribe, caste or religion. It may also have to take a position on the role of public versus private provision of health care, and whether some level of health care should be a basic entitlement. So far, many of these issues have not become pressing for VBP advocates because in the UK many of these values are, at least formally, excluded from the clinical encounter, and every citizen has a formal entitlement to health care when in need of it.

I have argued elsewhere (Venkatapuram, 2011) for a theory of health justice that is applicable across all societies and which is centred on the entitlement of every human being to a capability to be healthy. The present discussion on the VBA is not the appropriate place to advocate such a theory. However, VBP may have much to gain from drawing on such theories of health justice, of which there are a few alternatives (Daniels, 2008; Powers and Faden, 2008; Segall, 2009). By being grounded in moral and political philosophical foundations such as those offered in these theories, VBP may become better equipped at dealing with various criticisms, such as value imperialism or cultural relativism, as well as contributing to furthering global health equity, human rights, and global justice. In turn, VBP may also have much to offer theorists of health justice. VBP offers a richer set of procedural and substantive principles for the clinical encounter than the bioethics principles which most health justice theorists accept as the best available option.

VBP also offers an interesting alternative to the habit of 'thinking big' in global health while working with generalisable scientific evidence and implementing standardised intervention programmes. In the same vein as or, perhaps, in solidarity with those who see an alternative vision of global health where most of the sustainable improvements in health happen locally informed by local contexts, VBP applied carefully and integrated with local contexts may provide new insights for the global health movement. VBP may have the potential to show that good governance at the clinical level could in turn impact the governance at the global level.

References

Anand, S. (2002) The concern for equity in health. *Journal of Epidemiology and Community Health*, **56**, 485–487.

Berkman, L. F. and Kawachi, I. O. (2000) *Social Epidemiology*. New York: Oxford University Press.

Commission on Social Determinants of Health (2008) Closing the gap in a generation: Health equity through action on the social determinants of health. *Final Report of the Commission on Social Determinants of Health*. Geneva: World Health Organization.

Daniels, N. (2008) *Just Health: Meeting Health Needs Fairly*. Cambridge: Cambridge University Press.

Deaton, A. (2003) Health, inequality, and economic development. *Journal of Economic Literature*, **41**, 113–158.

Editors (2011) Global mental health. *Lancet*, **378**, 1439–1526.

Frenk, J. and Moon, S. (2013) Governance challenges in global health. *New England Journal of Medicine*, **368**, 936–942.

Fulford, K. W. M., Peile, E. and Carroll, H. (2012) *Essential Values-Based Practice: clinical stories linking science with people.* Cambridge: Cambridge University Press.

Kawachi, I., Subramanian, S. V. and Almeida-Filho, N. (2002) A glossary for health inequalities. *Journal of Epidemiology and Community Health*, **56**, 647–652.

Krieger, N. and Birn, A. E. (1998) A vision of social justice as the foundation of public health: commemorating 150 years of the spirit of 1848. *American Journal of Public Health*, **88**, 1603–1606.

Macintyre, S. (1997) The Black Report and beyond: what are the issues? *Social Science & Medicine*, **44**, 723–745.

Marmot, M. (2006) Health in an unequal world: social circumstances, biology and disease. *Clinical Medicine*, **6**, 559–572.

Marmot, M. G. and Wilkinson, R. G. (1999) *Social Determinants of Health.* Oxford: Oxford University Press.

Marmot, M., Ryff, C. D., Bumpass, L. L., Shipley, M. and Marks, N. F. (1997) Social inequalities in health: next questions and converging evidence. *Social Science & Medicine*, **44**, 901–910.

Mccoy, D., Kembhavi, G., Patel, J. and Luintel, A. (2009) The Bill & Melinda Gates Foundation's grant-making programme for global health. *Lancet*, **373**, 1645–1653.

Pang, T., Daulaire, N., Keusch, G. *et al.* (2010) The new age of global health governance holds promise. *Nature Medicine*, **16**, 1181.

Powers, M. and Faden, R. R. (2008) *Social Justice: the moral foundations of public health and health policy.* Oxford: Oxford University Press.

Ravishankar, N., Gubbins, P., Cooley, R. J. *et al.* (2009) Financing of global health: tracking development assistance for health from 1990 to 2007. *Lancet*, **373**, 2113–2124.

Ruger, J. P. (2007) Health, health care, and incompletely theorized agreements: a normative theory of health policy decision making. *Journal of Health Politics Policy and Law*, **32**, 51–87.

Segall, S. (2009) *Health, Luck, and Justice.* Princeton, NJ: Princeton University Press.

Sen, A. (2002) Why health equity? *Health Economics*, **11**, 659–566.

Sen, A. (2009) *The Idea of Justice.* London: Allen Lane.

Sunstein, C. R. (1995) Incompletely theorized agreements. *Harvard Law Review*, **108**, 1733–1772.

Venkatapuram, S. (2011) *Health Justice. An Argument from the Capabilities Approach.* Cambridge: Polity Press.

Wilkinson, R. G. and Pickett, K. (2009) *The Spirit Level: why more equal societies almost always do better.* London: Allen Lane.

Wolff, J. (2012). *The Human Right to Health.* New York: W.W. Norton.

World Health Organization and Commission on Social Determinants of Health (2008) Closing the gap in a generation. *Health Equity Through Action on the Social Determinants of Health.* Geneva: World Health Organization.

Chapter 12

Is values-based practice useful in psychiatry? – a practitioner's view

Alistair Stewart

Values-based practice is a theoretical approach, first advanced by Fulford and others, to working with the complex and conflicting values at play in encounters between people seeking help and psychiatrists and other mental health professionals. It has been claimed that

> Philosophy, through a new model linking values with evidence, called values-based practice (VBP), gives us specific tools to help make science work for us in a more patient centred way. (Fulford, 2008)

and further, that

> Values-based practice is the philosophy-into-practice cutting edge of the new interdisciplinary field of philosophy of psychiatry. (Fulford *et al.*, 2004)

It is proposed that VBP is complementary to evidence-based practice, which involves the systematic synthesis of the available evidence on any particular clinical question. VBP has been taken up in various forms by the Department of Health in the UK, and was used in training materials for the introduction of the revised MHA 2007. There are also claims that its effectiveness in improving practice has been shown by semi-quantitative research (Altamirano-Bustamante *et al.*, 2013). VBP is often described in terms of ten principles or pointers. I will not elaborate these here, but it is the form of description as a list of ten which I find most interesting.

In order to use VBP in practice, we need to have answers to the following questions.

Debates in Values-Based Practice, ed. Michael Loughlin. Published by Cambridge University Press. © Cambridge University Press 2014.

(1) What conception do we have of values? How stable are anybody's values? Are they hermetically sealed off from the world around us or are they maintained by dialogue with other people in the world around us? (See Chapters 5, 7 and 8.)

(2) How valid are the claims made for the status of VBP? Does it really represent anything new? If it does, is it actually an achievement for philosophy? (See Chapter 3.)

(3) How far is illness an evaluative or value-laden concept? (See Chapters 4, 6, 7 and 19.)

(4) What about clashes of values, prior to the involvement of any psychiatrist or mental health professional? (See Chapter 10.)

(5) Are there some values which are 'right values'? It is clear that there are values which certain people in particular roles are expected to keep to, but are there values which are right for everyone? (See Chapters 4, 5 and 6.)

Some general points about values

The concept of values is rather vague and that is not necessarily a bad thing (Fulford, 2013), but we can perhaps define values as those things which a particular person or community hold as important and which guide their choices and actions. This suggests that values are demonstrated through behaviour rather than through assertion. We know that the way people vote in elections is often different to what might be concluded from their answers to questionnaires about what they consider the most important issues. To put it bluntly, they may answer the researcher from their heart and vote with their wallet.

If I hold certain values seriously, then they will be exemplified in my behaviour. I will stand up for them against a degree of resistance, and I may also seek to inculcate them in other people around me. My values will determine to what I give priority. Certain life changes – think of a serious illness or the arrival of parenthood – may prompt me to reconsider my order of priorities and so revaluate my values. Our values are also developed, not in isolation but through our experience and interchanges with other people, so that someone's values may change as a result of prolonged reflection and debate.

A model for taking account of values

Before I touch on the problems I find with the concept of values-based practice, I would like to describe a tradition of working in a therapeutic way with people who are in the kinds of psychological distress or predicament which tend to be described as mental illness. Now, someone in this situation is very often at a point of no longer being able to carry on their life in the old way, no longer being able to guard themselves from harm as they normally would; perhaps they have a great fear of losing their mental integrity or their mind, or of losing their memory; or they are paralysed by depression, tormented by hallucinations, perhaps contemplating suicide. They are at their most vulnerable and to some extent at the mercy of those to whom they turn for help. They may have friends and family to support them and accompany them as they seek this help, but sometimes either their attitudes and behaviour have caused a rift or breach with their family or friends, or their social circle itself has played an important part in bringing on their problems. Since social isolation itself is a very important risk factor for mental breakdown, it is not surprising that some people we meet on this basis are literally un-befriended.

Sometimes a person may have no complaint or distress and they come to attention because of someone else's concern for their welfare or fear of their behaviour, but then in most cases there are features of how they act and express themselves which lead other people, not usually specialists, to guide them towards the mental health service or something similar.

At a time like this, any one of us will hold on as tight as we can to what is most important to us, our sanity, our identity, our pride, our self-esteem, people who matter to us, often our home, our familiar surroundings, our mode of dress, our toilet habits, our favourite music, our mobile phone, our sustaining beliefs, our religion, our political commitments and our first language. It will only be natural for someone in this position to fear any threat to these aspects of themselves and it is only too easy for those in a helping role, through arrogance, prejudice, impatience, intolerance or clumsiness, to injure us in these respects.

What the psychiatrist needs to bring is something of the experience and openness described by the poet Rainer Maria Rilke as necessary for writing a poem:

> For the sake of a line of poetry one must see many people, cities and things, one must know animals, must feel how the birds fly, and know the gestures with which small flowers open in the morning. One must be able to think back to paths in unknown regions, to unexpected meetings and to partings one long saw coming; to childhood days that are still not understood; to parents one had to hurt when they brought one a joy and one did not understand it (it was a joy to someone else); to childhood illnesses that set in so strangely with so many profound and heavy transformations; to days in quiet, muted rooms, and to mornings by the sea, the sea altogether, to nights travelling that rushed up and away and flew with all the stars; and if one can think of all that it is still not enough. One must have memories of many nights of love, none of which resembled another; of screams in the delivery room and of easy, pale, sleeping women, who are closing themselves. But one must also have been with the dying, have sat by the dead in the room with the open window and the spasmodic noises. (Rilke, 1910, pp. 13–14)

Rilke's words were proposed by the late Robert Hobson as applying 'to every understanding intervention in psychotherapy' (Hobson, 1985), and they are a useful catechism. It is important for psychiatrists and other mental health professions to explore, understand and take into account the values held by people they are trying to help, particularly because of the imbalance of power in this relationship. The imbalance arises partly from the legal powers which the psychiatrist is able at times to exercise, partly from the socially privileged position of the doctor and partly from the fact that the person seeking help is by definition at a particularly vulnerable point in their own life.

One of the drivers behind the idea of values-based practice is the concern, which has a strong historical foundation, that psychiatry and medicine have a propensity to be practised in an extremely authoritarian way. This is related to the sociology of the professions and to the legacy of positivist views of science (Fulford, 2013; see Chapters 4, 16 and 18).

The status of values-based practice

The point is that in order to engage and understand someone who is in the throes of some form of mental illness, we have to understand as much as possible about them, about what they are experiencing now and about what makes them who they are, what makes them tick. I am not claiming that this necessarily reflects the actual practice all or even much of the time in psychiatry, but within reason it is an achievable aim and one which has been an aspiration well before the introduction of VBP.

This is why I have difficulty with the claim made by Fulford and others that values-based practice represents an achievement for philosophy or indeed a new approach to working with 'complex and conflicting values in medicine' (Fulford, 2008; see Chapter 3). It may well be useful as a way of presenting reminders or of systemising best practice but it hardly represents a breakthrough. In particular, why it should result in ten principles rather than nine, or eleven, or four, is difficult to understand in philosophical terms, although this structure may well have some use as a teaching aid, reminder or even checklist. Checklists certainly have their place in medicine, as a way of ensuring the retention and recall of crucial sequences of information, such as the causes of atrial fibrillation, or the elements of a reliable examination of cognitive functions, or the instruments used in a surgical operation which need to be accounted for at the end. However, the analogous use of checklists when considering less concrete matters, while it may be thought to appeal to doctors and those with similar training, gives a spurious impression that matters are more straightforward than they really are. The codification of ethical principles *and* of approaches to integrating values, echo in an unhelpful way approaches which are better adapted to dealing with uncontroversial matters.

Values-based practice has the definite merit of being oriented towards making a practical difference for the better to the way in which mental health professionals and others work with and care for the people who come to them for help. It is notorious that medical students and doctors tend to focus their attention on matters which are subject to formal examination, often in the form of some variant of multiple choice questions. This poses a real challenge for teachers who want to demonstrate meaningful changes in their students' practice resulting from training in the field of ethics, broadly considered.

In this context, a recent study carried out in Mexico (Altamirano-Bustamante *et al.*, 2013) is of considerable interest. The researchers demonstrated that an educational intervention derived from the theory of values-based practice was successful in bringing about positive changes among a large group of health care professionals in certain higher order values – described as openness and self-transcendence – thought to be relevant to improved patient-centred practice. The study is an impressive achievement, and at least points the way to how the impact on practitioners' behaviour of an intervention based on VBP could be evaluated using the principles of evidence-based medicine. It would be necessary to show a connection between changes in the subjective views of trial participants and their behaviour with patients, but this would not be impossible. However, because the only control condition in the study was the attitudes of the participants before the intervention, the possibility remains that similar changes could have been brought about by an educational intervention based on a quite different theoretical approach.

How far, and in what ways, is diagnosis in psychiatry value-laden?

Values-based practice seeks to make explicit the value-laden nature of judgements, including diagnostic judgements, in psychiatry and in medicine more generally. It is noted that in many situations this value-laden aspect goes unrecognised because certain basic values are so widely shared. For example, most of the time we all value being alive, being able to move around independently, having the power of speech and communication, being able to see and hear, and being free of pain. Only in certain situations will these values be in question, for example if someone finds life unbearable because of pain or disability. Psychiatry is seen as an area where the value-laden nature of judgements is more obvious, because it is 'concerned with areas of human experience and behaviour, such as emotion, desire, volition and belief, where people's values are particularly highly diverse' (Thornton, 2011).

For example, withdrawing from much human social contact may represent a valid and rational choice within a particular religious world-view; or it may be a natural option for someone who is by nature happily solitary and not in need of company; or it may be a reflection of a pervasive and morbidly depressed mood state; or it may be an adaptive way of avoiding, say, drug-dealers, who are after my blood; or it may be a response to frightening delusional ideas.

It is recognised that many people experience hallucinations of voices which do not handicap them in everyday life, and which may be integrated into their sense of themselves, becoming a source of comfort and strength. We know something about these people thanks to the work of Iris Sommer and others (Daalman *et al.*, 2011), who have demonstrated that the quality of the hallucinations they experience are different from those which affect people suffering from illnesses like schizophrenia. However, even though all diagnoses in psychiatry are value laden, it is not the case that the range of values which are in play is always equally wide.

That DSM-5 would sanction the diagnosis of major depressive disorder in someone with certain symptoms for more than two weeks after a bereavement should certainly give us pause for thought. There are statues all over Britain of a woman whose grief over the loss of her husband resulted in a process of mourning which was well known to the whole population and went on for many years. Where are the rules for the right amount of mourning, or the right intensity of grief? Again, post-traumatic stress disorder is a particularly vexed concept because it fails to take account of the many ways in which people and communities may respond to a major trauma and make sense of it in the context of their overall life experience and their values.

On the other hand the progressive loss of short term memory and then other faculties which occurs in Alzheimer's disease would probably be accepted by most people as a serious illness and loss of a critical faculty; there are simply fewer options available for construing it otherwise. Dyslexia can be viewed as a socially determined disorder in that it might present no problem in a society where literacy is not important, but it *is* a problem for most affected people in today's world where being unable to read is a major disadvantage (see Chapter 11).

People suffering from schizophrenia do not typically experience benign hallucinations but ones which are unpleasant and distressing and are also accompanied by other phenomena such as disturbances in self-experience, incoherence of thinking, impairment of motivation and planning and delusional thinking. These clusters of features are associated with poor physical health, premature death, difficulties in negotiating friendships and family relationships, reduced chances of finding work, increased risks of being the victim of assaults, increased risk of suicide, and not surprisingly with a great deal of suffering. Whilst many of these consequences can be influenced for the better by intelligent social measures, there is again a more limited range of values which can reasonably be brought into consideration in considering diagnosis.

Take another example. A man plans to kill or injure his baby child because he is convinced that it is possessed by evil and threatens him and his family. Now we know that in some value systems it is held that a child may become possessed by evil and is then a legitimate target for fear, rejection and even for being physically abused or killed. This was one element in the case of Victoria Climbié and it has featured in other cases of child abuse or murder since then. However, in this case no one in the family or community shares the beliefs, which arise after the man comes across a newspaper article which he believes refers in some oblique way to his baby and its malign influence. He hears voices telling him to kill the child. His emotional attitude is incongruously calm and indifferent. The diagnosis of mental illness in such a case is not necessarily more value laden or more obviously value laden, than a diagnosis of myocardial infarction in someone with chest pain. The recognition of diminished responsibility in someone who commits a crime when mentally ill may not be universal but it is at least widespread in most societies with a minimum degree of civilised standards. While this observation is by no means incompatible with VBP, it is not clear how VBP brings anything to light that was not already known by many who have practised without it for a long time. But perhaps VBP really comes into its own when dealing not with shared values but with values that are in conflict.

Values in conflict

Values-based practice highlights the difference between the value system of the patient and that of the doctor as particularly important. Mental health professionals, as noted before, are in a powerful position with respect to their patients, and the potential for doing harm is significant. Questions relating to values can easily be overlooked. Apart from their own personal values, these professionals may be under various pressures to conform to, or enforce, the requirements of society at large, and so to neglect those of their patients.

Differences and clashes between values are very often at play well before the psychiatrist becomes involved. There may be a conflict between the values of an individual and the society around them or between the values held by one group of people and wider society, or between an individual and members of their own family, or indeed there may be an internal conflict within one individual involving irreconcilable values which they are trying to hold at the same time. So I may hold to a set of values according to which I am entitled to take whatever I want for myself. If I am unsuccessful in doing this I may find myself subject to sanctions or punishment from society at large which leave me feeling persecuted and resentful. I may be torn between my desire to escape from and expose abuse which I am suffering at the hands of members of my family and my strong sense of duty and loyalty to my family which makes me dread creating a shameful scandal for them. I may be a violent young offender in prison with no overt qualms of conscience but tormented by disturbing memories of a violent act I have committed. I may be a man with a fierce commitment to being strong and independent, now disabled following a stroke and having to learn the hard way that sometimes independence is not possible. I may hold certain strong religious views which cause me turmoil over my unshakable sexual attraction to people of my own gender. Following bereavement I may be torn between my strong sense of injury and personal resentment over how my relative has treated me and my equally strong sense that I should respect and defend their memory and not diminish them in the eyes of other members of the family. I may hold it as an article of faith that it is important for everyone to like me and be aware that I am always choking back my own aspirations and desires in order to achieve this.

Part of the psychiatrist's job then, may be not simply to understand the person's values but to help them resolve the conflicting values which are contributing to their distress. This challenge is common as part of any psychotherapeutic exploration which aims at increasing someone's awareness of their own feelings and motivations, in order to help them get free of patterns of relating to other people and to themselves which are paralysing or the source of unnecessary suffering. This kind of understanding certainly predates values-based practice, and it is not clear that VBP adds anything useful to it. The checklist approach may give the impression that the process of working with conflicting values has been (or could be) reduced to an applied science, when its intuitive nature, involving morally contentious and unresolved issues, remains unaddressed by VBP's emphasis on 'process'. Is it possible to avoid the question of which values are 'right' when values conflict? (See Chapters 4, 6 and 8.)

The right values – unavoidable questions

There remains the question of whether there are in fact some values which are to be generally preferred over others. Clearly for particular social and professional groups there are particular sets of values to which they are expected to adhere – doctors obviously, also teachers, accountants, sports people, perhaps soldiers, even politicians. But what of the preferred values for society at large?

Thornton and Lucas (2010) raise a very useful question in their paper 'On the very idea of a recovery model for mental health', where they consider the set of values which might shape the aspirations of people moving forward from an experience of mental disorder. They contrast a hedonic approach with a eudaimonic approach, the latter being derived from Aristotle and his description of 'activity in accordance with virtue'. This is further elaborated as 'values connected to human flourishing' (see Chapter 6). The contrast recalls a line from a Bob Dylan song: 'she says your debutante knows what you need, but I know what you want'. We are left with the question of what constitutes human flourishing. Some people might say that human flourishing depends on such things as social inclusion, whereas others would say that it depends on conditions which promote the highest possible degree of self-actualisation by the most gifted and talented people.

Where values are based on the following ideas, to what extent should we take them on board or respect them or factor them in to our decision-making? Someone feels that they should only be interested in looking after number one; or that they are entitled to take whatever they want from other people; or that it is laid down in scripture that men and women have assigned roles in life and that they should keep to them; or that homosexuality is a grievous sin; or that foreigners are all scroungers and not to be trusted; or that my family's honour makes it acceptable for me to punish my children if I think they threaten it; or that anyone who thwarts me or challenges any aspect of my behaviour is disrespecting me; or that the world owes me a living. Is there a line to be drawn and where do we draw it? (See Chapter 3.)

Such questions are fundamentally political, but they cannot for that reason be avoided, or resolved by the balancing of 'legitimately different perspectives' (Fulford, 2008) – the term used in the fifth principle of values-based practice. The question is what can be considered 'legitimate'? (See Chapters 5, 6 and 8.) With the exception of certain values – Fulford (2013) specifically mentions racism – it seems that all values are equally legitimate, and the problem of how to resolve them is left to participants in the VBP process. How can this guarantee an outcome that is genuinely good? The process does not even give us a method for determining which outcomes are good or bad, better or worse than others.

With respect to particular professional groups, it is clear that behaviour grounded in some basic human values is essential and not always to be found. Professional codes go some way to ensuring at least minimum standards of ethical behaviour. However, if we consider the Francis enquiry into events in Mid-Staffordshire, published in 2013, it is clear that the absence of decent values is an issue for all health care professionals, not just those working in the field of mental health. Not only that, but it appears that in some respects standards have sometimes been better in the past than they are now. My own touchstone for the practice of psychiatry in a humane, patient-centred and intelligent way is the experience I had of working on a locked intensive care ward in a hospital in South London in the mid-1970s.

The trick for any attempt to improve our practice now may not be to import a new approach, whether or not it is philosophically driven, but to capture what has already been practised at certain times and in certain places (see Chapter 7). Practitioners may learn and embrace a values-sensitive approach more by observing good role models who demonstrate how to do things in practice, than by formal training. How we generate and sustain professionals who can act as those role models is another question.

Acknowledgements

This piece is based on a talk I gave at the Philosophy of Psychiatry workshop held at Lancaster University on 10 June 2013 and organised by Dr Rachel Cooper. I am grateful to her and to all the participants for their helpful comments.

References

Altamirano-Bustamante, M. M., Altamirano-Bustamante, N. F., Lifshitz, A. et al. (2013) Promoting networks between evidence-based medicine and values-based medicine in continuing medical education. *BMC Medicine*, 11(1), 39.

Daalman, K., Boks, M. P. M., Diederen, K. M. J., de Weijer, A. D., Blom, J. D. and Sommer, I. E. (2011) The same or different? A phenomenological comparison of auditory verbal hallucinations in healthy and psychotic individuals. *Journal of Clinical Psychiatry*, 72(3), 320–325.

Fulford, K. W. M. (2008) Values-based practice: a new partner to evidence-based practice and a first for psychiatry? *Mens Sana Monographs*, 6(1), 10–21.

Fulford, K. W. M. (2013) Values-based practice: Fulford's dangerous idea. *Journal of Evaluation in Clinical Practice*, 19, 537–546.

Fulford, K. W. M., Stanghellini, G. and Broome, M. (2004) What can philosophy do for psychiatry? *World Psychiatry*, 3(3), 130–135.

Hobson, R. (1985) *Forms of Feeling*, Chapter 3. London: Tavistock.

Rilke, R. M. (1910) *The Notebooks of Malte Laurids Brigge*. Translated by Pike, B., Dalkey Archive edition, 2008.

Thornton, T. (2011) Radical liberal values-based practice. *Journal of Evaluation in Clinical Practice*, 17(5), 988–991.

Thornton, T. and Lucas, P. (2010) On the very idea of a recovery model for mental health. *Journal of Medical Ethics*, 37, 24–28.

Chapter 13

Living with uncertainty: a first-person plural response to eleven commentaries on values-based practice

K. W. M. (Bill) Fulford

It is conventional in articles of this kind to thank one's commentators, friends and foes alike. In this case, however, my thanks are substantive. Friends and foes alike have offered a series of helpful critiques that severally and together illuminate and deepen our understanding of both the strengths and limitations of values-based practice.

In this chapter I indicate what I for one have learned from these commentaries across a range of topics in two main sections covering respectively the practice of values-based practice and its underpinning theory. In a brief concluding section I return to the theme of my title, indicating how values-based practice helps us in the circumstances of contemporary health care to live with uncertainty without being paralysed by hesitation. I start with a brief 'first impressions' and indication of my overall approach.

First impressions and my approach

My first impression of the commentaries can be summed up in one word, 'diversity'. As series editor (with Ed Peile) I was already aware that Michael Loughlin had done a great job in drawing together a set of very different disciplinary perspectives, both philosophical and practical. It is perhaps worth emphasising that although Michael's proposal went through the normal processes of editorial and peer review, Ed and I had no direct say in who was invited to contribute. So it was all the more welcome to find when I finally saw the commentaries as such that they indeed covered widely diverse views about the overall practical usefulness of values-based practice and about the merits or otherwise of the various elements of which it is composed.

Debates in Values-Based Practice, ed. Michael Loughlin. Published by Cambridge University Press. © Cambridge University Press 2014.

We can learn from this diversity of views in various ways. In some cases the relevant learning point is to find a balance: the extent to which values-based practice represents a novel approach falls somewhere between the extremes of the (Gupta/Stewart) 'nothing essentially new' view and the (Thornton) 'all a bit too radical' view. In other cases the relevant learning point is simply that with so many different views they cannot all be right: Gupta's and Stewart's assimilations of values-based practice to their respective disciplines of clinical ethics and of a particular way of practising psychotherapy, cannot both be right. In yet other cases the learning point is to recognise that the different views are indeed all correct but for different aspects of values-based practice. Peile's claim that values-based practice may illuminate and Brecher's claim that it may obfuscate are both right: Peile is right that values-based practice may illuminate aspects of clinical practice (as in the move from ICE to ICEStAR in communication skills for example); but Brecher is also right that the emphasis on process in values-based practice risks obfuscating its own underlying values.

In what follows I will be drawing on the commentaries in all these ways through what I hope will do justice to our respective positions. It is in this sense that although the selection of points and the treatment of them are of course my own, the voice of my response is not first-person singular but first-person plural.

The practice of values-based practice

A key learning point for me is that a number of commentators have gained an impression that values-based practice claims to be better than, or at any rate a competitor to, other ways of working with values in health care, notably ethics. Well, *mea culpa*: it is true that in the early days I did occasionally and not wholly tongue-in-cheek introduce values-based practice as 'anti-ethics'. As Tim Thornton notes (Chapter 4) it is sometimes helpful to locate something by reference to what it is not. And values-based practice is certainly 'anti' what might be called cut-price ethics: Thornton gives principlism as an example of this, a cut-price version of principles reasoning that *contra* Gupta (Chapter 7) he finds all-too-prevalent in health care. Values-based practice is also 'anti' cut-price evidence-based medicine (as I indicate below). Gupta, responding to my metaphor of the 'tool kit', suggests that further work needs to be done to explain exactly how values-based practice is distinct from other values-tools in focusing on individual values: 'no more tools!' she rightly says, unless they really are doing something distinctive and worthwhile.

It is this further work that I will try to do in this section. I will look first by way of context at how values-based practice grew out of engagement between my original theoretical work in philosophical value theory and an early programme in what might now be called clinical ethics (the Oxford Practice Skills Project, Hope et al., 1996). I will then outline how these origins play out in contemporary values-based practice in its relationships (of partnership) between, respectively, clinical ethics and evidence-based medicine.

Origins

Values-based practice, although appearing on the scene early in the present century, grew out of developments in medicine in the 1990s. This was a period, as Gupta reminds us, of growing concern at the increasing dominance of principles-based approaches. I had published *Moral Theory and Medical Practice*, the primary source code for values-based practice (see below), at the beginning of this period (Fulford, 1989). At the time though, I saw this as being relevant mainly to the development of philosophy of psychiatry which was (and remains) the focus of my research interests. My point of access to the 1990s debates in medical ethics was instead by way of the work that Tony (A. R.) Hope and I did in setting up the Oxford Practice Skills Project (OPSP) as part of our teaching responsibilities as clinical lecturers in psychiatry (Hope *et al.*, 1996).

The OPSP, like values-based practice, focused on clinical decision-making. It made clear the importance of using a range of methods of ethical reasoning including case-based reasoning (identified by Gupta as a defining characteristic of clinical ethics) as well as principles reasoning, it was process driven (and specifically clinical-skills process driven) rather than outcomes driven (it was we believe the first programme to bring together communication skills with ethics and law in clinical decision-making), and it emphasised the importance of best evidence as a full partner to ethical reasoning in clinical decision-making.

Given these parallels it will be clear why Gupta is right to point to overlaps between value-based practice and what she and others now call clinical ethics. The OPSP was indeed an early form of clinical ethics (as helpfully defined by Gupta as the application of academic ethics to clinical practice); Tony Hope as Oxford's first Professor of Medical Ethics has continued to work in the nuanced and case-oriented way Gupta describes; and one of Tony's former PhD students, the general practitioner and ethicist Anne-Marie Slowther, has gone on to establish a programme in clinical ethics at Warwick University Medical School. All of us meanwhile, in our post-OPSP lives, have continued to work closely in ethics and values-based practice: Anne-Marie for example wrote the first curriculum statement in clinical ethics and values-based practice for the UK's Royal College of General Practitioners; and Ed Peile (Chapter 2) and I are both contributing to Anne-Marie's innovative cross-cutting VLE (Values, Law and Ethics) theme for Warwick Medical School's new undergraduate curriculum.

From clinical ethics to values-based practice

But the story of values-based practice does not end with clinical ethics. In the 1990s I was among those arguing the need for a diversity of approaches to ethical decision-making in medicine (Fulford, 1994). But through my work in philosophy of psychiatry I now came to see the challenge for clinical reasoning, at least in mental health, to be both wider and deeper than was widely perceived in the ethics of the day: wider in that a whole raft of values in addition to ethical values were involved in clinical decision-making (Fulford *et al.*, 2002); deeper in that the conceptual issues went much deeper in psychiatry than was generally assumed (Dickenson and Fulford, 2000).

The immediate clinical need therefore, as I and others had come to see it by the end of the 1990s, was to break out of the increasingly narrow model constraining the engagement of academic ethics with practice. As Gupta rightly emphasises, academic ethics was at the time and remains a rich resource of theory and practice for tackling ethical issues: philosophical value theory after all (underpinning values-based practice, see Chapter 1) is one such resource. The problem, however, was not academic ethics but the increasingly narrow way in which academic ethics was being translated *into practice*. We might debate the merits or otherwise of this cut-price narrowing of the practical engagement of ethics with medicine in general (again, I return to this point in the next section). But in my own field of psychiatry at least, cut-price ethics was by the end of the 1990s already driving an increasingly defensive and risk-averse approach to practice directly inimical to the recovery-oriented model of best practice then starting to emerge. The term 'recovery' as used here means focusing on quality of life rather than (just) symptom control and developing self-management skills (rather than remaining reliant on services) through co-production (an equal partnership) between service users and service providers. And values (broadly not narrowly construed) were key to this model: one of the lead figures in recovery called it 'values in action' (personal communication, see also Allott et al., 2005).

It is perhaps surprising therefore that it was not until early in the new millennium that the obvious point finally hit me: why not bring together the work I had done in psychiatry using philosophical value theory with my by now growing understanding of the practical demands of clinical ethics? I remember sketching the first outlines of values-based practice over two days of rare stillness sitting beside Lake Lucerne in the summer of 2001. It all seemed to fit. From the point of view of practice, philosophical value theory,

(1) was consistent with much that I had learned from Tony Hope and others about best practice in clinical ethics including the importance of clinical skills, yet with some distinctive twists (such as specific ways of raising awareness of values, and the extension of values to diagnosis as well as treatment);

(2) it added a broader way of thinking about values in medicine that (importantly in psychiatry at least) was wider than, though it included, ethical values; and

(3) its emphasis on form (language) rather than content led to a corresponding reliance on process rather than outcomes, thus making values-based practice a natural partner to (the also process-based) evidence-based practice as a support tool for clinical decision-making.

Additionally, and from a more theoretical point of view, philosophical value theory,

(1) suggested an analytic premise for values-based practice that acted as an in principle counter to the rule-oriented drift of ethics in its then dominant cut-price connections with practice, and

(2) connected naturally (as a branch of ordinary language philosophy) with other philosophical and empirical resources for medicine as a research-led discipline.

Values-based practice today

Values-based practice has come a long way since the 2001 'Lucerne protocol' as I perhaps rather fancifully called my original (unpublished) draft. It has been through the educational and service developments in mental health described in Chapter 1, with products including the training manual 'Whose Values?', the NIMHE Values Framework, the '3 Keys Programme' (on assessment in mental health), and the Foundation Module for the training materials supporting the UK Mental Health Act 2007. As Gupta points out, these developments have thus far been mainly in mental health, although in the UK at least this includes primary care. But latterly there have been early moves out of mental health and primary care into other areas of medicine (see the VBP website, www.go.warwick.ac.uk/values-basedpractice, Chapter 1).

The series in which this book falls is an important resource for the further development of values-based practice in medicine. The launch volume for the series, *Essential Value-Based Practice* (Fulford, Peile and Carroll, 2012), explores through a series of clinical stories a number of aspects of the distinctive contributions of values-based practice across a range of representative clinical areas in secondary as well as primary care (breast surgery, acute abdomen, IVF, etc). The story in Chapter 2 of *Essentials* (which is about the management of chronic low back pain) illustrates how values-based practice, in focusing on individual values, fits together with and complements other support tools for clinical decision-making. One particular place where values-based practice 'kicks in', as Ed Peile shows in this book with his concept of 'squaring down' (Chapter 2), is at the point of individual decision-making. As Peile emphasises, the use of values-based practice in 'squaring down' on a clinical problem depends critically (as the use of values-based practice in any other context depends critically) on it being exercised in partnership with evidence-based practice (see also below).

It will be worth looking in a little more detail at a further story in *Essentials*, this one from Chapter 5 illustrating one particular way in which values-based practice brings something new to the partnership with clinical ethics, in this case specifically with casuistry and its role in communication skills. The chapter is called 'Teenage acne: widening our values horizons'.

Teenage acne

The story in Chapter 5 of *Essentials* shows how a brief casuistic reflection helps a GP, Dr Mangate, to manage a consultation with a teenage patient, Jane Brewer, who is concerned about recent onset of acne and is asking for a proprietary treatment not available on the NHS. In this chapter, we run the consultation twice, first without and then with the pre-consultation case-based reflection. On the first run of the consultation, Dr Mangate's implicit values drive him off course. On the re-run his brief casuistic reflection has made him aware of how his own values are influencing the way he responds to Jane Brewer's concerns, with the result that the consultation now runs well. And what 'runs well' means here is this: Dr Mangate uses the *same clinical (notably his well-developed communication) skills* as before, he draws on the *same values* (aesthetic and economic as well as ethical) as before, and he and Jane Brewer come to the *same decision* (she does not get the non-proprietary product). The difference is that when Dr Mangate employs his communication skills with awareness of his own values, the result is an entirely *different process* and hence better outcome *for them both*. On the first run Jane Brewer, denied her request, ends up feeling patronised and misunderstood while Dr Mangate is painfully conscious that he has alienated his young patient (it is the first time she has consulted him on her own without her mother). On the re-run, Dr Mangate, aware now of his own values, is better able to relate to Jane Brewer's values, the net result being that she comes to understand and indeed ends up convinced by his reasons for not agreeing to give her the proprietary product for which she was asking.

Casuistry, as Mark Tonelli emphasises in Section 2 of this book (Chapter 19), is important in all aspects of clinical reasoning whether or not, as in this case, concerned directly with values. As such casuistry provides one of the many links between values-based and evidence-based practice. I return to the wider relationship between values-based practice and ethics below (in the section on philosophy and practice) but it is to the relationship between values-based practice and evidence-based practice that I turn next.

Values-based practice and evidence-based medicine

In contrast with 'anti-ethics', it seems clear from the commentaries that I have been successful in getting across the message that values-based practice is 'pro-EBM'. Richard

Hamilton (p. 96), referring to the name 'values-based practice', calls it 'skilful marketing'. It is rather 'clear marking', that is to say a deliberate and intentionally unambiguous marking of the close partnership between values-based practice and evidence-based medicine as process-focused rather than outcome-focused clinical support tools made necessary by the increasing complexity respectively of the values-base and evidence-base of clinical decision-making.

Hutchinson and Read (Chapter 6) suggest indeed that I am rather *too* close to evidence-based medicine, having as it were taken on the values equivalent of the 'colours of the enemy'. I make no apology for this. It reflects (as discussed further below) my own values too. Before going into psychiatry I did several years of lab-based research working on the immunology and bacteriology of sexually transmitted diseases. It was a great experience and I moved into psychiatry only because my conceptual research interests narrowly trumped my interests in empirical research (I have still unfulfilled research ambitions to work further on the biology of *Treponema pallidum* the paradoxical features of which make it, as I used to call it, the 'philosopher's bacterium'!). So it was definitely a 'plus' for me when, as I described above, the original ('Lucerne protocol') sketch of values-based practice suggested that there were deep links between it and evidence-based medicine.

As to our shared values, however, these are certainly not the shared values of the 'cut-price EBM' that is now evident in so much of practice. As Peile (Chapter 2) describes, EBM properly understood involves a carefully reasoned distillation and weighing of relevant evidence employing tacit as well as explicit clinical skills together with an understanding of relevant values (of clinician and patient) in a process of decision-making that is fully attuned to the particular circumstances of the case in question. So this is a million miles from the cut-price one-size-fits-all rule-book use of evidence-based medicine all too familiar in contemporary practice. The 'positivist' values identified by Hutchinson and Read are the values of this cut-price EBM. Whereas by contrast the very definition of evidence-based medicine given by David Sackett and others in the early days of its development makes clear that cut-price EBM was very far from what he and other trail blazers of the day had in mind: Sackett you will recall from Chapter 1 defined EBM as combining best research evidence with clinical experience and patients' values. And the best of evidence-based practice continues actively to resist cut-pricism: the UK's NICE for example (National Institute for Health and Care Excellence), which is responsible for establishing evidence-based clinical guidelines for the National Health Service, emphasises the importance of making decisions 'appropriate to the circumstances of the individual' which includes their 'individual needs and preferences' (see NICE, 2009, pp. 2 and 4 respectively; reproduced in the context of decision-making in breast cancer in *Essentials*, Chapter 8, Figure 8.2, p. 109).

The partnership in practice

The partnership between values-based practice and evidence-based medicine is reflected in various ways and at different levels in values-based practice. It is actually demanded by the account of values it derives from R. M. Hare: as Thornton (Chapter 4) reminds us, Hare pointed out that the criteria for the value judgements expressed by value terms are *descriptive* criteria. For this if no other reason, therefore, value judgements require the best of evidence. (I return to Hare and values-based practice in the next section.)

Conversely, as Gupta (Chapter 7) points out, evidence-based medicine is deeply value laden. She suggests that I am insensitive to this. But the two feet principle of values-based practice (Chapter 1) is that all decisions are values-based as well as evidence-based. And *all* decisions includes all the decisions that go into the research and development processes with which evidence-based medicine is concerned: these decisions run from the initial selection of research topics through the choice of methods (including controls) to the selection and analysis of data in the generation of 'results' and the derivation from these results of clinical guidelines and the implementation of those guidelines in practice. None of this is news to evidence-based medicine. As I have several times indicated, David Sackett actually defined evidence-based medicine as incorporating patients' values (Chapter 1). Values-based practice extends our understanding of the range and variety of values involved in clinical decision-making (see *Essentials*, Chapter 2). And Gupta underplays the extent to which Sackett follows through on the values part of his definition: whole sections of his book use a version of decision analysis to connect values with evidence in clinical decision-making.

Despite its in-principle importance, there is much still to do in working out exactly how the partnership between values-based and evidence-based approaches should work in practice. This is not for lack of collaboration it should be said. NICE (see above) has been a good partner to values-based practice from the start; and their Citizens' Council represents an innovative approach to incorporating social values into their processes of guideline production. Mila Petrova's work (noted in Chapter 1) on methods for retrieving research literature on health-related values was strongly supported by among others Paul Sutcliffe as an expert on evidence-based medicine and the work was published not in a philosophy or ethics journal but in the *Journal of the American Medical Informatics Association* (Petrova *et al.*, 2011). Iain Chalmers (one of the founders of evidence-based medicine) has a current programme exploring the role of patients in decisions about the initial choice of research priorities (see the James Lind Alliance at www.lindalliance.org). Iain and I both contribute to the philosopher Jeremy Howick's Masters level programme on the history and philosophy of evidence-based medicine (www.conted.ox.ac.uk/B900-77) based on his corresponding book (Howick, 2011). And specifically on implementation (the final stage of the process summarised in the preceding paragraph) there have been substantive developments in both the theory and practice of combining values with evidence in clinical commissioning (Heginbotham, 2012).

The MMR story

An example of the importance of partnership between evidence-based and values-based approaches is Hutchinson and Read's account of the story of the MMR vaccine (Chapter 6, this book). Their account runs essentially thus: the evidence in the MMR story is at least with hindsight overwhelmingly clear; it is true, they point out, that there may have been legitimate concerns at the time; but this they say is just the kind of case where a deliberative forum could support decision-making; and adopting a '*via negativa*' (precautionary) first principle, they continue, would make it 'merely sane' (p. 83) to opt for the MMR triple vaccine.

I do not have space here (nor do I have the knowledge) to go into the pros and cons of this case. But the specifically values-based 'two feet' point goes to Hutchinson and Read's own conclusion that *based on a precautionary first principle* ('first do no harm') there can be no reasonable doubt about the right thing to do. The conclusion is persuasive because the evidence in this case with hindsight really *is* clear. But the 'two feet' point is simply that it is precisely where the evidence *is* clear that it is even more important to look carefully at the operative values. 'Think evidence, think values too!' was the way we summed up its clinical implications in *Essentials* (Chapter 10). There are clearly many values in play in cases such as these. But the 'two feet' point to make about Hutchinson and Read's presentation is that, persuaded as they are by the evidence, they lose sight of how their values (their own precautionary first principle) would have played out at the time from the perspective of those actually concerned, i.e. the parents who on behalf of their children were, literally, on the sharp end of the decision. Far from it being the 'merely sane' conclusion to accept vaccination, if you or I were the parent restraining your own child while a white-coated operative injects them with a foreign substance, the precautionary principle itself would say 'don't do it' unless you really can be sure that whatever good it may do, it will at any rate do no harm. And at the time, as Hutchinson and Read say, you really could not be sure that you (as the child's parent) would not do harm.

Again, to be clear, I am not arguing the case as such. My point is the 'two feet' point about the 'values blindness' that can arise when a persuasive body of evidence is in play. Hutchinson and Read's readiness to call their own view 'merely sane' (and by implication views contrary to their own 'just insane') reflects the fact that, deeply persuaded as they are by the evidence, they lose clear sight of the operative values, including in this case the operation of their own precautionary first principle. Hutchinson and Read will say (they do say, p. 82) that the anti-authoritarian Bill Fulford will resist them on this. And I do. Hutchinson and Read's introduction of deliberative democracy is a welcome illustration of the potential of political philosophy as a resource for values-based practice; and their 'deliberative fora' look in many respects like the 'shared value frameworks' of values-based practice (Chapter 1). But their proposals for the use of 'deliberate force' (p. 80) certainly did raise my anti-authoritarian antenna! And as Thornton notes on my behalf (Chapter 4) at least in mental health the historical evidence is that the use of 'deliberate force' in the exercise of well-intentioned authority has led to some of the worst abuses of psychiatric power (Fulford *et al.*, 2003).

Philosophy and practice

In this section I shift the emphasis of my comments from practice to theory. The shift is only one of emphasis, however, since as will become evident the theme of the section is 'partnership writ large'. The relationship between philosophy and practice, that is to say, is a larger scale version of the two-way partnership by which, as indicated in the preceding section, the relationship between values-based practice and other support tools for clinical decision-making (both evaluative and evidential) is properly characterised.

I will illustrate this partnership-writ-large theme, first with the role of philosophy as a powerful ally in the development of reflective practice, second with the role specifically of ordinary language philosophy as a partner in research and, third, with an indication of how philosophical value theory (as the philosophy most directly underpinning values-based practice) both contributes to and in turn is informed by its partnership with practice.

Philosophy and reflective practice

For many practitioners philosophy seems irrelevant to practice. Stewart (Chapter 12) says values-based practice is 'just' a particular form of psychotherapy. Kingma and Banner (Chapter 3), both professionally trained philosophers, are robust in their rejection not just of the role of philosophy in values-based practice but of philosophy (or at any rate moral philosophy) in practice as a whole: it is just, they say, referring to ethical problem-solving in practice, a matter of looking closely enough at the details of the case in question.

It would be easy to fall into stereotypes here. The engaged physician clear-eyed and confident in decision and action and the withdrawn metaphysician speculating outside the contingent constraints of the way the world actually is, have little to say to each other. Both have their place. But it was a larger place in the nineteenth than in the twentieth let alone the twenty-first century. The complexity (scientific, social and political) of contemporary health care practice means that the reality of today's clinical decision-making is more often uncertainty than clear-eyed certainty. And the failure of foundationalism in philosophy means that contingency (the way the world is) instead of being a constraint on metaphysical speculation is a resource for today's more empirically engaged philosopher. Indeed 'failure' as I have argued elsewhere (Fulford *et al.*, 2013) is the wrong word here: it was instead a *success* for philosophy in the middle decades of the twentieth century (with the work of Wittgenstein, Gödel and others) to show that its own programme of establishing foundations was (not just in practice but in principle) incapable of completion.

This shift of perspective, from failure to success, is important for health care when it comes to 'living with uncertainty' (see below). The net result though of the perceived failure of foundationalism was that the second half of the twentieth century saw the emergence of a whole series of philosophies *of* this or that practical discipline: philosophy of psychiatry was in the 1990s a relative late-comer to the empirical party. The rationale for the turn to practice is neatly captured in what Hutchinson and Read (Chapter 6) say about medicine as a practical discipline not being 'philosophy free': practical disciplines are shaped by largely implicit conceptual frameworks; and to the extent that the framework in question contributes to the complexity of a given field it may be helpful to make the framework explicit and thereby to understand and work with it more effectively (including in some cases changing it). This is part at least of what philosophers working in partnership with practitioners can do. In a sense they are still working on foundations (conceptual rather than metaphysical foundations) but now as a partner with rather than as a precursor to empirical disciplines. This way of working indeed is directly reflected in the 'modest foundationalism' of Miles Little's FAP version of values-based medicine (see our joint concluding Chapter 22).

So today's practitioner struggling with complexity and today's philosopher studying the conceptual contributions to that complexity have a great deal to say to each other. And there are pay-offs from the conversation both ways. As to the pay-off for philosophy, the philosopher Stephen Toulmin (1982) went so far as to say that medicine actually saved the life of ethics: and I return below to the pay-off from the conversation specifically for philosophical value theory. Among pay-offs from the conversation for practice, not the least is the extent to which philosophy supports reflective practice. Faced with an urgent clinical decision there is no time for reflection let alone philosophical reflection. But as Donald Schön (1983) was among the first to point out, the complexities of contemporary health care practice mean that our capacity to act decisively when decisiveness is needed is enhanced by reflection on practice. Reflection and action cannot always go hand in hand. But both are needed. R. M. Hare (1981) made much the same point as a philosopher with his distinction between level-1 (reflective) thinking about moral problems and level-2 (reflexive) decisions and action.

Casuistry and values in clinical care

The importance of reflection to decision and action is illustrated by the role of casuistry in the story outlined above of how values-based practice grew out of engagement between philosophy (my 1980s work in philosophical value theory) and practice (the clinical ethics of the 1990s OPSP). As Gupta notes (Chapter 7), casuistry became prominent in medical ethics over this period. We owe the reintroduction of casuistry into medical ethics to the philosopher Stephen Toulmin (above) and the theologian Albert Jonsen (Jonsen and Toulmin, 1988). Working together in the USA on the National Commission for the Protection of Human Subjects of Biomedical and Behavioral Research, they noted that, consistently with Kingma and Banner's characterisation of ethical problem-solving (above), while there was often wide disagreement on theory, when it came to actual cases everyone was usually in agreement. So far so good: medical ethics, they concluded, should work bottom-up from cases not top-down from theory. As Gupta describes, casuistry has correspondingly become a characteristic feature of clinical ethics. It was also, you will recall, a key component of the OPSP.

But, and this is the key 'but' for reflective practice, even as casuistry was gaining ground in the 1990s the American philosopher Loretta Kopelman (1994, also cited by Gupta) pointed out a snag. There was, she said, a problem of bias, namely that the very effectiveness of casuistry in driving agreement on cases reflected and was dependent on those concerned already having shared albeit usually implicit values. I met Loretta Kopelman at about this time and her ideas as reflected in this paper were a major influence on my own thinking. Her central point, that without an awareness of values the very effectiveness of casuistry in driving agreement on cases puts it at risk of self-confirming bias, goes to the heart of the partnership between clinical ethics and values-based practice: values-based practice needs case-based reasoning as one among other important resources for reasoning about values; but (if Kopelman's point about bias is right) case-based reasoning in turn needs values-based practice to support an explicit attention to the values (the ethical and other values) embedded in and driving any given instance of the use of casuistry in practice.

Bringing the story up to date then, Banner and Kingma are right to point to the power of case-based reasoning. But their proposal to limit reflection on cases to a philosophically uninformed reflection risks leaving us with a cut-price casuistry not fit for purpose in the complexities of contemporary clinical practice. Kingma and Banner's challenge though is not just to moral philosophy but to ordinary language philosophy. So where does ordinary language philosophy fit into the picture?

Ordinary language philosophy and research in health care

Ordinary language philosophy as I described in Chapter 1 starts from the observation well made here by Brecher of the limitations of definition as a guide to meaning. Brecher's example (p. 63) makes the point with neat economy: the 'pint' as a measure of fluid volume is (operationally at least) readily definable; but there is a good deal more to its meaning when used in a context such as 'fancy a pint?'. A 'philosophy of pints', correspondingly, concerned to explore the concept of 'a pint' and limiting itself to definition, would be working with an artificially restricted data set likely to lead to a narrow or distorted understanding of its full meaning. So, as Austin and others of the ordinary language school might have put it, one way to get started with a 'philosophy of pints' is to explore the ordinary use of the term: the idea is to get out of the armchair of philosophical reflection on meaning (understood as an extended exercise in definition) and to expand the data set for a 'philosophy of pints' by starting with a study of how 'pint' is actually used across a range of everyday non-philosophical contexts.

This is the essence of Austin's 'philosophical fieldwork' (Fulford and van Staden, 2013). It is the essence too of why as I argued in my (1990) article on the 'Oxford connection' ordinary language philosophy is a natural partner to empirical research. We have moreover at least one 'proof of product' of such mixed methods research in Colombo's work (Colombo *et al.*, 2003, see Chapter 1; the contribution of philosophy to that work is described in our paper, Fulford and Colombo, 2004). Why, then, it is natural to ask, are Kingma and Banner so un-persuaded?

Kicked upstairs?

Austin once complained that philosophy was unfairly stigmatised as being practically ineffective because whenever it threw off a practically effective product its role as progenitor was conveniently forgotten: it was as he put it 'kicked upstairs' (Warnock, 1989, p. 4; Austin had in mind such high profile spin-offs from philosophy as mathematics and natural science).

There is something of philosophy being 'kicked upstairs' in the dismissive line that Banner and Kingma and indeed others (Stewart) take on its role in values-based practice. I hope I have filled in enough of the story of values-based practice to indicate the extent to which values-based practice has been in Austin's terms 'thrown off' by philosophy. There are no doubt other routes to values-based practice: the philosopher Roger Crisp (2013) has made just this point in respect of the resources of Ancient Philosophy, a resource that is also drawn on to rather different effect by Hamilton in this volume (Chapter 8); there is to my mind an interesting and potentially fruitful route to values-based practice via the philosophy of science (see below); and there are non-philosophical routes as well (via decision analysis for example). But these different routes enrich rather than diminish values-based practice. Sure, my route was via the ordinary language philosophy of the language of values applied to the language of medicine. But it is a characteristic of any open and developing research-led field of enquiry that to any given 'product' there will be more than one route. That there is currently an expanding range of theories of gravity in no way diminishes the theory of relativity and to the contrary enriches physics. And whatever the role of ordinary language philosophy in the origins of values-based practice, it is as a contribution to the future of the field as an open and research-led discipline that I believe it has a continuing and indeed decisive role to play.

New horizons

The role of ordinary language philosophy, it is important to say straight away, is limited. I emphasised this in Chapter 1 and have spelled out the message in many other places (see e.g. Fulford and van Staden, 2013). But the point bears emphasis if only because, as I indicate in this section, it is as much through its self-set limitations as through any positive virtues that ordinary language philosophy makes a good partner in research. Thus, ordinary language philosophy is limited in that it is appropriate only for problems of or including conceptual issues (problems of meaning and understanding); for any such problem it is a 'first step' only; methodologically it works best with partners bringing skills and experience relevant to the area in which the problem in question arises (mixed methods are the norm); and its outputs are always a 'more complete' rather than 'full and final' understanding of the conceptual issues in question.

Each of these limitations of ordinary language philosophy will be important in future mixed methods studies if we are to meet the challenges presented by the particular Austinian 'field' of working with values in health care. And the challenges are to my mind scary: they are scarily complex and scarily life-threatening. This is directly illustrated by the new horizons for research opened up by two of the commentators in this book.

Unconscious values

A scarily complex new horizon is opened up by Harry Lesser's chapter (Chapter 10) on unconscious values. The environment of values-based practice as it has developed to date, namely the consultation between clinician and patient, recognises and indeed focuses on what might be called pre-conscious values: in *Essentials*, in Chapter 1, we called these 'background' as opposed to foreground values; and the story line of that chapter (and later episodes in the same story, in Chapters 2 and 14) illustrate how critical it may be to balanced clinical decision-making to move these background values from the pre-conscious to consciousness. Lesser, however, takes us to a whole new level of difficulty with values that are not merely pre-conscious but unconscious and hence subject to denial and other active defence mechanisms.

That the issues here are (in part but crucially) conceptual in nature is shown by the psychoanalyst Robert Hinshelwood's work on the implications for ethics of the Kleinian concepts of identification, introjection and projection (Hinshelwood, 1995, 1997). But what Lesser's chapter and Hinshelwood's work both show is that while conceptual research on unconscious values is necessary, it will not be sufficient unless carried out in a mixed methods partnership with analysts, a partnership of the kind to which ordinary language philosophy is particularly well suited.

Global values

Scary indeed, then, are the conceptual issues raised by unconscious values. But they are not half as scarily life-threatening as the issues for values-based practice in global health raised by Sridhar Venkatapuram (Chapter 11). Venkatapuram starts from the fact that values-based practice has developed to date mainly as a resource for clinical decision-making in the individual clinician-patient consultation. But the action in health care he points out is moving away from the individual to society. He draws here, as he puts it in his book *Health Justice* (Venkatapuram, 2011, p. 80), on the shoulders of giants: giants in epidemiology (like Michael Marmot) and giants in philosophically informed economics (like the collaboration between Martha Nussbaum and Amartya Sen). The message of these giants is that any sufficient theory of health justice must start from the brute if inconvenient fact that best evidence now strongly suggests that the burden of disease is predominantly a social-collective rather than biological-individual burden. Correspondingly therefore if values-based practice is to contribute to its own bottom line as a health-related discipline it too must shift (or at any rate widen) its focus from the individual to the collective.

Clearly I do not have space here to respond adequately to Venkatapuram any more than to Lesser. But by way of a promissory note towards future collaboration I welcome Venkatapuram's encouraging comments to the effect that values-based practice, notwithstanding its focus to date on the individual, could have a role in global health. There are indications that a partnership between our programmes may be timely. First, the issues with which he is concerned are in part conceptual and hence appropriate in principle for ordinary language philosophy as a partner in a mixed methods research paradigm: in his *Health Justice* for example he zeros in on concepts of disorder. Second, there are initiatives in values-based practice itself that are starting to move beyond the individual to the collective: in the UK there have been the developments in values-based commissioning (noted above); Stewart (Chapter 12) notes recent encouraging educational work in Mexico (Altamirano-Bustamante *et al.*, 2013); Ed Peile and David Davies from Warwick Medical School have used values-based methods in their work in Malawi training non-clinical workers in obstetric care (the training materials can be viewed on the project website at http://etatmba.org); and Werdie van Staden is working with colleagues in Africa to develop a distinctively African values-based practice ('Batho Pele') that, building as it does on African philosophies and practices, is distinctive precisely in that it is a social-collective rather than individual form of values-based practice (van Staden and Fulford, forthcoming).

A third encouraging development for collaborative work on health justice is in what might be called values-based economics. The Department of Health in the UK for example has a health economics based programme actually called value-based pricing (www.2020selection.co.uk/images/pdfs/value-based-pricing.pdf). Internationally, too, there is a growing move away from the traditional GDP (Gross Domestic Product) as a measure of economic progress to broader metrics such as the Genuine Progress Indicator (GPI, see e.g. Anielski and Soskolne, 2001). The GDP reflects only the volume of money in circulation. The GPI and similar measures are more broadly values-based in that they incorporate and balance a wide range of both environmental and social costs and benefits of economic growth as key aspects of wellbeing. Flourishing, to anticipate the discussion of Miles Little's values-based medicine in Section 2 of this book, is absent from the GDP but at the very heart of the GPI.

Philosophical value theory and its two-way relationship with practice

Understood as ordinary language philosophy applied to the language of values, everything in the above two subsections applies equally to philosophical value theory. There are however two additional points to make arising from the commentaries, respectively about (1) the values in values-based practice, and (2) the premise of values-based practice.

The values in values-based practice

Bob Brecher, mindful of the limitations of definition (above), asks for at least a 'minimal characterisation' (p. 63) of the values in values-based practice. It is this that philosophical value theory provides. Indeed every 'three words that mean values to you' exercise (see Chapter 1) produces a (locally) minimal characterisation of the values in values-based practice, a local 'logical geography' as the Oxford philosopher Gilbert Ryle (1963, p. 10) might have called it. Clearly, and consistently with the limited aims of ordinary language philosophy, such local logical geographies are very far from being a *complete* characterisation of the meaning of 'values' still less a definition of the term. But just in being 'local' they are fit for purpose in that as training exercises they allow trainer and trainees to start from where any given group 'is at'.

Where groups are 'at' furthermore is, as Figure 1.2 (Chapter 1) illustrates, a wide range of meanings of 'values': I have never yet run a training group where the range of meanings of 'values' the group came up with was any less diverse than that shown in Figure 1.2. It is thus appropriate that this ordinary (i.e. non-philosophical) multi-faceted use of the term 'values' is also the way the term is used in values-based practice. For values-based practice too engages at the level of ordinary usage: it is concerned with balanced decision-making in ordinary health care (not philosophical) contexts. For this reason therefore if for no other the 'values' in values-based practice is a generic use of the term covering a diverse range of meanings rather than being restricted for example to 'virtues' (as suggested by Hamilton, Chapter 8).

Generic use but also action guiding

A natural question that groups always come up with faced with this diversity of meanings is 'so just what *are* values?' This is why without attempting to define the term as such, in values-based practice values are further characterised following R. M. Hare as being 'prescriptive' or action guiding (Hare, 1952). While not exhaustive, this part of the meaning of 'values' makes sense to action-oriented health care practitioners and it is consistent with the way the term is used with other decision support tools (clinical ethics, decision analysis, health economics and Sacket's non-cut-price version of evidence-based practice). As Thornton describes (Chapter 4), Hare's characterisation of values makes sense in a number of further health care respects: one example, noted earlier, is the way Hare's observation that value terms express (implicit or explicit) value judgements the criteria for which are descriptive in nature, links values-based practice semantically with evidence-based medicine.

Generic use and inclusive practice

It is on the 'generic rather than specific' that I both agree and disagree with Hamilton on virtues. I agree (as most would agree) that the virtues are important in health care and not just as it were contemporary head-line virtues such as 'truth' and 'justice'. Understood as aspects of a practitioner's personality or character, virtues such as the capacity for empathy are widely and appropriately valued in health care and correspondingly have been among the entry requirements for and/or aims of professional training (see for example Hilton and Slotnick, 2005). But as the philosopher William May pointed out many years ago, mediaeval theology offers a sophisticated understanding of and tradition of working with a whole range of other and now neglected virtues with *prima facie* relevance to the demands of contemporary health care (May, 1994). May notes for example virtues such as 'memoria' meaning '. . . being true to the past', 'docility' which in this tradition is '. . .openness to the present, the ability to be still, to be silent, to listen' and 'solertia' meaning 'readiness for the unexpected' (May, 1994, pp. 85–86). The Anglican theologian Robert Atwell has made a similar point about the resources of the Christian tradition of spiritual direction (Atwell and Fulford, 2006). Furthermore, the virtues noted by Atwell illustrate the deep connections between virtue theory and values-based practice. The virtue of 'discernment' in spiritual direction, for example, as it comes into one of the stories in *Essentials* (Chapter 12), is the key to the way an ex-Benedictine parish priest, Benedict Brown, helps a couple through the traumas of IVF treatment.

So like Hamilton I say 'three cheers' for virtues in health care. But the 'three cheers' of values-based practice is both more inclusive and less exclusive than Hamilton would have us be. It is more inclusive in that, as just noted, it extends well beyond the virtues on which bioethics has tended to focus. This is indeed a somewhat under-developed aspect of the extended values-awareness of values-based practice, i.e. that awareness should extend also to values other than those traditionally recognised to be important in health care. Hare for example included aesthetic values as being action guiding. Later work however in such areas as 'connective aesthetics' (Gablik, 1992) and 'social sculpture' (Sacks, 2011) suggests that aesthetic values are better understood as enlarging the reflective framework of action. Aesthetic values that is to say, in enlarging our powers of perception, help us to come to a richer understanding of ourselves and others that goes beyond intellectual knowledge alone. Characterised by the psychiatrist and artist Helena Fox as moving us on 'from anaesthetic to aesthetic' (see http://inter-disciplinary.net/probing-the-boundaries/wp-content/uploads/2013/02/Fox.pdf), this richer understanding has potential clinical applications in improving empathic care (Musalek, 2010; Hughes and Beatty, 2013).

The generic use of 'values', furthermore, is also less exclusive in that it renders values-based practice open to learning from the way values are worked with in other non-health care disciplines. Hamilton is dismissive in particular of grocers and stock market traders. I have never been either. But (again, working with partners) I do have substantive (i.e. risk sharing) experience in other areas of commerce and this has taught me first-hand that the knowledge, skills and application required to 'turn a profit' are at least equal to their counterparts in health care. There are moreover among stock market traders those who have given thought to what amounts to a values-based approach that aims to build profits from value rather than value-less profits (Williams, 2011). Certainly, health care in general and values-based practice in particular has much to learn from business in areas such as conflict resolution (Fulford and Bennington, 2004).

Not values-free

The observation that the term 'values' is used in the generic sense just outlined might be taken to mean (as Brecher for example suggests) that values-based practice is or assumes itself to be somehow values neutral. This would be wrong. I come to the value-status of the premise of values-based practice below. But the premise aside, as Calder (p. 118) rightly points out, there are self-evident value commitments shaping values-based practice such as 'openness towards outcomes [and] sensitivity to context'.

I agree with Calder and I own just those values. They are though epistemic values not special to values-based practice but shared by any open and undogmatic heuristic including (in any non-cut-price version) evidence-based medicine. So it is indeed the case as Calder says that to the extent of such epistemic values values-based practice is *not* value-free. The point is rather (as I have said elsewhere, Fulford, 2013) that there is nothing in values-based practice itself that requires you to sign up to these values. It offers a process for balanced decision-making where complex and conflicting values are in play: this process includes the contingent constraints of the locally defined frameworks of shared values described in Chapter 1 and the analytic constraints of its premise. But there is nothing in values-based practice itself requiring anyone to sign up to its own epistemic values. If you sign up to these values well and good; if you do not sign up to them you cannot be a values-based practitioner, but neither can you be an evidence-based practitioner.

Expertise and competence

This feature of values-based practice makes problematic, as Calder also points out, the notion of good and bad values-based practice. Limitations of space mean that I must offer a second promissory note here rather than being able to take up adequately the implications of his careful development of the distinction between expertise and competence in relation to training in values-based practice. This is a promissory note on which Ed Peile as a medical educator is anyway better qualified to deliver. But the distinction certainly looks helpful to me. It makes clear in particular why, as Peile says, practitioners may find they have many of the skills of values-based practice already. This is not just a 'word of encouragement' as Calder (p. 118) generously puts it. It is true that many practitioners are naturally competent in this or that aspect of values-based practice. And not just practitioners: the most comprehensively competent values-based practitioner in *Essentials* is the (real life) 'cleaner who cared' in our postscript (p. 203). Indeed values-based practice as we emphasise in *Essentials* (p. 202) is all about building on good practice as thus exemplified. This is why the initial response of practitioners is often to say 'but that's just what we do!' Stewart (Chapter 12) sees in values-based practice nothing more than what from his description sounds like the very best of psychotherapeutic practice. Palliative care clinicians see their own best practice in values-based practice (Fulford and Cooper, 2013).

There is still room for the expert, however. Expertise in values-based practice includes expertise in building on and extending these exemplars: it thus involves expertise in such areas as recognising good practice (balanced decision-making) when you see it; joining exemplars up in a coherent overall framework; seeing how the framework fits with other aspects of practice; understanding the underlying (philosophical and empirical) theory; knowing how to extend good practice through training; and so forth. And if values-based practice were indeed 'just' best practice in this or that discipline, best practice is surely far from the norm. So if the values-based expert achieved nothing more than helping to advance best practice, he or she would have earned their crust.

Fulford and Hare

So there is a good deal to Brecher's (rightly) required minimal characterisation of 'values' that we can take from R. M. Hare and indeed others of the Oxford School. It is not true though, as several commentators suggest, that I am a Hare-man through and through. It is what might be called the small print in Hare's work on which values-based practice draws (as above; see also Thornton, Chapter 4, on the important link between diverse values and visible values) rather than the large print of his 'universal prescription' account of moral values. This brings us directly to the premise of values-based practice.

The premise of values-based practice

My personal biggest learning point from the commentaries is a significant shift (from the particular to the general) in how the premise of values-based practice (in mutual respect for differences of values) is derived (analytically) from the moves and counter-moves in theoretical ethics on the nature of values in general, usually called the 'is-ought' debate.

Sadly, all I have space to offer here on this learning point is a third promissory note towards future collaborative R&D. 'Sadly', because, besides being my personal biggest learning point,

(1) the premise in question is the theoretical heart of value-based practice,

(2) as such it is also at the heart of an Ariadne golden thread running through this book as a whole about the need in practice for 'answers' (I get back to this in my conclusions below and Miles Little and I return to it in our joint concluding chapter, Chapter 22),

(3) the R&D in question brings me back to my own philosophical research roots in philosophical value theory, and

(4) the outcomes of it are (potentially) a win-win for philosophy and practice in that not only does practice benefit from engagement with philosophy but philosophy also benefits from engagement with practice.

One instance of that collaboration is a further stage in a long-standing dialogue with Tim Thornton: see for example Tim's special issue of the journal I edit (*Philosophy, Psychiatry and Psychology*, Thornton, 2008) and Michael Loughlin's earlier edited collection in the *Journal of Evaluation in Clinical Practice* (Loughlin, 2011). As in his chapter in this book, Tim takes a more 'world responsive' line on values in contrast to my more 'world independent' view. Both views fit within the 'is-ought' debate, dating back as it does to the eighteenth century empiricist philosopher David Hume's (world independent) position 'no ought from an is'. Two centuries on I became directly involved in the debate during my DPhil with two terms of supervision in the care of R. M. Hare (world independent, as in Hare, 1952) followed by three terms with Hare's immediate (world responsive) opponent G. J. Warnock (as in Warnock, 1971). Chapter 3 in *Moral Theory and Medical Practice* (Fulford, 1989) presents in the form of a debate what I learned from this unique (and wonderful) experience. Several chapters in this book draw directly or indirectly on the is-ought debate (for example in the various discussions of emotivism).

The fact that the debate continues with salient points on both sides but without any promise of a near end is itself, however, both significant and a good thing too! Yes, a good thing for practice and a good thing for philosophy, a win-win indeed as I put it above. But to see exactly why, you will need to read more of the continuing story. The cast includes Putnam, Quine and Strawson; the setting is an agentic (action-based) as opposed to function-based account of mental disorder; and the (ordinary language) hero is the descriptive psychopathology of delusion. In the story, philosophy benefits from partnership with practice because the descriptive psychopathology of delusion turns out not only to keep the is-ought debate open and undecided but to propel it in new directions including the philosophy of science, the nature of rationality and theories of personal identity. So there is a win here for philosophy. But there is a win for practice (or at any rate values-based practice) too. For it allows the premise of values-based practice to be grounded not (as I have previously argued, as in Fulford, 2013) on the failure of descriptivism within the is-ought debate, but rather on the undecided (hence still open) status of the is-ought debate as a whole. And like any good serial, the last episode ends with a tantaliser: the possibility that a particular feature of the descriptive psychopathology of delusion, to wit the paradoxical delusion of mental illness, points Gödel-like to the possibility that the is-ought debate may be not merely contingently but essentially undecidable.

Living with uncertainty

Bertrand Russell, summing up the message of his monumental *The History of Western Philosophy* completed soon after the end of the Second World War, wrote that 'To teach how to live without certainty, and yet without being paralysed by hesitation, is perhaps the chief thing that philosophy, in our age, can still do for those who study it' (Russell, 1946, p. 14). As a young man Russell was among what in the *Oxford Textbook of Philosophy and Psychiatry* were called, in virtue of their grandiose foundational claims for philosophy (Russell, 1912), 'manic philosophers' (Fulford, *et al.*, 2006, p. 114). But the young Russell was a Russell who had not yet hit the full turmoil of his personal life, nor in the public realm the realities of Nazism; and this was the Russell too who as a philosopher still believed that he and A. N. Whitehead had finally got to 'the truth' about the foundations of mathematics (Gödel's incompleteness theorems were still nearly twenty years off). The Russell of *The History of Western Philosophy* then, the 'living with uncertainty' Russell, had hit, just as values-based practice hits, what Stewart (p. 147) calls the 'turmoil' of life.

Russell's message in *The History of Western Philosophy* has not been widely heard. This is important for values-based practice since it contains a warning that it too, and for the same reason, may not be widely heard. This is essentially because the shift from the early Russell-of-foundations to the later Russell-of-uncertainty is a shift, as values-based practice is a shift, from answers (the foundations of *x* are *y*) to process ('to teach (learn?) how to live . . .'). And the one thing that a majority of commentators have in common is a shared concern precisely about the shift in values-based practice from foundations (the right way to practice *x* is *y*) to process (a process based on learnable clinical skills). This concern indeed is shared equally by friends as by foes: it underpins for example Thornton's 'all a bit *too* radical' view; and it leads Venkatapuram to call for values-based practice to 'take a position' (p. 140) in global health contexts. And I may well have reinforced everyone's concerns with the Gödel-linked undecidability end point reached at the end of the last section.

There are though reasons to hope that within health care at least values-based practice *will* be heard. The operative point is that values-based practice contrary to the 'anything goes' claims of some of the commentators, in fact *does* give answers. True, the answers given by values-based practice, as my examples in Chapter 1 illustrate (such as the training materials for the UK's Mental health Act 2007), are 'little and local' rather than universally applicable but they are answers nonetheless. Also, the circumstances in which values-based practice gives its little-and-local answers are just those envisaged by Russell, namely of 'living with uncertainty'. As I indicated earlier, uncertainty, not certainty, is the norm in contemporary health care practice. Uncertainty in the evidence-base of practice is why we need the processes of evidence-based practice to support clinical decision-making. Uncertainty in the values-base of clinical decision-making is why we need the processes of values-based practice to support clinical decision-making. Advances in science and technology furthermore, as I indicated in my discussion of the 'science driven' principle in Chapter 1, far from resolving either kind of uncertainty will inevitably increase both.

The urgent need in contemporary health care practice is therefore precisely anticipated by Russell. The need is for nothing more nor less than 'to live without certainty, and yet without being paralysed by hesitation'. This may not be as Russell believed the chief thing that philosophy has to teach us. But it is what values-based practice teaches us. And judged by the needs of contemporary health care practice it is, to this little-and-local extent, a good thing.

First-person plural

As I indicated at the start of this chapter, if there is one word that sums up the commentaries on values-based practice in this section it is 'diversity'. This is why my response has inevitably amounted to what may seem something of a scatter-gram. I have picked up many but not all of the substantive points made by the commentators: and I have responded to some points more fully than to others. There are further points, practical and theoretical, that others may feel are missing altogether: 'do we have time for all this?' is a commonly asked question among practitioners that as far as I can see has not been raised in this predominantly philosopher-focused context.

Clearly, my selection of topics and extent of their respective treatments reflects my own particular perspective. My response is in this sense necessarily a first-person response. But that it is also a first-person plural response will be evident in the extent of my debt to the commentators, not only for many important points of clarification but also in no less than three promissory notes towards future R&D collaborations with partners with very different knowledge and skills from my own. Such collaborations, it is worth adding, have been the hall-mark of the story of values-based practice as (partly) recounted here. There is indeed almost nothing in this story to which I can claim unique intellectual property rights. I believe I was the first to spot the conceptual significance of evaluative delusions (Fulford, 1989, Chapter 10). But beyond that even the initial and key step of applying philosophical value theory to the language of medicine I owe to my DPhil supervisor Mary Warnock. It was (I think) in our very first supervision that she suggested this. I had, as many of us do when starting a doctorate, grandiose plans to 'solve' the is-ought debate and I remember my reply was something on the lines of 'yes, that would make a good first chapter'. Some first chapter!

References

Allott, P., Fulford, K. W. M., Fleming, B., Williamson, T. and Woodbridge, K. (2005) Recovery, values and e-learning. *Mental Health Review*, **10**(4), 34–38.

Altamirano-Bustamante, M. M., Altamirano-Bustamante, N. F. and Lifshitz, A. *et al.* (2013) Promoting networks between evidence-based medicine and values-based medicine in continuing medical education. *BMC Medicine*, **11**(1), 39.

Anielski, M. and Soskolne, C. (2001) Genuine progress indicator (GPI) accounting: relating ecological integrity to human health and well-being. In Miller, P. and Westra, L. (editors), *Just Ecological Integrity: The Ethics of Maintaining Planetary Life*, Chapter 9, pp. 83–97. Lanham, MD: Rowman and Littlefield.

Atwell, R. and Fulford, K. W. M. (2006) The Christian tradition of spiritual direction as a sketch for a strong theology of diversity. In Cox, J., Campbell, A. V. and

Fulford, K. W. M. (editors), *Medicine of the Person: Faith, Science and Values in Health Care Provision*, Chapter 6, pp. 83–95. London: Jessica Kingsley Publishers.

Colombo, A., Bendelow, G., Fulford, K. W. M. and Williams, S. (2003) Evaluating the influence of implicit models of mental disorder on processes of shared decision making within community-based multidisciplinary teams. *Social Science & Medicine*, **56**, 1557–1570.

Crisp, R. (2013) Commentary: values-based practice by a different route. In Fulford, K. W. M., Davies, M., Gipps, R., Graham, G., Sadler, J., Stanghellini, G. and Thornton, T. (editors), *The Oxford Handbook of Philosophy and Psychiatry*, pp. 411–412. Oxford: Oxford University Press.

Dickenson, D. and Fulford, K. W. M. (2000) *In Two Minds: A Casebook of Psychiatric Ethics*. Oxford: Oxford University Press.

Fulford, K. W. M. (1989, reprinted 1995 and 1999) *Moral Theory and Medical Practice*. Cambridge: Cambridge University Press.

Fulford, K. W. M. (1990) Philosophy and medicine: the Oxford connection. *British Journal of Psychiatry*, **157**, 111–115.

Fulford, K. W. M. (1994) Diverse ethics. In Fulford, K. W. M., Gillett, G. and Soskice, J. (editors), *Medicine and Moral Reasoning*. Cambridge: Cambridge University Press.

Fulford, K. W. M. (2013) Values-based practice: Fulford's dangerous idea. *Journal of Evaluation in Clinical Practice*, **19**(3), 537–546.

Fulford, K. W. M. and Benington, J. (2004) VBM²: a collaborative values-based model of healthcare decision-making combining medical and management perspectives. In Williams, R. and Kerfoot, M. (editors), *Child and Adolescent Mental Health Services: Strategy, Planning, Delivery, and Evaluation*, pp. 89–102. Oxford: Oxford University Press.

Fulford, K. W. M. and Colombo, A. (2004) Six models of mental disorder: a study combining linguistic-analytic and empirical methods. *Philosophy, Psychiatry, and Psychology*, **11**(2), 129–144.

Fulford, K. W. M. and Cooper, J. (2013) 'Why me?' and 'Whose good death?': anger and values-based practice in end of life care. In Gilbert, P. (editor), *Spirituality and End of Life Care*, Chapter 3, pp. 61–70. Hove: Pavilion House and Media.

Fulford, K. W. M. and van Staden, W. (2013) Values-based practice: topsy-turvy take home messages from ordinary language philosophy (and a few next steps). In Fulford, K. W. M., Davies, M., Gipps, R., Graham, G., Sadler, J., Stanghellini, G. and Thornton, T. (editors), *The Oxford Handbook of Philosophy and Psychiatry*, Chapter 26, pp. 385–412. Oxford: Oxford University Press.

Fulford, K. W. M., Dickenson, D. and Murray, T. H. (editors) (2002) *Healthcare Ethics and Human Values: An Introductory Text with Readings and Case Studies*. Oxford: Blackwell Publishers.

Fulford, K. W. M., Morris, K. J., Sadler, J. Z. and Stanghellini, G. (2003) Past improbable, future possible: the renaissance in philosophy and psychiatry. In

Fulford, K. W. M., Morris, K. J., Sadler, J. Z. and Stanghellini, G. (editors), *Nature and Narrative: an Introduction to the New Philosophy of Psychiatry*, Chapter 1, pp. 1–41. Oxford: Oxford University Press.

Fulford, K. W. M., Thornton, T. and Graham, G. (2006) *The Oxford Textbook of Philosophy and Psychiatry*. Oxford: Oxford University Press.

Fulford, K. W. M., Peile, E. and Carroll, H. (2012) *Essential Values-Based Practice: clinical stories linking science with people*. Cambridge: Cambridge University Press.

Fulford K. W. M., Davies, M., Gipps, R. *et al.* (2013) The next hundred years: watching our ps and qs. In Fulford, K. W. M., Davies, M., Gipps, R., Graham, G., Sadler, J., Stanghellini, G. and Thornton, T. (editors), *The Oxford Handbook of Philosophy and Psychiatry*, Chapter 1, pp. 1–11. Oxford: Oxford University Press.

Gablik, S. (1992) Connective aesthetics. *American Art*, **6**(2), 2–7.

Hare, R. M. (1952) *The Language of Morals*. Oxford: Oxford University Press.

Hare, R. M. (1981) *Moral Thinking: its Levels, Method, and Point*. Oxford: Clarendon Press.

Heginbotham, C. (2012) *Values-Based Commissioning of Health and Social Care*. Cambridge: Cambridge University Press.

Hilton, S. R. and Slotnick, H. B. (2005) Proto-professionalism – how professionalism occurs across the continuum of medical education. *Medical Education* **39**(1), 58–65.

Hinshelwood, R. D. (1995) The social relocation of personal identity as shown by psychoanalytic observations of splitting, projection and introjection. *Philosophy, Psychiatry, and Psychology*, **2**, 185–204.

Hinshelwood, R. D. (1997) Primitive mental processes: psychoanalysis and the ethics of integration. *Philosophy, Psychiatry, and Psychology*, **4**(2), 121–144.

Hope, T., Fulford, K. W. M. and Yates, A. (1996) *The Oxford Practice Skills Course: Ethics, Law and Communication Skills in Health Care Education*. Oxford: Oxford University Press.

Howick, J. (2011) *The Philosophy of Evidence-Based Medicine: a philosophical inquiry*. Oxford: Blackwell-Wiley.

Hughes, J. C. and Beatty, A. (2013) Understanding the person with dementia: a clinicophilosophical case discussion.

Advances in Psychiatric Treatment, **19**, 337–343.

Jonsen, A. R. and Toulmin, S. (1988) *The Abuse of Casuistry: a History of Moral Reasoning.* California: University of California Press.

Kopelman, L. M. (1994) Case method and casuistry: the problem of bias. *Theoretical Medicine*, **15**(1), 21–38.

Loughlin, M. (editor) (2011) Special issue. *Journal of Evaluation and Clinical Practice*, **17**(5).

May, W. F. (1994) The virtues in a professional setting. In Fulford, K. W. M., Gillett, G. R., and Soskice, J. M. (editors), *Medicine and Moral Reasoning*, Chapter 7, pp. 75–90. Cambridge: Cambridge University Press.

Musalek, M. (2010) Social aesthetics and the management of addiction. *Current Opinion in Psychiatry*, **23**, 530–535.

NICE (2009) *Early and Locally Advanced Breast Cancer: Diagnosis and Treatment.* NICE Clinical Guidelines 80. London: National Institute for Health and Clinical Excellence. (Renamed, National Institute for Health and Care Excellence.)

Perry/James/NSUN, Report on VBC. Available at: www.nsun.org.uk/news/taking-nsun-values-to-oxford-and-cambridge/.

Petrova, M., Sutcliffe, P., Fulford, K. W. M. and Dale, J. (2011) Search terms and a validated brief search filter to retrieve publications on health-related values in Medline: a word frequency analysis study. *Journal of the American Medical Informatics Association*, doi:10.1136/amiajnl-2011-000243.

Ryle, G. (1963, first published 1949) *The Concept of Mind.* London: Penguin Books.

Russell, B. (1912) The value of philosophy. *The Problems of Philosophy*, Chapter XV, pp. 237–250. London: Williams and Norgate.

Russell, B. (1946) *The History of Western Philosophy.* London: George Allen and Unwin.

Sacks, S. (2011) Social sculpture and new organs of perception: new practices and new pedagogy for a humane and ecologically viable future. In Lerm-Hays, L. I. Y. (editor), *Beuysian Legacies in Ireland and Beyond, European Studies in Culture and Policy*, pp. 80–98.

Schön, D. A. (1983) *The Reflective Practitioner: How Professionals Think in Action.* London: Maurice Temple Smith.

Thornton, T. (editor) (2008) Special issue on evidence-based and values-based practice. *Philosophy, Psychiatry, and Psychology*, **15**(2).

Toulmin, S. (1982) How medicine saved the life of ethics. *Perspectives in Biology and Medicine*, **25**, 736–750.

van Staden, W. and Fulford, K. W. M. (forthcoming) In Sadler, J. Z., Fulford, K. W. M. and Van Staden, W. (editors), *The Oxford Handbook of Psychiatric Ethics.* Oxford: Oxford University Press.

Venkatapuram, S. (2011) *Health Justice: an Argument from the Capabilities Approach.* Cambridge: Polity Press.

Warnock, G. J. (1971) *The Object of Morality.* London: Methuen.

Warnock, G. J. (1989) *J. L. Austin.* London: Routledge.

Williams, G. (2011) *Slow Finance: Why Investment Miles Matter.* London: Bloomsbury Publishing.

Chapter

14 Values, foundations and being human

Miles Little

Values

The word 'values' is widely used, and it is usually assumed that everyone knows what you mean when you use it. It refers to certain commitments to which you hold, certain attributes that guide behaviour and underpin your judgements. Your values are important, and when you are asked to do something that contradicts those values, you feel uneasy. You may make a stand, refuse to act, or you may act in ways that are personally inconvenient, threatening or risky in order to stick to your values, to be consistent with their demands.

That seems simple enough, but there are already some uncertainties. How do values, construed in these terms, differ from virtues or altruism or ethical behaviour? Does the branch of philosophy called axiology have anything more to say about our judgements than ethics and aesthetics reveal? Why has axiology waxed and waned in fashion and importance over the years? Is there any value for the philosophy or practice of medicine in exploring axiology? I think there is, and in this chapter I want to explore four things:

(1) a particular view of values as 'first philosophy' of social organisation and interaction;
(2) a formulation of foundationalism that is descriptive and pre-normative, rather than prescriptive and normative;
(3) a way to understand health care as grounded in foundational values that are expressed in different ways in different cultures and societies; and

Debates in Values-Based Practice, ed. Michael Loughlin. Published by Cambridge University Press. © Cambridge University Press 2014.

(4) an explanation of the potential contributions that a values-based medicine of this kind might make to medical philosophy, practice, policy and education.

Values as first social philosophy

I need to explain what I mean by the word values, as I and my colleagues have done elsewhere (Little *et al.*, 2012). They are not the same as preferences. Preferences may express values, but preferences are not values *per se*. Values for me are the end-points of iterative enquiry, a series of questions that keep asking for justifications until there is no answer except something like 'Because that is the way humans are', or 'Because societies cannot function any other way.' This leads to a naturalistic conception of values, and it follows the method of Hume's enquiry into the justifications of activities like exercise (Hume, 1991):

> Ask a man *why he uses exercise*; he will answer, *because he desires to keep his health*. If you then enquire, *why he desires health*, he will readily reply, *because sickness is painful*. If you push your enquiries further, and desire a reason *why he hates pain*, it is impossible that he can ever give any. This is an ultimate end, and is never referred to any other object...And beyond this it is an absurdity to ask for a reason. It is impossible that there can be a progress *in infinitum*; and that one thing can always be a reason why another is desired. Something must be desirable on its own account, and because of its immediate accord or agreement with human sentiment and affection. (Hume, 2004 (1777), p. 293)

It is also naturalistic in the Darwinian sense because it acknowledges that what allows us to survive and even flourish is what we do to make us fit best into the contexts of our world (Darwin, 1999).

Biographical interviews tell us a great deal about the things that people value, give great importance to, use to sustain their lives at critical times, to establish their identities, to guide them through ethical and other quandaries, and they reveal, directly and indirectly, the things they hold important. Analysis of such interviews over many years suggests that values might best be understood as processual, rather than as static personal attributes or psychosocial entities (Little *et al.*, 2012). To understand this better, it may be useful to trace an example of values-as-process, using a Humean iterative approach, asking questions until there appears to be no further than we can usefully go.

Most will agree that our Western societies value health services. Why? Because they provide ways and means for preserving and regaining good health. Who cares about good health? We all do, because illness and disease are unpleasant, painful, dangerous and potentially expensive to individuals and to society. They involve suffering. But why is suffering important? Because it robs individuals and groups of people of their potential to survive, their sense of security and their capacity to flourish. It robs them of their capabilities. Why does that matter? Because robbed of these foundational resources, we cannot survive or evolve as persons or peoples. It is tautological to say that we cannot survive without surviving, form stable groups without security, or enlarge our individual and group identities without access to means that allow us to transcend our quotidian lives. Holocaust survivors give us convincing testimony about these truths. So do survivors of cancer, victims of torture and sufferers from chronic diseases. So do doctors, lawyers, businessmen, tissue donors and those who suffer from chronic diseases.

So, we may begin with survival, security and flourishing (SSF) as foundational values. (I will return to the word 'foundational' later, because I know it causes trouble for anti-foundationalists.) Survival, security and flourishing might be thought of as *a priori* necessities for a culture or society to continue and to evolve – but it does not say how they must play out in each culture or society. All may agree that there is a concept of good health, and that there is a contemporary need to provide health services. But the philosophy behind the services may differ significantly from culture to culture, as they do, say, between the USA and the UK. In a sense, those differing systems can be appraised by the way that they fit into the prevailing beliefs and ideologies of the societies that house them. People will judge them according to different axioms that express their commitments, but those who construct and maintain them will defend them because they believe that their system is the 'best' way to insure maximum rates of survival, secure resources for those in trouble, and the capacity to restore the disabled to the potential to flourish.

Survival, security and flourishing are pre-normative, descriptive categories. To acknowledge them as being important in any culture is not to prescribe how they shall play out in every culture, nor is it to insist that the ways in which they play out should not change with time and context. The systems, institutions and procedures which express them (public health, hospitals, medical care services, community care and so on) express beliefs and the realities of resource availability, and they change with medical developments, economic circumstances, community pressures and political ideologies.

The three chosen foundations can be further justified.

(1) If humankind as a collective and humans as individuals did not value survival, we would not be here to debate the validity of some kind of foundationalism, or we would have no interest in debating. But we are here, and we do debate, so denying that we value survival makes no sense. We survive.

(2) No valuation of security is equivalent to tolerance of unpredictability. We all have to tolerate some unpredictability in nature, societies, other people and ourselves, but we need some statistical warrant for trust in our daily rounds. Countries that do not have security, or have lost it, plead to have it or have it back. Jean Améry described what unpredictability did to an individual imprisoned by the Gestapo (Améry, 1980). But security inevitably means accepting some impositions on untrammelled freedom (Berlin, 1958 (1969)). East Germans found 'freedom' unsettling after years of social control – which, with all its obvious injustice, had come to equal security, predictability, known rules for some citizens at least. T. S. Eliot wrote that 'Humankind cannot bear very much reality' (Eliot, 1943), nor is it comfortable with too much freedom. If we did not value security, we would break traffic and other laws as it suited us, and we would cease to have a functioning society. The unregulated Hobbesian community would soon destroy its own pluralism, and even the resulting elites would eventually divide and generate internecine war (Mosca, 1939; Michels, 1962; Pareto, 1966).

(3) No valuation of flourishing is equivalent to denial of individual and social development. Without access to flourishing, a culture dwindles to a purely instrumental grouping of indistinguishable members. Even in uniform-wearing societies, people still have ambitions, still seek self-expression, compete to show

loyalty, consciously comply with ideologies, and so on. People in many countries go to art galleries, sporting events, films, concerts, join voluntary groups. Even in prison camps, there are some who worship, paint, compose, dance, tell stories (Langer, 1982). If flourishing were not valued, none of these phenomena would be evident. But they are, and it makes no sense to deny that dependence on flourishing is in some sense a deeply situated attribute of being a person.

There is, therefore, an argument to suggest that a world that does not value the SSF complex *does* not exist, and that, in that case, a recognisable world peopled with recognisable humans *could* not exist. Something else no doubt could exist, but not one populated with persons as we know them. By the time we have eliminated SSF, we have a world that is either self-destructive or other-than-human. A society without foundational values is an incoherent concept.

Now, it is quite possible to talk about values anywhere along a continuum. At one end, we have the set of foundational values – we might call them F-values; at the other, we have the systems that give practical expression to these values in culturally appropriate ways – call them P-values. We value (or deprecate) the medical services and practices of our own countries; we are appreciative (or critical) of the health systems under which the services operate; we applaud (or denigrate) the social philosophies that inform our health systems. But in the end, we evaluate these things implicitly by assessing how far they go to insure individual and group survival, security and flourishing. And the elites who govern us justify them in the same way. However different our appraisals of our own and other health services, their evaluation and justification depend on the same foundational values.

The F-values are pre-normative, and to bring them to normative realisation implies that we adopt axioms that will once again differ from society to society and from individual to individual. These axioms are like intuitions, developed through enculturation, education, experience and reflection, and deployed as justifications for choices and evaluations (Hammond, 1996). Social axiom theory has been developed by others to examine social adaptations of migrants, establishment of individual and group identity, human flourishing and happiness. Interested readers are referred to the available literature (Leung *et al.*, 2002; Kurman and Ronen-Eilon, 2004; Cheung *et al.*, 2006; Hui *et al.*, 2006; Lai *et al.*, 2007; Joshanloo *et al.*, 2010), where they will find this definition (Leung *et al.*, 2002): 'Social axioms are generalized beliefs about oneself (i.e., personhood), the social and physical environment, or the spiritual world, and are in the form of an assertion about the relationship between two entities or concepts.' There is not enough space in this chapter to develop a comprehensive argument about axioms within the values continuum, and I simply offer one example from many hundreds drawn from qualitative interviews with clinicians. An experienced general practitioner says during her interview:

> 8.58. But it's mainly been when people have either allowed harm to come to others, or risked harm to others, because they haven't had the courage to either admit a mistake or they've tried to actually neglect or bully someone, when clearly it's not just lack of bullying, it's lack of actually being proactive, to help another person in trouble.

There are several axioms embedded in this quote. 'Good doctors should practice non-maleficence, should admit mistakes, not exploit their power, and help those in need of their services.'

If I declare some of my own axioms, by which I evaluate the ways in which societies (including my own) express their recognitions of foundational values, they look something like this.

(1) Societal survival and progress demands an open Darwinian pool. To disadvantage a section of a community, to rob it of opportunity, is to rob the whole community of the capabilities of the disadvantaged.

(2) A capabilities and functions approach recognises human needs and abilities better than an econometric one (Sen, 1993).

(3) Individuals and groups matter.

(4) A functioning society must, in these terms, enhance and protect appropriate opportunities for survival, security and flourishing.

(5) Both *zeit* and *geist* relate to a society's survival and progress. Axioms and their expressions in practice will – and need to – change with the times.

Your axioms may be quite different, but you will have them (without them you can make no judgements), and you may think of them too as values (Hammond, 1996). I am happy with that construal, but want to point out that they are in fact uninferred axioms that *guide* the 'right' expression and evaluation of foundational values, the conversion of F-values to P-values. They are norms that are reinforced by our experiences. They are an integral part of our values-based reasoning, and it seems reasonable to label them as A-values. Foundational values are logically prior to them, and it is worth distinguishing between the pre-normative and the normative in this dynamic relationship. By all means call a commitment to human rights a value, but it is a practical value derived from foundational values, and *justified* by certain axioms that make our assessment of human rights normative. Foundational values, axioms and practical values need to be distinguished in discussions, because it is much harder to secure agreement on the axioms and practical expressions of values than it is on the foundational ones. I will refer to this model of values as the 'FAP model'. It avoids the deterministic rigidity of classic foundationalism, and the acknowledgement of the role of axioms keeps us from the perils of extreme relativism. To interpret the preferences of another person, we need to acknowledge common foundational values, elicit the axioms that translate these into daily life, and frame our respect for the enactments that follow from this translational process. The only real difference between the VBM model that I support, and that of Fulford, lies in my suggesting that a full account of a values-base should include the F-values. We agree otherwise on the importance of the A-values and P-values. Indeed, Fulford helpfully lists a series of axioms that define the stance of his version of values-based medicine (Fulford, 2004).

A-values and P-values are perhaps the most talked about when values in general are used as a category of discourse. We say that we value such things as justice, fairness, compassion, kindness and courtesy in individuals, and characteristics such as law-abidingness, humanitarianism and cultural development in institutions and societies. It seems perfectly logical to use values to refer to such axioms and virtues as these because we value them, and so do many others, but they are particular A-values and P-values that express in distinctive ways the underlying F-values.

For these reasons, I want to urge that values be defined in any discourse at least according to whether they are F-values, A-values or P-values. F-values are not normative in the sense that they can be expressed in different ways in different cultural contexts, and their A-value and P-value expressions may change in response to context – witness the

UK's change from a mixed charity and private system to a National Health Scheme, or Australia's change to a national insurance scheme in the 1970s. The USA seems currently to be wrestling with a similar change under Obama, having worked with a largely private scheme for many years. But why did the UK change to a socialist scheme so long before the USA modified its private enterprise approach? It would be rash to offer any single or simple explanation. It is enough to say that these schemes ran in parallel in English speaking countries for over 50 years, apparently producing very similar health outcomes. Both could claim to be serving the same foundational values, but refracting them quite differently through the prisms of different political ideologies as different P-values. The same could be said of Chinese or Indian or Russian or German health services – significant differences in the delivery systems but the same foundational values. They express differences in culture, just as individual preferences express individual differences, but difference is underpinned by similar foundational evaluations. People want the same kinds of pre-conditions for their individual and corporate lives, the same F-values, but not necessarily the same universal realisations or P-values because they have inherited or developed different A-values.

Modest foundationalism and axioms

So far, this chapter has been about foundational values, and that will have annoyed anti-foundationalists (Uebel, 1996). I want to stress that I agree with anti-foundationalism when it takes issue with the strict, Cartesian form of foundationalism (Descartes, 1989). The Cartesian enterprise has had its critics since the day it was first formulated, and the post-modernists have effectively destroyed the idea that one can begin with an unquestionable truth and build an entire intellectual system from that point. The Humean (Hume, 1991) and twentieth century starting point is far more modest (Kaplan, 2003; Little *et al.*, 2012). It points out that there are some statements that we accept as propositions without being able to infer them from other unquestioned truths. If we ask why we accept the proposition that language has exchangeable meaning, for instance, we can only say that that is the way it is, that human communication relies on that proposition for its interchanges, its diplomacy, its cultures, and so on. Foundationalism in most of its forms attempts to avoid the problems of circularity and infinite regress. If asked to justify health, I may say, health is a good. Why is it a good? Because illness is bad, and illness is bad because health is good. That argument rapidly becomes circular. Alternatively, I can answer that health is good because it makes us feel well, and feeling well matters because that allows us to do productive things which means that other people benefit, and the benefit of others matters because everyone should interact productively in a society, and so on into an infinite regress.

Modest foundationalism differs quite significantly from the Cartesian version. It offers a more pragmatic, heuristic approach. It asks us to accept what appear to be tautological propositions as descriptions, not as normative declarations, nor as unmodifiable truths. We value survival because it makes no evolutionary sense to value our individual or group destruction. We value security because, as Jean Améry wrote (Améry, 1980), predictability is fundamental to our sense of identity. We strive to find ways to flourish, to transcend our daily lives by prayer or music, art or sport, or bushwalking, bird-watching, quilt making, and so on. Many Jews continued to worship in groups in the concentration camps of World War II. Australian prisoners played cricket or football in Japanese camps. Survival, security and flourishing are intimately connected, and essential to us as persons and peoples. But that makes no normative demands on how those things *should* be constructed in a functioning society.

This kind of foundationalism is much closer to Susan Haack's 'foundherentism' (Haack, 1993) than it is to Descartes' system (Descartes, 1989). Haack has deplored the opposition between foundationalism and coherentism as rival theories of knowledge. In reality, she argues, we use both systems. Consciously or unconsciously, we accept as a matter of experience certain uninferred propositions – language conveys meaning, life is worth living, friendship is good, security is desirable, suffering is undesirable. From this melange of culturally and individually developed axioms, we evolve an epistemological crossword (the analogy is Haack's), where our experiences, both direct and acquired from others (our experiential and credal foundations), are the clues and our answers (our reasoned beliefs) are justified by the fact that they fit the puzzle. The axioms represent the language, the vocabulary, the grammar and the semantics that distinguish us as individuals and members of groups. The crossword analogy does not demand that our answers be the only right ones, merely that they fit the puzzle, and that they cohere with one another, while addressing the clues appropriately in a language that is semantically and grammatically intelligible.

Values-based medicine

We now have rudimentary accounts of values and a particular kind of modest or aetiological foundationalism, and can try bringing them together in an examination and justification of values-based medicine. It seems necessary to do this because there is an influential movement, identified particularly with person-centred medicine, that is anti-foundationalist (Upshur, 2002). Medicine, it claims, is an emergent practice that needs no base, and that claim has been made repeatedly in the person-centred medicine literature (Miles and Mezzich, 2011a; Miles and Mezzich, 2011b). Furthermore, various authors explicitly insist that the act of basing on some foundation is intellectually constraining, and that a post-modern refutation of foundationalism is necessary to advance medicine. Person-centred medicine, the claim goes, seeks no foundations. At the same time, it argues its case on the grounds that it recognises the primacy of persons and people, and the importance of working from theories of personhood. The denial of a need for foundations and the insistence on justification by theories of personhood seems to me to be incoherent, and is perhaps itself based on an outmoded version of foundationalism. The building of grand systems from a single 'indisputable' base has been discredited by the post-modernists, but modest or aetiological foundationalism has not. Without accepting that there are uninferred beliefs and propositions embedded in our intellectual lives, it is very difficult to avoid circular reasoning or infinite regress. And every claim we make for intellectual priority (including those of modest foundationalism or person-centred medicine) rests on 'truths' pragmatically framed as being expressions of 'warranted assertability' (Dewey, 1941). I have argued the case for modest foundationalism and for a values-base for medicine elsewhere, and want to recapitulate those arguments in this chapter.

To begin, we need to ask what 'medicine' means in this discourse. Medicine has a philosophy with its own literature and journals. It has theories of disease and bodily function, of mind, of social impact, of health care delivery, of ethics and so on. It has a vitally important knowledge-base, a complex body of skills and techniques that translate knowledge into practice. It has an etiquette of relationships, comportment and communications. It has public and private components, and the capacity to attract large resources of people, material and money. It is sustained by an education system that is supposed to continue throughout a practising life. So when we claim that 'medicine' needs or does not need a base, we make a claim about an extremely complex system that is an integral part of the societies in which we live.

But its complexity does nothing to rule out the desirability of defining a base – quite the reverse. To understand why so much money, so many resources, so much commitment of time and human capital, so much media attention, so much political involvement are all invested in health care (of which medicine constitutes so important a part), we need to understand how foundational are the values that justify so much investment. Medicine's size, importance, cost, complexity, and above all its growth demand justification in the face of the other competing interests in the industrial-population complex that dominates the modern (or even post-modern) social order. Basing the system in the FAP model of values allows us to understand why medicine survives and even flourishes in a *zeit* of such financial, spiritual and social instability. In this sense, it provides a clearer insight into the relationship it has to foundational values that are necessary (although possibly not sufficient) for the past, present and future of humankind than other models, including evidence-based medicine, patient-centred care, person-centred medicine, narrative medicine and so on (and on). This model of VBM is no more or less prescriptive than any other model of how medicine should be. The foundational values are descriptive acknowledgements of what preconditions we appear to need as a species to survive and flourish. The axioms and their practical expressions are normative in the same way that privileging personhood or evidence is normative. But those axioms and resulting practices are available for review and revision in the face of change and the demands of context.

And what is the alternative to some such foundational model? The word that appears regularly in the person-centred medicine literature is 'emergence' (Upshur, 2002). Now emergence is an interesting concept with different definitions (O'Connor, 1994; Spencer-Smith, 1995), and so far the PCM literature gives no clear indication of the definition it favours. Emergence covers the unpredicted, the unanticipated properties of a sub-system that forms from a parent system. Thus, we could say that mind is emergent from the complex brain, or that language is emergent from social intercourse. But we can make these claims in three ways (Spencer-Smith, 1995). Emergence can be used to say that what emerges is mysterious and inexplicable; or it can claim simply that knowledge of properties is made possible by recognition of the link (unexplained) between the system and the sub-system; or, more benignly, that it acknowledges the link, but also acknowledges that present knowledge or understanding does not provide an adequate explanation. The third version expects that advances in understanding will provide better understanding of causal mechanisms, just as brain imaging increases our understanding of the functions of mind in relation to the matter of brain. Whether we will ever have complete understanding of the emergent phenomenon and its genesis from the underlying system remains an open question.

If we accept any of these definitions, how much does it help to say that medicine is simply emergent, in all its complexity? I suspect that it helps very little. We are first of all left with the question of what it emerges from. Is it society, or sociation? Is it from language and the ability to communicate and educate? Or is it from a human propensity for opportunism, the chance to gain power and possessions by exploiting the vulnerable?

Emergence is supervenience, and supervenience implies subvenience. Second, we need to ask whether the simple claim that medicine is emergent is sufficient reason to dismiss further enquiry into medicine's persistence and flourishing? War is presumably also an 'emergent phenomenon', but that gives no reason to cease enquiry into its causes and prevention. Third, if medicine is emergent, does that help us to understand how medicine fits into the hierarchy of welfares in modern cultures and societies? We can, of course, just go on accepting that *zeit* and *geist* will change the practice and the A-values and P-values of medicine, and we can accept those changes passively. Alternatively, we can iteratively question the validity of proposed changes by testing them against the F-values, seeking ways to practise that maintain the foundational telos of medicine as agent of foundational values.

So what?

I have no illusions that the FAP model of values-based medicine will produce a revolution in medical thinking, policy or practice. It is unlikely even to affect medical education in the form that I commit to. Fulford's is a more practical approach than mine, and I endorse his campaign to teach skills that will encourage recognition of and respect for personhood, individuality and cultural difference. My contribution, I hope, will simply add a justification for Fulford's privileging of preferences, and some further insight into what it is that preferences actually express.

Those acknowledgements aside, there are some possible inherent virtues in offering VBM as a resource at various levels of medicine and medical education. First, it provides a relatively stable reference point in times of rapid and unsettling change. Referring back to the F-values serves to remind us of the roles we are fulfilling in a foundational way. Medicine is important to society and its continuation. When that claim becomes untrue, we will have reached either Utopia or the end of days. Second, we are at the edge of an era when declining marginal benefit will compel us to evaluate with increasing care the commitment of resources to fit in with our cultural axioms about fairness, equity, capability and cost-benefit. Reference back to the F-values may be increasingly useful to remind us of the evolutionary requirements necessary for species survival. Health and welfare are not all about medicine. Survival of the fittest means survival of the creatures best fitted to the context of the time.

Let us take a brief look at how VBM and the FAP model might look in practice.

> The use of activated recombinant Factor VII to help control bleeding has been controversial (Yank *et al.*, 2011). There is enough evidence to support its use in the presence of Factor VII deficiency and in haemophilia with Factor VIII antibodies, but in other situations studies have produced differing conclusions. EBM's approach to this aporia has been a meta-analysis, itself producing inconclusive results, but broadly finding no or weak evidence to support its off-label use. Inconclusive results are interpreted as evidence *against* continuing use. The drug is very expensive (about $10,000 per ampoule), and on-label prescribing in most countries is restricted to the rare situations in which there is well-documented statistical evidence of benefit. That, however, has not stopped its widespread use in emergencies in obstetrics, cardio-thoracic surgery, urological surgery, intracranial bleeding and trauma. Indeed, in the USA 97% of usage has been off-label, and the editors of the *Annals of Internal Medicine*, which published the meta-analysis, went so far as to suggest that anyone practising off-label use would be open to litigation by patients who survived or

by the families of those who died (Avorn and Kesselheim, 2011). Their condemnation of its use was thus forthright, and it elicited a variety of defensive and justificatory responses. The place of observation and anecdote was defended as justification for desperate measures under desperate circumstances. How does this set of circumstances look through the perspective of VBM?

First, let us deploy the F-values. From a doctor's viewpoint, the patient's survival is paramount. In emergencies, as conditions deteriorate, there is strong pressure to try anything that may help. Anecdotes of benefit are plentiful enough, and there are some series that suggest benefit in various circumstances. Cost becomes an issue only when there is not enough money to make the drug available. The fact that there is not clear high level evidence of benefit does not outweigh the demands of a critical set of circumstances. For the continued security and flourishing of the doctor too, it is reasonable that he or she can say with conviction 'I did everything I could.' From society's point of view as well, every possible step should be taken, because life is precious, and the use of Factor VII is still within the means of most Western societies. That may change, but holds true for the moment. Faith in our own security implies that all reasonable means will be used by medicine when death threatens. Death is the end of flourishing. We want to feel secure that medicine does what it can to rescue us from vulnerability. It is thus easy enough to *understand* why doctors and the general public might want to see off-label use supported in the present state of knowledge.

Then let us look at A-values. What axioms might be deployed by interested people and groups at a time of crisis? Patients and their families might think that it is the task of medicine to do everything that is reasonable and possible. Doctors may feel that while there's life there's hope, while there remains something that might work we should continue to use any means that might produce a benefit. Administrators, bureaucrats and politicians may adhere to a set of maxims about costs and benefits, while balancing these against axioms of political expedience. EBM adherents have demonstrated their antagonism to something that does not fit the demands of their ideology. Their axioms seem to rule out as immoral any treatment that is not supported by high level evidence, to discount anecdote, and to override desperate responses to desperate circumstances. We can see that substantive disagreement begins at the A level, and eliciting the implicit axioms of participants becomes centrally important if there is to be dialectic rather than adversarial debate.

And so the F-A complex leads to valued practices that may be in sharp conflict. Opposing actions may be valued validly and powerfully by people with different axioms. There is likely to be agreement, as a starting point for dialectic, about the F-values. Everyone will claim that they are acting to maximise survival, to provide a secure expectation for the vulnerable, and to enable the maximum degree of flourishing for one and all. They will use arguments about costs and benefits, resource constraints, autonomy, the realities of experience, the expectations of individuals and social groups to explain how their axioms secure the best assurance for F-values. But the axioms are constructed from ideologies, from intellectual and political commitments, and unless they are made explicit, they cannot be the objects of dialectic. Nor can disjunctions be identified until the implicit agreement about F-values has been examined.

In the case of Factor VII, the disagreement at the level of axioms can be reduced to a disagreement about the verdict that follows inconclusive evidence. To demonstrate that there is *probably* no benefit required a massive and complex meta-analysis. Buried within that study were indicators that in *some* cases there might be some benefit. Meticulous though the study was by EBM's standards, the evidence was not overwhelming against off-label use.

An FAP approach suggests that the Not Proven verdict should be interpreted in context, and should not rule out the continued use of the drug under careful observation to find out whether the anecdotal and even numerical evidence for its occasional effectiveness can be further reduced to effectiveness in particular circumstances and sub-groups. Until social circumstances change, a values-based approach would suggest a continued search for value somewhere along the FAP continuum, because those who make claims for effectiveness are people working within a values-based and values-driven system for the benefit of the vulnerable. If population pressures, economic decline, climate change, epidemics, wars or natural disasters change the context in which values-based medicine is delivered, then we have at least some idea about how we might think about adapting our systems to serve the F-values as well as we can.

VBM in this form seems to have advantages (and no great disadvantages) as a part of medical education, bioethics, policy-making, medical practice and medical communication. Grounding medical education in the FAP model demands no impractical curricular reform. One can still teach EBM or PCM or mindful practice as before, but grounded and justified by recognisable, debatable and contextual values. Bioethics can still be taught using the familiar structure, but informed by values-based reasons for principles, rights, duties and virtues. Similarly, policy-making and policy advice can be tempered by reference back to F-values, and the implications of changes to A-values and P-values can be examined as contexts evolve and change. Medical *practice* may be emergent, but its demands still need explanation, and the FAP model allows this, and provides the tools by which practitioners can reflect on the demands and quandaries of practice. Medical communication will probably always be imperfect because of the constraints of language and the impossibility of communicating personal experience, but interpretation of patient narrative, media representations and complaints is facilitated by a values-based belief and practice system.

People are people, and Kant's dictum remains as true as it was in the eighteenth century – '. . .out of wood so crooked and perverse as that which man is made of, nothing absolutely straight can ever be wrought' (Kant, 1824). The wonder is that the species, warlike, spiteful, inconstant and capricious, has survived at all. Presumably, hidden among the knots and wandering grain of human timber are survival mechanisms that we might acknowledge with benefit and without loss. We all have values. The more we know about them, recognise them, discuss them and acknowledge how sustaining they are, the better our medical and social discourse is likely to be. VBM is another reflective means to add to the repertoire of wide reflective equilibrium (Daniels, 1980; Daniels, 1996; DePaul, 2001).

References

Améry, J. (1980) *At the Mind's Limits: Contemplations by a Survivor on Auschwitz and its Realities.* Bloomington and Indianapolis, IN: Indiana University Press.

Avorn, J. and Kesselheim, A. (2011) Editorial: a hemorrhage of off-label use. *Annals of Internal Medicine,* **154**, 566–567.

Berlin, I. (1958 (1969)) Two concepts of liberty. *Four Essays on Liberty.* Oxford: Oxford University Press.

Cheung, M. W. L., Leung, K. and Au, K. (2006) Evaluating multilevel models in cross-cultural research: an illustration with social axioms. *Journal of Cross-Cultural Psychology,* **37**, 522–541.

Daniels, N. (1980) Reflective equilibrium and Archimedian points. *Canadian Journal of Philosophy,* **10**, 83–103.

Daniels, N. (1996) *Justice and Justification: Reflective Equilibrium in Theory and Practice.* Cambridge: Cambridge University Press.

Darwin, C. (1999 (1859)) *The Origin of Species.* New York: Random House.

DePaul, M. R. (2001) *Balance and Refinement: Beyond Coherence Methods of Moral Inquiry.* London: Routledge.

Descartes, R. (1989) *Discourse on Method and the Meditations.* New York: Prometheus Books.

Dewey, J. (1941) Propositions, warranted assertibility, and truth. *Journal of Philosophy,* **38**, 169–186.

Eliot, T. S. (1943) Burnt Norton. *Four Quartets.* San Diego, CA: Harcourt.

Fulford, K. W. M. (2004) Ten principles of values-based medicine. In Radden, J. (editor), *The Philosophy of Psychiatry: A Companion,* pp. 205–234. Oxford: Oxford University Press.

Haack, S. (1993) *Evidence and Inquiry.* Oxford: Blackwell Publishers.

Hammond, K. R. (1996) *Human Judgement and Social Policy: Irreducible Uncertainty, Inevitable Error, Unavoidable Injustice.* Oxford: Oxford University Press.

Hui, V. K., Bond, M. H. and Ng, T. S. (2006) General beliefs about the world as defensive mechanisms against death anxiety. *Omega (Westport),* **54**, 199–214.

Hume, D. (1991) *An Enquiry Concerning Human Understanding.* Oxford: Clarendon Press.

Hume, D. (2004 (1777)) *An Enquiry Concerning the Principles of Morals.* New York: Prometheus Books.

Joshanloo, M., Afshari, S., Rastegar, P. *et al.* (2010) Linking social axioms with indicators of positive interpersonal, social and environmental functioning in Iran: an exploratory study; culture-level dimensions of social axioms and their correlates across 41 cultures; general beliefs about the world as defensive mechanisms against death anxiety; evaluating multilevel models in cross-cultural research: an illustration with social axioms. *CORD Conference Proceedings,* **45**, 303–310.

Kant, I. (1824) Idea of a universal history on a cosmo-political plan. *London Magazine,* 385–393.

Kaplan, M. (2003) Who cares what you know? *Philosophical Quarterly,* **53**, 105–116.

Kurman, J. and Ronen-Eilon, C. (2004) Lack of knowledge of a culture's social axioms and adaptation difficulties among immigrants. *Journal of Cross-Cultural Psychology,* **35**, 192–208.

Lai, J., Bond, M. and Hui, N. (2007) The role of social axioms in predicting life satisfaction: a longitudinal study. *Journal of Happiness Studies,* **8**, 517–535.

Langer, L. (1982) *Versions of Survival: The Holocaust and the Human Spirit.* Albany, NY: State University of New York Press.

Leung, K., Bond, M. H., DeCarrasquel, S. R. *et al.* (2002) Social axioms: the search for universal dimensions of general beliefs about how the world functions. *Journal of Cross-Cultural Psychology,* **33**, 286–302.

Little, M., Lipworth, W., Gordon, J. et al. (2012) Values-based medicine and modest foundationalism. *Journal of Evaluation in Clinical Practice,* **18**, 1020–1026.

Michels, R. (1962) *Political Parties: A Sociological Study of the Oligarchical Tendencies of Modern Democracy.* New York: The Free Press.

Miles, A. and Mezzich, J. E. (2011a) The care of the patient and the soul of the clinic: person centered medicine as an emergent model of modern clinical practice. *International Journal of Person Centered Medicine,* **1**, 207–222.

Miles, A. and Mezzich, J. E. (2011b) Person-centered medicine: advancing methods, promoting implementation. *International Journal of Person Centered Medicine,* **1**, 423–428.

Mosca, G. (1939) *The Ruling Class.* New York: McGraw Hill.

O'Connor, T. (1994) Emergent properties. *American Philosophical Quarterly,* **31**, 91–104.

Pareto, V. (1966) *Sociological Writings – Selected and introduced by S. E. Finer.* London: Pall Mall Press.

Sen, A. (1993) Capability and well-being. In Nussbaum, M. and Sen, A. (editors), *The Quality of Life,* pp. 30–53. Oxford: Clarendon Press.

Spencer-Smith, R. (1995) Reductionism and emergent properties. *Proceedings of the Aristotelian Society,* **95**, 113–129.

Uebel, T. E. (1996) Anti-foundationalism and the Vienna Circle's revolution in philosophy.

British Journal for the Philosophy of Science, **47**, 415–440.

Upshur, R. E. G. (2002) If not evidence, then what? Or does medicine really need a base? *Journal of Evaluation in Clinical Practice,* **8**, 113–119.

Yank, V., Tuohy, C. V., Logan, A. C. *et al.* (2011) Systematic review: benefits and harms of in-hospital use of recombinant factor VIIa for off-label indications. *Annals of Internal Medicine,* **154**, 529–540.

Chapter 15

Eliciting axioms to enrich debates about the pharmaceutical industry

Wendy Lipworth and Kathleen Montgomery

Background and rationale

The study described in this chapter illustrates the utility of Little's model of values (Chapter 14) as a way of interpreting the discourse of professional groups – in this case, the discourse of employees of the pharmaceutical industry – and as a way of enriching debates about controversial professional issues.

The problem with debates about the pharmaceutical industry

In recent years, the pharmaceutical industry has come under fire for what is perceived to be pervasive misconduct, including developing medicines that are likely to be commercially beneficial even if they do not address genuine unmet needs, carrying out research without sufficient concern for the wellbeing of research participants, distorting the design, conduct, interpretation and presentation of research in order to produce more positive results, overstating the costs involved in research and development in order to over-price medicines, abusing intellectual property laws, and engaging in ethically suspect marketing practices (Angell, 2004; Elliot, 2010).

Clinicians, researchers, journal editors, educators and regulators are well aware of these actions on the part of the pharmaceutical industry, and steps have been taken to try to minimise the pharmaceutical industry's influence over research, publication, policy-making, education and practice. For the most part, these steps have taken the form of regulations that either prohibit certain activities and relationships (e.g. companies

Debates in Values-Based Practice, ed. Michael Loughlin. Published by Cambridge University Press. © Cambridge University Press 2014.

providing doctors with lavish gifts) or demand disclosure of such relationships and activities (DeMartino, 2012; Lo, 2012; Raad and Appelbaum, 2012).

At the same time, however, many health and biomedical professionals collaborate with industry in, for example, early drug development and clinical research. Indeed, academic basic scientists and clinical researchers are now actively encouraged, if not mandated, by their institutions to form such relationships (Schulman *et al.*, 2002; Bekelman *et al.*, 2003).

Under these circumstances, one might expect that there would be a great deal of ambivalence towards the pharmaceutical industry and rich debate about the pros and cons of industry engagement. But instead, publicly stated views about the industry tend to be polarised with people being either strongly critical (e.g. Angell, 2004; Elliot, 2010) or defensive (e.g. Stossel and Stell, 2011) of the industry and its activities. For the most part, academics and clinicians in the public sphere tend be highly critical of the industry, despite their ever more complex entanglements with it.

While such a critical stance might be a good basis for avoiding harm, in its most extreme forms it might also represent a state of 'hostile dependence' on the part of academics and clinicians – that is, a state of needing and wanting to engage with the pharmaceutical industry, at the same time as being deeply mistrustful of the industry and/or resentful of one's dependence. Relationships such as these are problematic because they tend to preclude dialogue and genuine cooperation. This is evident, for example, in debates about the disclosure of industry payments to clinicians and researchers, which are adversarial and lacking in genuine mutual recognition of alternative positions (e.g. Angell, 2004; Stossel and Stell, 2011).

This raises the question: how can we improve communication between health and biomedical professionals, regulators and employees of the pharmaceutical industry so that they can communicate more effectively and thus collaborate more genuinely in devising pharmaceutical policy?

Analysis of axioms as a route to more productive discourse

Theories of public discourse provide some help in this regard. Jurgen Habermas, for example, devised a set of rules of discourse, aimed at enhancing understanding and agreement in situations of unequal power and value pluralism. While many of Habermas' ideas have been criticised (Roberts, 2012), his rules of discourse do give us an idea of what might be necessary for greater dialogue and cooperation between those within the pharmaceutical industry and its external critics in health and bio-medicine. Importantly, one of Habermas' central concepts was that speakers should aspire to the mutual recognition of various kinds of 'validity claims'. This entails (among other things) a speaker:

> select(ing) an utterance that is right in the light of existing norms and values in order that the hearer can accept the utterance, so that both speaker and hearer can agree with one another in the utterance concerning a *recognised normative background*. (McCarthy, 1978, p. 288, emphasis added)

Communication between the pharmaceutical industry and its critics might, therefore, be improved if speakers on both sides could more consistently identify such a shared – or at least recognisable – 'normative background'.

Habermas' rules of discourse do not, however, tell us exactly what constitutes this 'normative background', and this is where Little's theory of values becomes useful.

According to Little, values exist on a continuum. An individual's or group's attitudes and actions are culturally appropriate, practical expressions (P-values) of the foundational values (F-values) survival, security and flourishing. In between F-values and P-values are a set of 'axioms' (A-values) that bring F-values to normative realisation and that can be deployed as justifications for choices and evaluations (Chapter 14). Little argues that:

> To interpret the preferences of another person, we need to acknowledge common
> foundational values, elicit the axioms that translate these into daily life, and frame our
> respect for the enactments that follow from this translational process. (Chapter 14, p. 175)

These A-values sound very much like Habermas' 'recognised normative background', which might, therefore, be reframed as the set of shared – or at least recognisable – axiom-level values of discourse participants, where axioms are the beliefs held to be 'self-evident' by discourse communities.

Much is known about the axioms (or A-values) underpinning the practices of academic science and clinical medicine. And much is known about the practices (or P-values) of the pharmaceutical industry – including various forms of malpractice in research, publishing, pricing, marketing and so on. But very little empirical work has been done to elicit the axioms that underpin the practices of pharmaceutical industry employees.

We believe that this is an important lacuna because lack of attention to pharmaceutical axioms could be one of the reasons why discourse between the pharmaceutical industry and other stakeholders is so adversarial and lacking in nuance. We therefore set out to elicit the axioms underpinning the practices of those who work in the pharmaceutical industry, with the goal of developing a framework that might be used to improve communication and collaboration between health and biomedical professionals, regulators and employees of the pharmaceutical industry. We focused on the axioms of people working in 'medical affairs' departments of pharmaceutical companies – that is, those responsible for clinical trials, regulatory affairs and applications to have medicines reimbursed by governments and insurance companies. We chose to focus on this group of industry employees because they are the group most likely to participate in policy-related dialogue with clinicians, academic scientists and regulators. Drawing on Little's values framework, our broad research question became: 'What axioms underpin the practices of those who work in medical affairs roles within the pharmaceutical industry?'

Methods

Fifteen face-to-face interviews were conducted with people working in 'medical affairs' departments of nine pharmaceutical companies in Sydney, Australia. In Australia, almost all pharmaceutical companies are local subsidiaries of global companies. Participants represented most of the major companies that have an Australian presence, as well as one manufacturer of generic medicines. Purposive sampling was used in order to include participants from as many different companies as possible, from a variety of (non-commercial) professional backgrounds, particularly academic research, clinical medicine and pharmacy, and with a variety of pharmaceutical company roles, including medical director, clinical research manager, regulatory affairs manager, and pricing and

Table 15.1 Sample characteristics

	Gender	Age	Previous profession	Current role
P1	M	50–60	Physician and medical researcher	Medical director
P2	M	30–40	Physician	Medical affairs manager
P3	F	50–60	Pharmacist	Senior manager in clinical research
P4	F	50–60	Pharmacist and biomedical researcher	Senior manager in regulatory affairs
P5	F	40–50	Pharmacist and biomedical researcher	Internal scientific advisory role
P6	M	50–60	Academic health economist	Senior manager in pricing and reimbursement
P7	M	60–70	Physician and clinical researcher	Medical director
P8	M	50–60	Physician	Medical director
P9	M	50–60	Pharmacist	Senior manager in pricing and reimbursement
P10	M	40–50	Pharmacist	Senior manager in clinical and regulatory affairs
P11	F	60–70	Biomedical researcher	Senior manager in clinical research
P12	M	50–60	Pharmacist and biomedical researcher	Medical director
P13	M	50–60	Pharmacist and biomedical researcher	Senior manager in pricing and reimbursement
P14	M	40–50	Pharmacist	Senior manager in pricing and reimbursement
P15	M	50–60	Pharmacist	Senior manager in clinical research

reimbursement manager; several participants currently or had previously held more than one of these positions (see Table 15.1). Interviewees were identified first through organisational websites and the professional contacts of the researchers and then via snowball sampling from the initial group. Sixteen people were approached in total and one declined to be interviewed.

Semi-structured interviews were conducted in late 2011 and early 2012, and lasted approximately one hour each. Participants were first asked to describe, in their own words, their decision to move out of science or clinical work and into industry, and their experiences of making the transition. They were asked how they learned to fulfil their new roles and responsibilities, and whether they had been influenced by any role models. They were asked to describe people they admired and people of whom they disapproved, and to discuss those aspects of their work they found most and least rewarding. Through this loosely structured format, participants were able to define and discuss their careers and working lives as they wished. Interviews were recorded (with interviewees' permission) and transcribed verbatim. Names were replaced with pseudonyms in the database and are referred to herein by numerical designations.

Data analysis drew both on Morse's outline of the cognitive basis of qualitative research (Morse, 1994) and on Charmaz's outline of data analysis in grounded theory (Charmaz, 2006). This procedure involved initial coding via line-by-line analysis, synthesising codes into categories until no new codes could be developed from the data, focused re-coding using these categories, and abstracting into concepts. A coding tree was generated. Throughout the data analysis, a process of constant comparison was employed. Existing codes, categories, and concepts were refined, enriched and reorganised as new codes; and categories and concepts were developed or as similarities and differences were recognised. Enough material was analysed to ensure that categories were saturated and all concepts were fully described and well understood. Thematic saturation was reached after approximately eight interviews. WL conducted the interviews and initial coding. Codes and their interpretation were then discussed and developed with KM, and agreement was reached on the major themes and categories. The study was approved by the university's research ethics committee. All participants signed consent forms and agreed to speak from their own (rather than their company's) perspective.

Results

It soon became evident that participants' talk was rich in descriptions of what it means to behave as a 'good' person in the context of pharmaceutical work. In other words, their talk was rich in descriptions of virtuous practices. Data were therefore re-read to elucidate the specific content of these statements, and it became clear that participants were driven by the beliefs that:

- to be virtuous is to be *altruistic (publicly oriented)* at times and *commercially self-interested* at other times,
- to be virtuous is to be *courageous* at times and *cautious* at other times,
- to be virtuous is to be *tenacious* at times and *flexible* at other times, and
- to be virtuous is to be *compliant* at times and *resistant* at other times.

There were, in other words, four sets of potentially competing virtue-oriented axioms ('virtue axioms') evident in our participants' talk. Participants also spoke at length about the need for knowledge and wisdom of various kinds.

Continuum 1: Altruism–commercial self-interest

The first set of competing 'virtue axioms' to be described is that of altruism and concern for the public versus concern about the company and its employees, which is referred to here as commercial self-interest.

Axiom 1: to be virtuous is to be altruistic

Concern for one's fellow humans was seen to be an important motivation for engaging in pharmaceutical work.

> P3: . . . Very often you do know somebody with one of these conditions, and it's a feel good factor that I think you can be proud of what you do, feeling like you're contributing to the wellbeing of your fellow humans. Really that's it.

Maintaining a focus on patients was seen to be a crucial part of the 'medical' role within a commercial environment.

> P12: I talked to a marketing person once and I said 'well where do you see your market for this product?' And he said 'everyone with a mouth' . . . They were half joking, but it's understanding that we are working with products that aren't fast-moving consumables, and decisions are made on behalf of people that aren't really capable of making the decision on their own.

A sense of public responsibility also played out in participants' relationships with other stakeholders. They saw it as their responsibility to collaborate with regulators in finding ways to improve the system for all concerned, to support academic researchers, and to respond to crises in such a way that all interests are accommodated.

> P4: I like the whole strategy of okay how can we get the best outcome for everyone, and not make the crisis not be a crisis, but well-planned, well-organised, so the [regulator] is happy with us, the global is happy with us internally, and I think most importantly the patient is protected.

Participants also thought it was important to consider national resources and to have a global perspective on the effects of Australian drug development.

> P13: . . . my feeling was that we, Australia, owe it to our cousins in Asia for example, to bear them in mind when we are making our own decisions, or when we develop our own processes, because what's good for Australia might have these ripples elsewhere, so we need to be conscious of that.

Axiom 2: to be virtuous is to be commercially self-interested

At the same time, participants were very frank about the fact that they worked for companies that had to consider the rights of shareholders as well as those of the public.

> P3: At the end of the day, we're not a philanthropic organisation. And I'm quite happy to say that. . . And then do we make a profit? Yes we do, we're a business.

P1 described his company's view of compassionate access programmes. While compassion was seen to be an important virtue, this could not be achieved to the detriment of the company's finances.

> P1: So that was applying compassion, but it was applying compassion while keeping an eye on the regulatory environment, keeping an eye on the reimbursement environment, keeping an eye on the evidence of the action of this drug in a particular disease, and also looking at what the financial impact might be on an organisation that has an obligation to its shareholders, to make sound business decisions.

P1 distinguished between the virtue of generosity, which could potentially harm the company, and the virtue of compassion, which was essential and not necessarily at odds with commercial goals.

> P1: We're a pharmaceutical company, and it's essential to make a healthy profit. So I wouldn't use the word generosity, but I would use the word compassion. We do need to be compassionate in what we do.

Continuum 2: courage–caution

A second set of competing 'virtue axioms' to emerge was that of courage, or adventurousness on the one hand, and caution on the other.

Axiom 3: to be virtuous is to be courageous

Participants emphasised the importance of companies being daring, particularly when making large financial decisions and taking financial risks.

> P12: I think why pharma is in so much trouble is they have lost their risk appetite.

Because of the firm's need for daring individuals, participants themselves were seen to need to have a risk appetite and a taste for entrepreneurship.

> P2: [Re why he is successful in industry] I was a bit of an entrepreneur at heart, I liked the idea of entrepreneurship, so I thought that just was a bit more appealing to me [than a medical career].

This, in turn, demanded a degree of calmness, level-headedness and the ability to respond strategically to crises

> P4: I think the...person I admired...(it) was just the way in which he, in difficult circumstances, remained so calm, so level-headed, was very strategic, didn't panic, just through this big mess just sort of came through ...

Axiom 4: to be virtuous is to be cautious

In contrast, in describing their efforts to ensure that their companies would be protected from financial harm, participants placed considerable emphasis on the need for caution, circumspection and self-control. This entailed, for example, doing thorough research before committing to any course of action, as well as having foresight and a long term vision.

> P8: One of the hassles in industry when dealing with some of the marketing guys, is they think very short term, whereas you should think long term ... And I mean if you think in most cases companies want to be around for a long time, so you don't want to do anything stupid today that you will regret in a year's time.

Caution also played out in interactions with other stakeholders and involved recognising what kinds of social interactions were, and were not, appropriate (for example relationships with regulators) and what information could, and could not, be disseminated publicly.

> P5: We have to get abstracts approved, or papers approved, but that's another step – nothing has ever happened to stop that, it's just always been checked.

Several participants emphasised the importance of caution as a means of pre-empting and preventing criticism of the company. In this context, objectivity and truthfulness were important related virtues.

> P6: [Discussing economic applications] they get hold of the data, they can review the data, it's embarrassing if you make mistakes, it's embarrassing, and it can go very much against you if you cause delays, if you actually leave out information.

Caution emerged as a virtue not only when participants were focused on their companies, but also when they were focused on obligations to patients and the general public. In this context, caution entailed demonstrating protectiveness towards research participants and patients. Protection of research participants primarily involved monitoring clinical trials extremely carefully and stopping trials if there was any concern about safety, while protection of patients involved not letting unsafe products go to market and withdrawing medicines from the market in the face of safety concerns.

> P10: It was just too difficult a drug to leave on the market as a [disease] drug, when GPs would be managing it ... and the company chose to pull it off the market pretty soon after its launch, and I think that was a good call.

Continuum 3: tenacity–flexibility

Another set of competing 'virtue axioms' was that of tenacity – the willingness and ability to commit to a course of action – versus flexibility – the ability to change course when appropriate.

Axiom 5: to be virtuous is to be tenacious

It was seen to be crucial to be sufficiently tenacious and assertive in achieving one's goals, to have a 'can do' attitude, and to be committed to one's product, while at the same time being sufficiently tough to tolerate knock-backs.

> P3: [Discussing clinical research] ... we're out there, we're passionate about the drug, and what we hope it's going to improve and how efficacious it's going to be ... there's a sense of ownership about the product that is developed.
> ...(But) It's quite challenging, they get a lot of knockbacks ... You need quite a lot of tenacity, patience, perseverance, you've got to have a little bit of a thick skin I have to say, because you can get quite a lot of knockbacks.

It was also seen to be important to make use of all available mechanisms for achieving one's goals, such as regulatory appeals processes.

> P4: [Discussing regulatory assessments] if we felt the evaluation was really poor, our responses would reflect that. There's also an advisory committee meeting process, then there's appeals. So there are mechanisms.

The communicative correlates of tenacity were assertiveness and rhetorical capacity, i.e. the ability to make the best possible case for one's product and persuade others of one's point of view.

> P10: It became very apparent that you were almost a lawyer for the drug. You're trying to put forward the best aspects of the drug, defend it where possible. ....

Axiom 6: to be virtuous is to be flexible

At the same time, it was acknowledged that it was sometimes important to give up on one's previously defined goals.

> P3: [Re why trials were shut down by her company] Some of them were lack of efficacy, there were a couple that were safety ... and then there were some that were just struggling, and really they'd taken so long, and we'd say we're still working on an injectable, and the competitor's already got an oral formulation, so that type of thing.

Adaptability and willingness to compromise were other related virtues, as was the ability to move on after disappointments.

P10: You could say it's similar to a barrister in court, they've got to put the best foot forward, and the person could be innocent and the person could be guilty, but you've got to do the best job that you can and you've got to, at the end of the day you've got to move on with the next drug and the next opportunity.

Just as tenacity demanded assertive communication, yielding required participants to defer to others, admit their mistakes and accept disagreements.

P8: you have to participate in many teams, and a lot of them with fairly robust discussion on 'I think it should be developed like this', 'no I think it should be developed like this'. You know what I mean. And you can end up with quite a robust scientific discussion, and there's no right and wrong, this person's process is quite okay, but in the end you have to make a decision.

Continuum 4: compliance–resistance

The final set of competing 'virtue axioms' we describe is that of movement between social compliance, or conformity, and resistance.

Axiom 7: to be virtuous is to be compliant

In the context of the pharmaceutical industry, compliance took several forms, including regulatory compliance, teamwork and procedural compliance.

Regulatory compliance: participants all went to great pains to describe their conformity with regulation at all levels including the law, industry guidelines and company rules and protocols.

P12. . . we operated in a highly professional way . . . our goal was always to be very highly compliant, not only with our legal and our industry standards, but from the moral and ethical point of view.

The combination of internal auditing [P11] and external policing [P13] was seen to be particularly valuable as mechanisms for supporting the virtuous compliance of individuals.

P11: . . . there's people that will always bend the rules, and you've got to really protect against fraud, you've got to really audit . . . Now we audit ourselves to make sure everything is hunky dory . . .

P13: [Re codes of conduct] I think they're a good thing. And they're applied, and the reason they're applied and work is because we dob on each other basically, so it's a small world and it's a bit incestuous, so if a company misbehaved, every other company would know about it within 24 hours and would make a complaint. So it's an internal self-policing sort of thing.

Teamwork: it was seen by all participants to be crucial to be comfortable working as part of a large national or global team.

P10: Australia contributes 1–3% of the world's patients, and knowing that the individual work you do contributes overall to a global knowledge base which is then used for registration around the world, so you need to be very comfortable at being a long term cog in a system of many wheels, and doing your job well.

This entailed being willing to prioritise the good of the team over one's own personal interests.

P11: I don't like people who are secretive and think knowledge is a sacred thing and that they all want the glory for themselves. So I won't associate with people like that . . . I don't like people that dob and say 'sorry, she did that and she didn't tick that box on that form'.

Procedural compliance (following protocols): finally, it was seen to be important to be disciplined, and rigorous in one's work, adhering closely to procedural protocols.

P3: We've got hundreds of SOPs, and we train people on GCP tool, they could probably recite it all verbatim. . . . That's probably something we wear internally more than anywhere else.

It was also seen to be important to put clear structures around decisions and have good reasons for deviating from standard processes.

P6: because the [PBS] process has very specific guidelines on how you should do things, what you must do, what you should do. And if you deviate from that you have to have a rationale for it. So it's a well-disciplined system.

Axiom 8: to be virtuous is to be resistant

At the same time, it was seen to be important to be sufficiently independent and not become 'trapped in dogma' or comply slavishly with regulation.

P12: I think the framework is pretty good. Sometimes you have to use your own intuition and own feeling . . .

With respect to teamwork, all participants emphasised the importance of showing courage and independence when the company did not seem to be doing the right thing, manifested in the ability and willingness to speak up within the company, whistle-blow where necessary and leave a company if one felt ethically compromised.

P1: A healthy organisation is one where people will challenge what might be the prevailing view, or what might be the view of the leader or the dominant individual, the alpha male, whatever it is. So that's courage. And so if you think that what we as a company are about to do might be wrong, you have an obligation to speak up and say so. That can require courage.

The meta-axiom: to be virtuous is to have knowledge and wisdom

In addition to isolating specific virtues, knowledge and skills of various kinds were highly valued by participants and this was necessary for the enactment of all other virtues. It was seen to be important to have an understanding of both science and commerce. The ability to reason academically, scientifically and/or clinically was also highly valued.

P5: In the day-to-day work, I use definitely the skills that I got during my PhD, and even honours and being a pharmacist is a foundation for that.

Both unique and specialised knowledge and skills and breadth of knowledge were seen to be valuable attributes.

P10: So I have a broad range of experience which I like as well, a lot of people in industry they are very narrow, they have only worked in industry, they have not had that, and they've got blinkers on, they can't think outside the square.

Attaining this wisdom, in turn, demanded that participants were open to learning – both through self-education and through formal training.

> P11: we've all got to be thoroughly trained, we have monthly training sessions, somebody like me has got to over(see) what the junior people are doing.

But knowledge and skills were not enough, and participants needed to have commercial, political and interpersonal acumen and shrewdness.

> P2: [Re who is likely to succeed in industry] I think people who think a bit commercially, who have a bit of commercial acumen or are interested in having commercial acumen.

They also needed to be intellectually curious, creative and strategic.

> P2: For me I like the strategic kind of things, I like being able to think creatively and come up with lots of different solutions and different approaches. I like to think through problems . . . I like(d) the company, I thought it was very strategic, it was sort of change-embraced creativity and innovation.

Discussion

Summary

The participants in this study were asked to reflect on their careers before and after entry into the pharmaceutical industry. They were asked to describe their own views and experiences, and to comment on other people they had encountered. They were asked to describe people they admired and people of whom they disapproved, and to discuss those aspects of their work they found most and least rewarding. When they did so, they tended to describe themselves and others with reference to virtuous practices.

Theoretical interpretation

Our results suggested that some of our participants' P-level values were underpinned by the axiom 'being virtuous allows one to flourish' and, more specifically, that to be virtuous was to have knowledge and wisdom and to be (at various times) altruistic and commercially self-interested, courageous and cautious, tenacious and flexible, and compliant and resistant. Participants' concerns about altruism and commercial self-interest, courage and caution, tenacity and flexibility, and compliance and resistance are all recognisable as virtues, and their desire to be knowledgeable and wise could correspond to the 'meta-virtue' of phronesis (practical wisdom).

It is not surprising that participants' A-level values were expressed in terms of axioms about what it means to be virtuous in particular situations. After all, we have known for millennia that virtues are linked causally or conceptually to eudaimonic (versus hedonic) human flourishing (MacIntyre, 1993; Pellegrino and Thomasma, 1993; Nussbaum, 1995). MacIntyre, for example, has argued that virtues can best be interpreted by way of the telos or purpose of any beneficent human practice. A good action is one that serves the purpose of promoting welfare according to the telos of the field in which it is carried out (MacIntyre, 1993).

Resonance with other research

These findings have resonance with the few other studies that have explored the values of those working in pharmaceutical and biotechnology companies. Emily Martin interviewed people involved in pharmaceutical sales and marketing departments, and concluded that despite increasingly ruthless profit seeking on the part of their corporations, contemporary pharmaceutical employees can still achieve a kind of 'moral microclimate' in which to carry out their work (Martin, 2006, p. 158) and that they do so by 'find(ing) ways of seeing their work as worthy according to old and enduring American ideas about virtue: pursuing a kind of "health altruism" in which science is harnessed to produce devices that can improve health' (Martin, 2006, p. 158). Steven Shapin interviewed scientists who had chosen to conduct their research in biotechnology companies rather than in academic laboratories. He found that such scientists emphasised a number of virtues, including their ability to compromise, and be flexible, with respect to their research agendas (including, where necessary, sacrificing accumulated intellectual capital). They also took pride in their willingness and ability to work in teams and give up individual credit for achievements, in their loyalty to their companies and willingness to defer to authority, and in their capacity to generate practical outcomes (Shapin, 2008). Although Martin and Shapin did not make the link between espoused virtuous practices (and associated P-values) and underlying guiding axioms (A-values), their research does add credence to the idea that some of the key axioms underpinning pharmaceutical practice take the form of propositions about what it means to be virtuous in particular situations.

Practical implications

The virtue-based axioms upon which participants' practices were based would be easily recognisable to those outside the industry, for there is nothing unique to the pharmaceutical industry about the need for knowledge and wisdom, or the need to balance altruism and commercial self-interest, courage and caution, tenacity and flexibility, and compliance and resistance. This means that, while those outside industry might not recognise or agree with industry's practices (and associated P-values), they are much more likely to share – or at the very least recognise – industry employees' virtue-based axioms (A-values). This, in turn, suggests that virtue-based axioms could form a significant part of the shared 'normative background' of those engaged in debates about the pharmaceutical industry, and that discourse between critics and proponents of the pharmaceutical industry might be improved by distinguishing between P-values – which are likely to differ substantially – and shared, or at least recognisable, axioms.

While such recognition will not solve practice-level disagreements in its own right, it might improve the overall quality of discourse and make it easier to address P-level differences. For example, as mentioned previously, there is an ongoing debate about the kinds of interactions between academic researchers and the pharmaceutical industry that need to be publicly disclosed. In general, debates about this issue have been adversarial, with critics of industry arguing for ever-more stringent disclosure requirements, and supporters of industry fighting back in order to minimise these requirements (Stossel and Stell, 2011). This is an example of a 'P-level' disagreement – i.e. a disagreement about practices.

It is conceivable that this discourse could be enriched if those outside industry were aware of, and able to reflect on, the axioms shaping the industry's P-level attitudes. First, those outside industry might question their assumption that those within industry are driven *only* by the axiom 'to be virtuous is to be commercially self-interested'. Instead they could try to acknowledge that industry employees are driven by a complex set of potentially competing axioms. In addition, doctors, scientists and regulators could acknowledge more frankly that they too hold the belief that 'to be virtuous is to be commercially self-interested', whether this relates to earning a living from caring for patients, funding research projects or establishing academic and clinical institutions. If nothing else, these acknowledgements might change the tenor and sophistication of debates over issues such as disclosing financial transactions.

This in no way absolves those in the pharmaceutical industry of responsibility for ensuring that the practice-level expressions of their deeper axioms are ethical, and for living up to their espoused virtue-based axioms. Nor is it meant to provide an argument for abolishing or relaxing regulation of the pharmaceutical industry. But it does suggest that there is little to be gained from demonising the pharmaceutical industry and being afraid of engaging directly in values-based discourse with those who work within it. In other words, none of this argues against a critical stance to industry, but it does suggest that attempts to deepen and enrich communication with industry by eliciting and reflecting on axioms might be more productive than hostile dependence, distance and suspicion, and may also be more in line with the contemporary realities of the pharmaceutical industry.

Limitations and future research

This was a small qualitative study, and one cannot be certain of the degree to which our findings are generalisable. Future qualitative research might usefully extend to commercial and research departments of pharmaceutical companies and to companies outside Australia, and it would also be useful to corroborate the findings quantitatively. It was also not possible to make fine distinctions between the sub-groups studied (e.g. clinical trial managers versus regulatory affairs managers versus medical directors). Future research might focus on teasing out any differences among these groups. It could also be argued that because this research reports the claims of industry, it is possible that participants were not being entirely honest and were trying to present themselves in a favourable light. Triangulation with other methods (e.g. ethnographic observation) might help to determine the veracity of these accounts. Nonetheless, *espoused* virtues are likely to be significant motivators of future behaviour irrespective of the degree to which they have been put into practice in the past.

Conclusion

Individuals working in the medical affairs departments of pharmaceutical companies spoke at length about the virtues to which they aspire. Little's framework usefully allowed this to be viewed as an expression of flourishing in terms of virtuous practices, underpinned by virtue-style axioms.

Current relationships between the pharmaceutical industry and other stakeholder groups can be described as a form of 'hostile dependence', and discourse among these groups is currently adversarial and lacking in nuance. But this situation might be improved if both groups could be more cognisant of Little's distinctions among different levels of values, and acknowledge the distinction between divergent practices, and the more convergent, or at least recognisable, axioms that underpin them. This could help to bring to light a 'shared normative background' and make discourse less antagonistic and more sophisticated.

Acknowledgement

This study was supported by a grant for values-based medicine research awarded by the Medical School Foundation, University of Sydney.

References

Angell, M. (2004) *The Truth About the Drug Companies: How they deceive us and what to do about it.* New York: Random House.

Bekelman, J., Li, Y. *et al.* (2003) Scope and impact of financial conflicts of interest in biomedical research: a systematic review. *Journal of the American Medical Association,* **289**(4), 454–465.

Charmaz, K. (2006) *Constructing Grounded Theory: A practical guide through qualitative analysis.* London: Sage.

DeMartino, J. K. (2012) The Physician Payment Sunshine Act. *Journal of the National Comprehensive Cancer Network,* **10**(3), 423–424.

Elliot, C. (2010) *White Coat, Black Hat: Adventures on the dark side of medicine.* Boston, MA: Beacon Press.

Lo, B. (2012) The future of conflicts of interest: a call for professional standards. *Journal of Law Medicine and Ethics,* **40**(3), 441–451.

MacIntyre, A. (editor) (1993) *After Virtue – A Study in Moral Theory.* London: Duckworth.

Martin, E. (2006) Pharmaceutical virtue. *Culture, Medicine and Psychiatry,* **30**, 157–174.

McCarthy, T. (1978) *The Critical Theory of Jurgen Habermas.* Cambridge, MA: MIT Press.

Morse, J. M. (1994) Emerging from the data: the cognitive processes of analysis in qualitative inquiry. *Critical Issues in Qualitative Research Methods,* pp. 23–42. Thousand Oaks: Sage.

Nussbaum, M. (1995) Non-relative virtues: an Aristotelian approach. In Nussbaum, M. and Sen, A. (editors), *The Quality of Life,* pp. 242–269. Oxford: Clarendon Press.

Pellegrino, E. and Thomasma, D. (1993) *The Virtues in Medical Practice.* New York: Oxford University Press.

Raad, R. and Appelbaum, P. S. (2012) Relationships between medicine and industry: approaches to the problem of conflicts of interest. *Annual Review of Medicine,* **63**, 465–477.

Roberts, J. M. (2012) Discourse or dialogue? Habermas, the Bakhtin Circle, and the question of concrete utterances. *Theory and Society,* **41**(4), 395–419.

Schulman, K., Seils, D. *et al.* (2002) A national survey of provisions in clinical trial agreements between medical schools and industry sponsors. *New England Journal of Medicine,* **347**(17), 1335–1341.

Shapin, S. (2008) *The Scientific Life: a moral history of a late modern vocation.* Chicago, IL: University of Chicago Press.

Stossel, T. P. and Stell, L. K. (2011) Time to 'walk the walk' about industry ties to enhance health. *Nature Medicine,* **17**(4), 437–438.

Chapter 16

Using the survival-security-flourishing model to explain the emergence and shape of the medical profession

Kathleen Montgomery and Wendy Lipworth

Introduction

In this chapter, we will explore the value of Little's theory of 'modest foundationalism' as a means of shedding a fresh perspective on the medical profession. In particular, we seek to determine whether we can explain why the medical profession exists, and persists, in the form it does in Western societies, without resorting to the almost taken-for-granted assumptions about self-interested striving for power and status that prevail in much of the sociological literature. We first review the development of theories about the emergence and maintenance of the medical profession, drawing primarily from sociological traditions in the USA and UK. Next, we articulate our understanding of the main elements of Little's theory, in which he identifies three pre-normative values – survival, security and flourishing – that, he argues, exist and are expressed in any culture or society. We then propose that a shift in the level of analysis from that of society to that of the collective – in this case the medical profession – can offer new insights into the nature of the profession and its role in society. We conclude with observations about the relevance of this wider perspective for theory and for medical education and governance.

Threads of sociological thought about the medical profession

The medical profession has long been studied as the prototypical model of professionalisation, and its study has formed the basis of many general theories of the professions. A central goal for these theorists has been to explain the high levels of autonomy and prestige held by professionals in society, relative to other occupations.

Debates in Values-Based Practice, ed. Michael Loughlin. Published by Cambridge University Press. © Cambridge University Press 2014.

The functionalist approach

Early work tended to characterise professions as a distinct type of occupational group, by delineating special 'traits' that set professions apart from, and above, other occupations (Carr-Saunders and Wilson, 1933). For several decades thereafter, sociologists devoted much attention to articulating the distinguishing characteristics of professions, including an elevated ethical sensibility, an advanced body of knowledge and esoteric theoretical base, an altruistic orientation, and a sense of professional community, among other traits (e.g., Parsons, 1939; Goode, 1957; Greenwood, 1957; Millerson, 1964; Vollmer and Mills, 1966). These scholars maintained that such traits justified the autonomy, status and power held by professions.

Power-based explanations

An alternative line of thought emerged in the 1970s, dismissing functionalism as little more than a defender of the power and prestige of professionals that resulted from professionals' perceived invaluable role in society. Sociologists began to question the 'attribute approach' as little more than a 'mixture of unproven and often unexamined claims' for professional control and autonomy (Roth, 1974; Hafferty, 1988, p. 203). Instead, these scholars were determined to shift the focus from examining what functions professional groups served and why they differed from other occupational groups, to examining how the groups gained and maintained their power and prestige.

Freidson, one of the leaders of this new perspective, did not deny that professions and occupations were different, but his focus was on the unique ability of professionals to 'exercise control over their work and its outcome' and to be the 'arbiters of their own work performance, justified by the claim that they are the only ones who know enough to be able to evaluate it properly' (Freidson, 1973, p. 30). His goal was to explain how such claims to professional autonomy and control were achieved and maintained. His seminal study of the profession of medicine (Freidson, 1970a) laid out the stages through which the organised profession had historically engendered state support for barriers to entry, such as licensing, based on attainment of higher education and expertise. Larson described these efforts as 'professionalisation projects' (Larson, 1977), which revealed the interdependence between professional claims to expertise and institutional reinforcement through state-supported 'labor market shelters' of licensing and credentialing (Freidson, 1986). Abbott (1988) explored how professional groups established 'jurisdictional niches' to which they claimed exclusive rights to practice, which in turn furthered the power and prestige of such groups.

Balancing functionalist and power-based perspectives

The popularity of this approach to examining – and challenging – professional powers quickly overshadowed the earlier functionalist explanations, with their focus on the essential role of professionals in society. Nevertheless, in recent years, there have been signs of a blending of the two perspectives, recognising that professions can in fact be distinguished from other occupational groups and that their autonomy claims and concomitant power are not wholly unjustified. In his later writings, Freidson (1994, 2001) espoused a more balanced view of professionals and professional powers, through what he labelled a 'third logic of professionalism' that has, at its core, a specialised knowledge that society values enough to want advanced and applied in socially useful ways. This specialised and valuable knowledge, he argued, largely justifies the jurisdictional protections and resulting professional power held by the medical profession.

Dingwall (Dingwall, 2004; Pilnick and Dingwall, 2011) struck a similar chord, highlighting the enduring asymmetrical relationship between patient and physician; others have also emphasised this asymmetry, which provokes an inevitable need for trust (Mechanic, 1998, 2004; Hall *et al.*, 2001; Broom, 2005). Dingwall drew from Adam Smith to illustrate the essence of trust in the medical profession and its relationship to prestige: 'We trust our health to the physician...Their reward must be such, therefore, as may give them that rank in society which so important a trust requires' (Smith, 1776 (1976), p. 118). Dingwall concluded that 'the place of professions in the modern world...uses more colours in its palette than the monochrome of occupational imperialism' (Dingwall, 2004, p. 10).

In this chapter, we pick up the threads of these more recent arguments – that the existence of the medical profession in its current form is better understood using both functional-based and power-based theories of professions. A linking mechanism, we will argue, can be found in Little's theory of foundational values and their expressions.

Foundational values and their expression

In Chapter 14, Little proposes an aetiological theory of foundationalism, in which he identifies three foundational values (F-values): survival, security and flourishing. We briefly summarise our understanding of his argument as follows.

The three F-values are pre-normative, descriptive, *a priori* necessities for a culture to continue and evolve. 'Survival' represents existence, without which a society and its people would disappear. 'Security' represents the need for stability, in order to facilitate survival. Security needs constitute the basis of our willingness to trust and to accept some forms of social control in exchange for predictability. 'Flourishing' represents the need for self-development and self-expression, beyond what is necessary for survival and security, that makes life worth living.

According to Little, these three F-values help to explain and justify our existence, as well as the specific patterns and institutions that give meaning to each society by enabling a sense of security and personal flourishing. While the three F-values exist in any context, their expression – that is, the beliefs, preferences, and practices that flow from the F-values – will differ over time and across cultures and societies. These are codified as axioms (A-values) and practices (P-values).

Axioms (A-values) are generalised principles or 'truths' that are espoused by a particular group in society. A-values often take the form of normative assertions of 'needs' that are derived from the three foundational F-values. They form the beginning of a normative ideology, or set of maxims, from which preferences and practices flow.

Practical values (P-values) are the practices that flow from the axiomatic principles, as a means for implementing the F-values. They are based on the preferences of a particular culture or society at a particular time. P-values thus represent translations of the A-values into actional 'shoulds'.

Explaining medicine using the survival-security-flourishing (SSF) framework

Little's model of survival-security-flourishing (SSF) focuses on the ways in which individuals come together to form societies that enable them to achieve survival, security and flourishing. Our goal is to explore the explanatory power of the SSF model within the health care context at three levels: the level of individuals in societies, the interactional level of patients and their physicians, and the collective level of the medical profession. It is through the combination of these three lenses that we believe a more nuanced understanding of the existence and shape of the medical profession can be advanced. We embrace Little's proposition that F-values are foundational and thus unvarying across societies and levels of analysis. We then propose that many, if not most, societies will espouse the following A-values related to the existence and shape of the medical profession.

• *An axiom that expresses the need for survival*: illness and disease threaten survival, so people need help to deal with illness and disease.
• *An axiom that expresses the need for security*: people who become sick need health services they can rely on and trust.
• *An axiom that expresses the need for flourishing*: people need expert health care so they can enhance their capabilities for self-development and self-expression.

We then propose that the above axioms can be turned into practical actions (P-values) at three levels of analysis: at the level of society, at the level of relationships among individuals, and at the level of collectives (Table 16.1). These three levels of analysis provide complementary explanations for the existence and shape of the medical profession in society.

The societal level of analysis

Survival

The key health care related axiom pertaining to survival (that people need help to deal with illness and disease) generates a societal-level P-value that 'a society should assure that sick people receive the help they need to survive'. More detailed societal-level P-values can be articulated beyond this general one, and their exact expression will depend on the health belief systems and the nature of medical knowledge available in a particular society at a particular time. For example, in one society, a P-value might be that 'people with fever should receive treatment with leeches'; in that same society at a more recent time, a P-value might be that 'people with fever should be treated with antibiotics'. Some societies might adhere to a P-value that 'people with breast cancer should be treated with herbal medicine', while in another society, at the same time, a P-value might be that 'people with breast cancer should be treated with radiation and surgery'.

Security

The key health care related axiom pertaining to security (that people who become sick need health services they can rely on and trust) might generate a societal level P-value that 'a society should assure that health services are appropriate, and that those

Table 16.1 F-values, A-values, and P-values representing relationships in health care at three levels

F-values	A-values	Societal level P-values	Interactional level P-values	Collective/professional level P-values
Survival	• **illness and disease threaten survival** • **people need help to deal with illness and disease**	• a society should assure that people receive the help they need to survive	• physicians should give priority to their patients' needs, as the *telos* of medicine	• a professional entity should exist to support a society's survival needs to manage illness and disease • a medical profession should establish jurisdictional boundaries and legal protections to assure its survival as a distinct entity
Security	• **people who become sick need health services they can rely on and trust**	• a society should assure that health services are appropriate for the needs of people in the society	• physicians should strive for the highest levels of competence, integrity and benevolence in caring for patients	• a medical profession should establish educational, licensing and credentialing requirements to practice medicine • a medical profession should create and enforce codes of conduct to assure ethical behaviour of its members
Flourishing	• **the expression of people's capabilities is restricted by illness** • **people need expert health care so they can enhance their capabilities for self-development and self-expression**	• a society should support research and advancement in medical knowledge, technology, and care provision	• physicians should respect the need for patients to restore their capabilities, and should apply their knowledge and expertise to facilitate that	• a medical profession should offer specialty training, and participate in biomedical and psychosocial research to enable its members to perform at the frontier of knowledge and care provision

allocating resources can be trusted to meet the needs of people in society'. While related somewhat to the discussion about survival needs, this P-value reveals the way in which societies can differ substantially in their system of health care services and providers, depending upon their view as to what is appropriate for the needs of people in their particular society. For example, one community's P-value might be that 'people should have open access to a 24-hour clinic', while in another, a P-value might be that 'people should be seen by specialist physicians through referral and appointment'. P-values relating to payment for health services can also be articulated and will distinguish among societies, such as, 'people should have access to health services regardless of ability to pay', in contrast to 'people should pay to have access to health services'.

Flourishing

The key health care related axiom pertaining to flourishing (that people need expert health care so they can enhance their capabilities for self-development and self-expression) generates a societal level P-value that a 'society should support research and advancement in medical knowledge, technology, and care provision'. This P-value explicitly addresses the evolutionary aspect of Little's model that goes beyond the instrumental P-values associated with mere survival and security; it focuses instead on an individual's or group's potential and capability for self-development and self-expression. It also acknowledges the potential that emergent diseases and epidemics are likely to require innovations in treatment. More specific societal level P-values might articulate an expectation that 'a society should devote a certain portion of GNP to investing in medical research', or that 'a society should foster private investments in technology and pharmaceuticals'. Such P-values are likely to shift over time even within the same society, depending on prevailing political and economic climates.

The interactional level of analysis

As noted earlier, while F-values and A-values might be stable across societal, interactional and collective levels of analysis, their expressions in P-values will be different for each level. We turn now to a more detailed discussion of the interactional level of analysis that involves patients and their physicians.

Survival

The key health care related survival axiom (that people need help to deal with illness and disease) might lead to an interaction-level P-value that 'physicians should give priority to their patients' needs'; this represents the *telos* or ultimate purpose of medicine. Implicit in this P-value is the belief that doctors should take the view that 'the health of (the) patient will be my first consideration' (Declaration of Geneva, 1948) and that 'physicians' self-interest should be secondary to the interest of patients'. Additional specific P-values might provide guidelines for the care of patients with serious disease or chronic illnesses in a way that, for example, incorporates tenets of patient-centred care, and have been shown to vary substantially across communities.

Security

The key health care related security axiom (that people who become sick need health services they can rely on and trust) might lead to an interaction-level P-value that 'physicians should strive for the highest levels of competence, integrity, and benevolence in caring for patients'. As studies of trust have shown (e.g., Hardin, 1996), these are characteristics of trustworthiness, which is considered essential for an optimal physician-patient relationship. Yet, interpretation and implementation of these characteristics can vary substantially between or within societies. A detailed P-value related to integrity might be that 'a physician should be completely honest and forthcoming in discussions with patients about their conditions'. In some societies, however, a different P-value might prevail, that 'a benevolent physician should protect patients by not telling them about a negative prognosis'.

Flourishing

The health-related flourishing axiom (that people need expert health care so they can enhance their capabilities for self-development and self-expression) might yield an interaction-level P-value that 'physicians should respect the need for patients to restore their capabilities, and should apply their knowledge and expertise to facilitate that'. This particular P-value aligns closely with the patient-centred care movement that emphasises respect for patients and patients' wishes. However, in some societies, a different P-value might be espoused that maintains a 'doctor-knows-best' approach to health care provision, with patients discouraged from expressing preferences or asking questions about their treatments.

The collective level of analysis

Thus far, we have detailed health-related P-values from the perspective of individuals in society (the societal level of analysis), and individuals interacting with their physicians (the interactional level of analysis). We turn now to the collective level of analysis to examine the explanatory power of Little's model in relation to the survival, security and flourishing of the medical profession itself. We suggest that this level of analysis both explains the existence of the medical profession as a collective, and reveals the indispensable connection that the survival, security and flourishing of the medical profession has to the survival, security and flourishing of individuals and societies.

Survival

The main health care related survival axiom (that people need help to deal with illness and disease) might generate a collective-level P-value that states that 'a professional entity should exist to support a society's need to survive by managing illness and disease'. This P-value is a likely practical expression of the need for society and individuals to receive the health care they need to survive, by identifying a group who can best serve that purpose.

A second collective-level P-value based on the survival axiom might state that 'a medical profession should establish jurisdictional boundaries and legal protections to assure its survival as a distinct entity'. This P-value shifts the focus from the survival needs of the community to the survival needs of the profession itself. As discussed earlier, there is a substantial body of literature devoted to the ways in which the medical profession has gained and maintained its exclusive legal jurisdiction to practice medicine (e.g., Freidson, 1970a, 1986; Larson, 1977; Abbott, 1988). Although non-physician health care providers, such as nurses and technicians, may have obtained a degree of legal authority also to offer health services, in most Western societies they have only limited authority to operate independently of the medical profession. Freidson (1970b) has referred to this arrangement as 'professional dominance', reflecting the asymmetry in the medical hierarchy where physicians remain legally in charge, overseeing the work of other health care workers. This ongoing dominance might be explained by a P-value (or set of P-values) that sustain such legal protections and help to assure the survival of the medical profession as an entity with distinct responsibilities.

Security

The main health care related security axiom (that people who become sick need health services they can rely on and trust) leads directly to collective/professional P-values that are designed to enhance the trust of individuals not only in their physicians but also in the medical profession as a collectivity. Notably, these P-values dictate the kind of standards that the profession should establish, such as 'a medical profession should establish educational, licensing, and credentialing requirements to practice medicine' and 'a medical profession should create and enforce codes of conduct to assure ethical behaviour of its members'.

The first of these P-values sets up barriers to entry, so that only appropriately educated and licensed practitioners can legally provide health care services. In so doing, this P-value (and more specific P-values that flow from this, outlining details of the nature of medical education, post-graduate training, licensing examinations, performance evaluations, and the like) signals to individuals in society and to patients that the medical practitioners caring for them have been vetted as having met the standards necessary to offer services.

At the same time that this P-value provides a signal of professional trustworthiness to individuals, it also serves the interests of the profession itself, by restricting the potential pool of practitioners and thus limiting competition. Such processes enable the profession to preserve its exclusivity, to heighten demand for its services, and thereby to enhance its power. All these factors strengthen the security for members of the profession as a lifelong career path, once they have successfully passed the barriers to entry.

A second collective-level P-value derived from the security axiom relates to the idea that 'members of the profession should conduct themselves ethically'. For individuals, this P-value is a valuable sign that their physicians can be trusted to exhibit the utmost ethical behaviour, because it is a widely espoused norm of the profession. For the profession itself, this P-value enables members to function with confidence in their own abilities and trust in their peers, and also serves as an important reinforcement of its claim to professional autonomy through practices of self-regulation. Similar to the profession's claim of autonomy and self-determination in setting educational, training and performance standards, the validity of the claim of self-regulation is demonstrated by endorsing and monitoring codes of conduct among members of the profession. Indeed, should a member of the profession engage in unethical conduct, the security of the entire profession may be threatened because of questions raised about the effectiveness of its self-regulation and, ultimately, justification for its claim to autonomy.

Flourishing

The key health care related flourishing axiom (that people need expert health care so they can enhance their capabilities for self-development and self-expression) might generate a P-value at the collective/professional level that states 'a medical profession should offer specialty training, and participate in biomedical and psychosocial research to enable its members to perform at the frontier of knowledge and care provision'. For individuals, this P-value helps to ensure that the profession will expand its knowledge base and expertise, thereby enabling individuals to continue to thrive in the face of emerging health issues that have the potential to threaten their capabilities.

For the profession itself, this P-value enables members of the profession also to expand their capabilities for self-development and self-expression through opportunities for specialisation and gaining advanced knowledge. In so doing, the profession enhances its value to individuals and societies, thus reinforcing the relationship between professional development and the survival and security of individuals and societies.

Discussion

Little has proposed that a set of three pre-normative foundational values underpins a set of axioms or 'truths' that a group or society may adhere to, and from which more specific preferences and practices become articulated and embraced. Although the foundational values are stable regardless of the context, the axioms may be different across societies and over time, and the practices will vary to an even greater extent. Little uses examples of individuals in societies to illustrate his argument.

We have drawn from the basics of Little's theory to explore the relevance of this framework at two other levels of analysis, namely, the interactional level and the collective level. We have identified the key survival, security and flourishing related axioms that pertain to health care; and, within that context, we have articulated several practical values that express these axioms. Our goal has been to use this approach to offer insights about the existence and shape of the medical profession that extend beyond purely functionalist or power-based theories.

Theoretical implications

We began by summarising two main strands of sociological thought about professions, one that justifies the long-standing power and prestige of the medical profession because of its value to society, and the other that challenges the power and prestige of the medical profession as having resulted from a self-interested process of negotiation with the state and other decision-making bodies to establish barriers to entry that has served to enhance professional powers in a variety of ways. We next identified some more recent writing to suggest there is merit in both perspectives, and set out to illustrate the validity of this more nuanced approach using Little's framework.

We have demonstrated how a society's need for survival, security and flourishing can be promoted when a group of experts – in this case a recognised medical profession – provides the health care that is needed for the survival of individuals in the society, serves as a reliable and trustworthy source for such care, and is well prepared to deal with emergent health challenges that may impinge on the flourishing of individuals. This interpretation aligns with the early understandings of a medical profession advanced by functionalist thought. Similarly, the medical profession fulfills a number of interpersonal roles whereby members of the profession help to promote survival, security and flourishing for their patients.

At the same time, when we employ Little's framework at the collective level and examine the relevant P-values, we can see how the medical profession's own survival, security and flourishing are enabled by the construction of professional boundaries, jurisdictional niches, barriers to entry, and opportunities for specialisation. These processes are all consistent with those identified by power-based theorists to explain professional power and its enduring autonomy and self-regulation.

Importantly, we show that these various views of the medical profession express the same health care related axioms which, in turn, are based on the same foundational needs for survival, security and flourishing. We also show that the survival, security and flourishing of a powerful medical collective can facilitate survival, security and flourishing at societal and interactional levels. Thus, our approach suggests that explanations of the existence and shape of the medical profession are richer when they engage in a complex, multi-level examination that neither rejects nor wholly embraces either of the two major streams of thought that have prevailed in sociology for many decades. As with the best theories, we find that Little's framework provides greater clarity and nuance, and has broad applicability and explanatory power.

Practical implications

This nuanced view of the existence and shape of the medical profession also has implications for medical education and governance. From an educational perspective, it highlights the importance of encouraging students to feel proud of the many important functions that their profession fulfils, while reminding them not to take for granted the acceptability or ongoing existence of their professional power.

Further, this framework can help medical students better to understand, and manage, disagreements that may arise in the practice of medicine, by revealing that the same foundational values of survival, security and flourishing underpin beliefs and preferences, even when those beliefs and preferences may differ substantially across communities and over time. Recognising the convergence of F-values and, often, A-values, despite widely varying P-values, can be a powerful insight, especially for those working across cultures.

Efforts to improve the quality of medical practice should similarly focus not only on curtailing abuses of professional power, but also on promoting the medical profession's collective strength so that it can fulfil its many important roles.

References

Abbott, A. (1988) *The System of Professions*. Chicago, IL: University of Chicago Press.

Broom, A. (2005) Medical specialists' accounts of the impact of the Internet on the doctor/patient relationship. *Health*, **9**, 319–338.

Carr-Saunders, A. and Wilson, P. (1933) *The Professions*. Oxford: Clarendon Press.

Declaration of Geneva (1948) World Medical Association, Geneva, Switzerland. Available at: www.wma.net, accessed 15 April 2013.

Dingwall, R. (2004) Professions and social order in a global society. *Revista Electrónica de Investigación Educativa*, **6**, 1–12.

Freidson, E. (1970a) *Profession of Medicine: A Study of the Sociology of Applied Knowledge*. New York: Dodd, Mead.

Freidson, E. (1970b) *Professional Dominance: The Social Structure of Medical Care*. New York: Atherton Press.

Freidson, E. (1973) Professions and the occupation principle. In Freidson, E. (editor), *The Professions and Their Prospects*, pp. 19–38. Beverly Hills, CA: Sage.

Freidson, E. (1986) *Professional Powers*. Chicago, IL: University of Chicago Press.

Freidson, E. (1994) *Professionalism Reborn*. Chicago, IL: University of Chicago Press.

Freidson, E. (2001) *Professionalism: The Third Logic*. Chicago, IL: University of Chicago Press.

Goode, W. (1957) Community within a community: the professions. *American Sociological Review*, **22**, 194–200.

Greenwood, E. (1957) Attributes of a profession. *Social Work*, **2**, 45–55.

Hafferty, F. (1988) Theories at the crossroads: a discussion of evolving views on medicine as a profession. *Milbank Quarterly*, **66**, 202–225.

Hall, M., Dugan, E., Zheng, B. and Mishra, A. (2001) Trust in physicians and medical institutions: what is it, can it be measured, and does it matter? *Milbank Quarterly*, **79**, 613–639.

Hardin, R. (1996) Trustworthiness. *Ethics*, **107**, 26–42.

Larson, M. (1977) *The Rise of Professionalism: A Sociological Analysis*. Berkeley, CA: University of California Press.

Mechanic, D. (1998) The functions and limitations of trust in the provision of medical care. *Journal of Health Politics, Policy and Law*, **23**, 661–686.

Mechanic, D. (2004) In my chosen doctor I trust. *British Medical Journal*, **329**, 1418–1419.

Millerson, G. (1964) *The Qualifying Associations: A Study in Professionalization.* London: Routledge and Kegan Paul.

Parsons, T. (1939) The professions and social structure. *Social Forces*, **17**, 457–467.

Pilnick, A. and Dingwall, R. (2011) On the remarkable persistence of asymmetry in doctor/patient interaction: a critical review. *Social Science and Medicine*, **72**, 1374–1382.

Roth, J. (1974) Professionalism: the sociologist's decoy. *Work and Occupations*, **1**, 6–23.

Smith, A. (1776/1976) *The Theory of Moral Sentiments.* Oxford: Clarendon Press.

Vollmer, H., and Mills, D. (editors) (1966) *Professionalization.* Englewood Cliffs, NJ: Prentice Hall.

Does medicine need a base? A critique of modest foundationalism

Ross E. G. Upshur

> But the scientific spirit requires a man to be at all times ready to dump his whole cartload of beliefs, the moment experience is against them. The desire to learn forbids him to be perfectly cocksure that he knows already. Besides, positive science can only rest on experience; and experience can never result in absolute certainty, exactitude, necessity or universality.
>
> *(C. S. Peirce, 1955, pp. 46–47)*

It is an honour and privilege to provide a commentary on Miles Little's thoughtful and provocative chapter (Chapter 14). In this chapter I will try to make amends for confusion created in some of my previous work that Little criticises. To that end I will clarify some of the terms that I have used in previous essays, particularly 'emergent'. I will, however, stand by my critique of foundationalism, rooted in either values or evidence. I will argue that it may be best to dispense with the concern for foundations entirely as unproductive and misleading. I will defend a version of fallibilism as most relevant to our understanding of evidence and values in medicine. After this, I will invert Little's FAP model and argue that what he has termed F-values are neither pre-normative nor foundational, but rather serve as regulative ideals. I will argue that there is nothing axiomatic about the A-values and that the P-values are where most of what is relevant to medicine transpires. In my chapter I will acknowledge sincere intellectual debts to Charles Taylor, Hilary Putnam and Peter Galison, though the animating spirit is largely Peircean.

Emergence and foundations

I would like to spend some time clarifying my position, apologising and, I hope, making amends for using the term 'emergence' in a confusing way and raising the issue of foundationalism in the first place. I will retrace my steps through a series of papers starting in the late 1990s to early 2000s where I sought to examine the conceptual bases of evidence-based medicine (EBM).

Debates in Values-Based Practice, ed. Michael Loughlin. Published by Cambridge University Press. © Cambridge University Press 2014.

It was clear from the advent of EBM that it would become influential and assume prominence in health care. The early writings of the Evidence-based Medicine Working Group were characterised by insouciance and iconoclasm that was no doubt attractive to many clinicians. However, as EBM evolved there was a distinct disinterest with respect to its conceptual base, from both a normative and an epistemological perspective.

Grateful of funding from a Canadian programme, Health Evidence and Application Linkage Network (HEALNet), I was tasked with examining how evidence might be considered in a more expanded set of disciplines related to health care beyond clinical epidemiology. It was evident from this work that EBM had no operative or agreed upon definition of evidence. Furthermore, there were conspicuous silences and gaps in the types of things considered evidential by EBM. The idea of an evidence hierarchy seemed problematic and we sought to conceptualise evidence in a non-hierarchical manner. We argued that there was no compelling reason to exclude qualitative and conceptual thinking from having status as evidence. We proposed a more dialectical vision of evidence where considerations of meaning and measurement are mediated by their origin and application in the context of care. The weight of consideration would vary depending on whether the application was at the individual or population level (Upshur et al., 2001).

Evidence was not the only problematic concept for EBM. From the beginning EBM has had an uneasy relationship to values. Ethical issues were eclipsed and there seemed to be little recognition of reflexivity in thinking about the relationship between the steps of EBM, the 'facts' that emerge from the types of research it endorses and the value neutrality of those practising EBM. Values, often in tandem with preferences, were to be elicited from patients and integrated into clinical decision-making in an as yet still unspecified manner. That this was an important element of EBM was oft acknowledged by its chief promoters. Little progress has been made and comparatively few efforts have been forthcoming from proponents of EBM to provide clinical tools to aid practising clinicians with this task.

My enquiries into evidence led me away from an approach based on seeking an essential definition of evidence but rather focused on characterising features of evidence as manifest in the life world of medicine. I identified, through reflection rather than systematic review, seven characteristics of evidence that I thought germane to discussions of what we might mean when we engage in discussions about evidence in relation to health care (Upshur, 2000). I will leave interested readers to pursue this paper on their own and I would welcome any additional thoughts regarding whether these characteristics are necessary, unnecessary, sufficient, incomplete or simply misguided.

Three characteristics of evidence are relevant to this discussion and perhaps lead to some of the misperception of my position as argued by Little. Evidence, in the form of published clinical research, I argued, is provisional, defeasible and emergent. I suspect that Little would have no issues with the first two properties, particularly given the tip of his hat to pragmatism. Provisionality and defeasibility simply attest to the well-experienced reality that clinical evidence can be overturned and discarded as relevant to practice as new, more 'adequate'[1] evidence arises. The example of peptic ulcer disease illustrates this point (and conveniently parallels my career in health care). As an undergraduate student, I

---

[1] I will not attempt here to examine what more adequate means in this context. It is a complicated story deserving of its own account.

was an orderly in a community hospital. One of my responsibilities was to ferry patients through the elaborate rituals of hospital admission and pre-operative assessment: cardiograms, chest x-rays and blood work were required for all patients prior to surgery. The most common operative procedure on Monday was vagotomy and pyloroplasty to treat the consequences of chronic duodenal ulceration. In the 1980s when I attended medical school, cimetidine was the breakthrough medication for treatment of ulcers. In the 1990s while studying infection control as a resident in public health, the landmark studies of Warren and Marshall demonstrating the bacterial basis of peptic ulcer disease were adapted and disseminated into effective treatment strategies based on the eradication of *Helicobacter pylori*.

Each of these approaches was based on the best evidence at the time. Technological and pharmaceutical innovations, as well as the application of established canons for assessing causation, were instrumental in the creation of an evidence-base. I will return to this example again below.

My choice of the term 'emergent' was perhaps unfortunate given the precise and technical meaning it has in other forms of discourse as explicated by Little. What I was trying to capture was the temporal horizon within which evidence emerges into medical practice. In my original paper I was trying to understand why research evidence may be ignored and how the provisional nature of evidence needed to be understood as it contributes to a wide range of uncertainties and differences of interpretation. As well, new evidence will often displace or disturb the creation of practice guidelines and patterns of care, often after considerable investment of human and financial resources. So, what I termed as emergence had little to do with complex dynamic systems or supervenience or parts and wholes, but this potential for new evidence to emerge over time and replace or displace established thinking. I will, therefore, no longer use the term 'emergence' in this context.

So my point was that evidence has a temporal dimension and often a limited horizon of utility and application. Perhaps, borrowing from Galison, I will suggest that evidence and clinical practice are often poorly intercalated (Galison, 1997). Galison, in his book *Image and Logic*, points out the many discontinuities within and between scientific discourses in the evolution of particle physics. In his view, rather than there being strong unity in science, there is rather, considerable disunity, typified by discordance and fractures. I think this aptly captures the state of 'evidence' in health care as there is no united and coherent approach to the development and creation of evidence in medicine, nor any common agreed upon structure for its uptake and translation into clinical practice, let alone any universal agreed upon structure for the delivery and evaluation of health services. There is also no reasonable means for a clinician to anticipate when new and relevant evidence will arise and no clear overarching process to ensure the temporal ordering of discoveries relative to needs and priorities, regardless of their ultimate merits. In short, we have an *aporia* of the highest order, one that consumes massive amounts of human and financial resources for which agreed upon goals are largely absent.

I hope I have rephrased and clarified the notion of emergence. I apologise for the confusion. It was no doubt misleading.

I will also try and make amends for the use of the term 'foundationalism'. In what follows I hope to clarify what I think is at stake in the discussion around foundations. I will also stick to my guns, so to speak, and argue that seeking to place medicine on foundations, however modest, is mistaken. The line of argumentation I will pursue here will lead back to epistemology to disavow certain claims about foundations, and to recast the project of what we hope to achieve by seeking foundations in a framework deriving and adapting arguments from Hilary Putnam, Charles Taylor and Peter Galison.

In the paper that Little cites, 'If not evidence, then what? Or does medicine really need a base?' I explore the concept of the 'base' that evidence provides (Upshur, 2002). I argue that for EBM, it would mean that evidence of the sort they endorse is at the ground, the most important element or a fundamental starting point for medicine. I then make the following claim:

> There has been a vigorous debate in the philosophy of science and epistemology concerning the foundations of knowledge. From the perspective of epistemology, EBM can be regarded as a species of foundationalism. Foundationalism is a general term for theories of knowledge that support the belief in the pursuit of incorrigible, secure or infallible knowledge. . . . For EBM advocates, evidence in the form of well-designed clinical studies, provides sufficient reason to support belief and action. It is in this sense, I believe, that the term 'base' is intended to operate in the name 'evidence based medicine'. (Upshur, 2002, p. 114)

I then go on to argue that evidence, given its characteristics as noted above, does not provide the sort of foundation sought by advocates of EBM. It is after the critical analysis that I introduce alternative accounts that are anti-foundationalist. The word emergent occurs again in this context, but not in the sense that I used it previously, but quoting from others. In my conclusion I wrote:

> It has been further shown, from an antifoundationalist standpoint, that medicine and health care are not in need of a single solid foundation, but can operate well in a dynamic emergent framework. (Upshur, 2002, p. 115)

So let me first recant my claims about EBM being foundationalist. It is not simply because EBM is not a theory of knowledge. Calling EBM foundationalist in the sense originally intended is to overstate the ambitions and purpose of EBM. As well, the foundationalism I accused EBM of espousing is a form of what is termed classical foundationalism. One prominent virtue of classical foundationalism is that it provides a response to the sort of infinite regress arguments for justification that Little wishes to forestall with his appeal to Hume. A second feature of foundationalism is the existence of non-inferentially justified beliefs.

I seriously doubt any advocate of EBM believed that the methods and practices of EBM lead to incorrigible and indubitable belief (even if it seemed like this sometimes!). As well, much of the discussion of foundationalism in standard accounts of epistemology bears little resemblance to the context and concerns of clinical medicine, and seldom uses medical examples.

Arguably, the more sophisticated EBM advocate may find common cause with Little in claiming a need for modest foundationalism. Modest foundationalism is subject to a range of formulations, but an apt definition comes from Poston:

> For purposes of terminological regimentation we shall take 'modest' foundationalism to be the claim that the basic beliefs possess knowledge adequate justification even though these beliefs may be fallible, corrigible, or dubitable. A corollary to modest foundationalism is the thesis that the basic beliefs can serve as premises for additional beliefs. The picture then the modest foundationalist offers us is that of knowledge (and justification) as resting on a

foundation of propositions whose positive epistemic status is sufficient to infer other beliefs but whose positive status may be undermined by further information. (Poston, 2010)

I think this definition coheres with what Little espouses, but it remains unclear to me how a modest foundationalism improves on accepting a non-foundational form of fallibilism that I have argued for elsewhere. Is there a psychological or normative advantage to come from wedding language about foundations or bases to an account of what it means to be engaged in medicine?

I think not, and in what remains I wish to move past discussion of foundations, modest or otherwise, and move towards sketching out what I think are promising means of achieving what EBM and VBM desire.

To achieve this I want to set out an argument about why we do not need foundations, explore the relationship between facts and values, and re-engage with the arguments made above about fractures and disunities in medical knowledge.

Grounds without foundations

Charles Taylor, in his paper 'Overcoming epistemology' argues how strategies rooted in attempts to ground knowledge in secure foundations fail because the knower and the known are intimately intertwined. As he argues:

> But once we take this point, then the entire epistemological position is undermined. Obviously foundationalism goes, since our representations of things – the kinds of objects we pick out as whole, enduring entities – are grounded in the way we deal with those things. These dealings are largely inarticulate, and the project of articulating them fully is an essentially incoherent one, just because any articulative project would itself rely on a background or horizon of non-explicit engagement with the world. (Taylor, 1995, p. 6)

I think this critique of foundationalism is relevant to medicine as it directs us to the fact that in medicine our understanding is intimately intertwined with what we seek to do and how we understand the meaning of this endeavour. In short, clinical medicine is not based on representational or propositional knowledge but on our engagement with practices and meaning structures. There is no external 'out there' that further justifies our beliefs. There is no doubt an 'other', which would be the patients to whose suffering, ailments, present and future wellbeing we seek to respond.

The second line of reasoning I would like to trace derives from Hilary Putnam's arguments concerning the collapse of the fact/value distinction (Putnam, 2004). Putnam, though addressing the pretensions of economics to be value neutral, argues that facts and values are intimately entangled. Putnam demonstrates how in sciences like physics, epistemic values pervade theory choice. Concerns for simplicity and elegance, for example, are not factual but normative. In medicine, factual claims are deeply entangled with the overarching purpose of medicine itself. For example, physiology, anatomy, genetics, immunology all have a set of structured 'facts' of interest and value in and of themselves, but the animating purpose as related to medicine is to understand human illness and wellbeing. In EBM any concern for precise diagnosis, effective therapy and accurate prognosis flows from a set of normative concerns. In this case both epistemic and normative values intertwine inextricably. What is important to note is that neither necessarily prevails. Facts and values are co-constitutive in medicine, and looking to disentangle them in any permanent or reliable manner is destined to failure.

I would like to draw together what I have said so far and suggest that rather than looking for something to base medicine on, or trying to locate its centre point, we should embrace a rather different approach and metaphor.

Following Taylor, and the 'interpretivists', the distinctly hermeneutic nature of clinical medicine should be acknowledged. Much effort has been devoted to 'objective' measurement, algorithms, risk tools, and other quantitative strategies largely blind to the inherent reflexivity of clinical medicine. However, as Horton has argued, medicine has an 'interpretive grammar' that is broadly neglected in medical training and thus goes underdeveloped in clinical practice (Horton, 1998). There is a mutual constitution of meaning in the clinical encounter which does not reduce to either factual or normative foundations (Upshur, 1999).

So rather than the pursuit of foundations, I suggest we devote more time to the evolution of medical ideas and trace the varied sources of knowledge and values that shape clinical practice and constitute and influence medicine's current self-understanding. Some of these have shown to be of enduring value, even if they have been subject to vicissitudes over time (Benatar and Upshur, 2013). Think of the evolution of diagnostic reasoning since the time of Hippocrates to the present and how each successive epoch has expanded nosology on the basis of clinical observation and advances in related sciences and technology. We are witnessing a veritable revolution in technology as it relates to diagnosis and patient management with the advent of advanced imaging, genomics and other assorted molecular approaches, computerisation and informatics. However tempting it may be to base or centre medicine in the gene or the brain or the computer for that matter, there will still be no 'out there' out there that transcends meaning, escapes the requirement of reflexivity and interpretation and therefore secures a foundation for medicine. The language we employ and the interpretive structures will no doubt alter. Taylor's historical search for the sources of the modern self seems like an appropriate strategy for modern clinical medicine (Taylor, 1989). Rather than looking for the foundation, we should trace back the multiple strands of science and ethics that have informed and shaped modern medicine. There may be sources worth retrieving and some worth preserving lest they be eclipsed by more totalising views of medicine and health under the banner of a foundation or base.

Building on Taylor and drawing on Galison, I think it important that we expose and explore the discontinuities and fractures in the modern vision of medicine. Medicine is an extremely complex undertaking. Clinical medicine is now informed by more epistemic and normative sources than ever, particularly given the forces of globalisation and the advent of concern for ecology and public health. These epistemic and normative sources are by no means completely aligned, aimed at the same ends or at the same stage of historical evolution. Furthermore they may never be. And it strikes me that in some fundamental way this alignment in either methods or purposes is required if something aspires to be foundational. This, to my mind is impossible and, therefore, so too is any argument for foundations.

Basing or centring medicine on any one thing, be it evidence, persons or patients, seems to me to be a mistaken enterprise. I am not sure what motivates the requirement for this and why, for example, evidence, values and persons or patients cannot be seen as mutually constitutive. In some circumstances evidence, however conceived, may hold more weight than values and vice versa. There are contexts where the interests of persons or patients, always deserving of respect, may take a subordinate role to the needs of a community or society. I have not provided any examples of these particular situations, but they are easily imagined.

I will conclude in the same vein as I did in my earlier paper. In critiquing evidence as the base for medicine, I used Peirce's metaphor of a cable to suggest that evidence is not a golden thread that has privilege over other threads in the cable that gives strength to the inferences of science. Similarly, values or persons or patients should not be privileged above evidence.

> The task of understanding knowledge in health care is to understand and appreciate how the intertwining disciplinary threads relate to and give strength to the modern enterprise of medicine. In this vision, the contexts of practice, experiences and narratives of practitioners and patients, the basic and clinical sciences, values and societal perspectives are not banished to subsidiary places beneath the throne of evidence, but conceived as integral elements of a larger process. (Upshur, 2002, p. 119)

The FAP model

Little starts his essay with an endorsement of an argument strategy employed by Hume to forestall infinite regress arguments. There is a time when questioning must stop. Once one has reached this stage, one is close to bedrock in terms of what can reasonably be stated. I trust that this is the manner in which Little desires us to interpret the two statements concerning values, which, so far as I can follow, he considers to be foundational. He writes:

> So, we may begin with survival, security and flourishing as foundational values. . . . Survival, security and flourishing might be thought of as a priori necessities for a culture or society to continue and to evolve – but it does not say how they must play out in each culture or society. All may agree that there is a concept of good health, and that there is a contemporary need to provide health services. But the philosophy behind the services may differ significantly from culture to culture, as they do, say, between the USA and the UK. In a sense, those differing systems can be appraised by the way that they fit into the prevailing beliefs and ideologies of the societies that house them. People will judge them according to different axioms that express their commitments, but those who construct and maintain them will defend them because they believe that their system is the 'best' way to insure maximum rates of survival, secure resources for those in trouble, and the capacity to restore the disabled to the potential to flourish. (Little, Chapter 14, p. 173)

Little argues that survival, security and flourishing are conjointly required. Yet it is unclear whether they are necessary or sufficient conditions to be met. My sense is that any one 'foundation' is insufficient to secure the conceptual framework that Little seeks. It is unclear whether these three *a priori* necessities are sufficient in themselves to provide the sort of modest foundation that Little desires.

On the basis of the survival, security and flourishing foundation, Little wishes to defend what he calls a FAP model. These three modes must be carefully distinguished from each other. If I have read him correctly the model works as follows.

(1) Foundational values (Little labels these F-values) are broadly shared across cultures and societies. The formulation of these foundational values does admit to variability.

(2) F-values are considered 'pre-normative'.

(3) Normativity is mediated by axioms that will then shape the practical manifestations of the foundational values.

(4) These practical manifestations of values are termed by Little P-values.

(5) There may be different modes of emphasis within and between cultures and societies and even amongst individuals with respect to the modes of emphasis or articulation of the axioms and P-values.

He provides a further articulation of his own specific axioms.

> If I declare some of my own axioms, by which I evaluate the ways in which societies (including my own) express their recognitions of foundational values, they look something like this.
>
> (1) Societal survival and progress demands an open Darwinian pool. To disadvantage a section of a community, to rob it of opportunity, is to rob the whole community of the capabilities of the disadvantaged.
>
> (2) A capabilities and functions approach recognises human needs and abilities better than an econometric one (Sen, 1993).
>
> (3) Individuals and groups matter.
>
> (4) A functioning society must, in these terms, enhance and protect appropriate opportunities for survival, security and flourishing.
>
> (5) Both *zeit* and *geist* relate to a society's survival and progress. Axioms and their expressions in practice will – and need to – change with the times.
>
> (Little, Chapter 14, p. 175)

To this point, I have simply explicated what I take to be the core of Little's argument.

I find it hard to understand survival, security and particularly flourishing as pre-normative. Indeed much of the evolving debate in ethics over the centuries concerns exactly what is meant by such terms. I do not see these as *a priori* necessities at all, but rather as regulative ideals that we strive, collectively, to ensure. Even then, history has demonstrated that such necessities have not been present in many manifestations of human culture, and survival has been prioritised to some but not all humans. Simply put, without an argument of a Kantian nature about the dignity of humans or the embrace of a cosmopolitan world view, some further justification regarding the survival criterion is needed, as large numbers of humans have spent massive amounts of time and effort to ensure that other humans do not survive.

Similarly, security would not be foundational in my account. It may be desirable, but from a fallibilist perspective, 'epistemic insecurity' is constitutive of human existence. We may aspire to trust in norms or knowledge, but this may be a grand delusion. The 'fact' that people crave certainty and stability in no way makes this notion of security foundational. It is more akin to a kind of metaphysical comfort. The Grand Inquisitor in Dostoyevski's Brothers Karamazov famously argues that humans cannot bear the weight of freedom. Freedom is exchanged for security. Similar to the quotation from Eliot that Little provides, the Inquisitor says to the returned Christ:

> You look meekly at me and do not deign even to be indignant with me? I want you to know that now – yes, today – these men are more than ever convinced that they are absolutely free, and yet, they themselves have brought their freedom to us and humbly laid it at our feet.
>
> (Dostoyevski, 1972, p. 294)

Freedom has been a foundational value in many modern cultures, but seems to play a limited role in Little's F-values. This account strikes me as needing a bit more on how to determine what counts as a legitimate range of freedoms and what constitutes 'untrammelled' freedom. I would like to see this issue spelled out more specifically with respect to health care. Is he suggesting that there must be some process in place to set limits on health care choices? Is he referring to controls on markets that foster health inequity? Would this limit on 'untrammelled' freedom not in some way impede the flourishing of some? If yes, then there must be some minimal norm regarding what is encapsulated in the concept of flourishing. It also seems to me that admitting that there are variable constructions of how this can be conceptualised is too plastic for even modest foundations.

Even though the axioms and P-values are consequent to these foundations, it strikes me that there is something that lies beneath these F-values relating to the value of persons. So, *prima facie* it strikes me that there are questions that can be raised at this stage and the F-values as stated may not be as foundational as Little may think.

The notion of humankind and individuals needs some further elaboration. Clearly these F-values relate to persons, and there must be some conception of persons operative in these F-values. Do the values of survival, security and flourishing apply to all humans and societies equally? That is, ought persons, *qua* persons, qualify for or share these values? If so, then they must be regarded as normative in some sense, otherwise they can be countered as non-necessary and therefore non-foundational.

I remain unconvinced by the axiomatic status of the A-values. In Little's scheme, axioms can vary considerably from society to society and person to person. Perhaps I am overly constrained by my training in mathematics and logic in that I consider an axiom to be a proposition that is so manifestly true that it compels assent without proof. The notion of social axioms and the sorts of statements that play the role of social axioms seem to be far from manifestly true and open to considerable need for discussion and justification. Little quotes from one source:

> Social axioms are generalized beliefs about oneself (i.e., personhood), the social and physical environment, or the spiritual world, and are in the form of an assertion about the relationship between two entities or concepts. (Little, Chapter 14, p. 174)

So a question I would ask is what is the meaning of axiom in this context? These generalised beliefs as stated in the quotation are expansive enough to cover virtually anything, and given the admitted variability of these axioms, they seem to do no specific work. As they can take on multiple guises, they seem ill suited to assisting in understanding much at all. Why are they constrained between two entities or concepts? Why not more? So I remain unconvinced that the A-values as stated can actually provide much substantive guidance as they no doubt will give rise to substantive disagreement as in many forms of discourse. I may be guilty of misinterpreting their true meaning and purpose.

I am grateful to Little for providing his own personal axioms as he at least makes clear where he stands on the matter. All I will say about them is that I do respect them, but they are far from self-evident. I will not say much about P-values except to say that it is an unfortunate nomenclature given the prominence of P-values in statistical hypothesis testing. My understanding is that the P-values are the practical or life world manifestations of the F-values and A-values.

In closing this section I would like to pose some questions that are latent in the application of the FAP model to the case of clotting factors. He writes:

From society's point of view as well, every possible step should be taken, because life is precious, and the use of Factor VII is still within the means of most Western societies. That may change, but holds true for the moment. Faith in our own security implies that all reasonable means will be used by medicine when death threatens. Death is the end of flourishing. We want to feel secure that medicine does what it can to rescue us from vulnerability. It is thus easy enough to *understand* why doctors and the general public might want to see off-label use supported in the present state of knowledge. (Little, Chapter 14, p. 180)

I would like to see in this model some sense of how to discuss limits and the end of life. Yes, death is indeed the end of flourishing, but I cannot accept that concern for security requires that all reasonable means be employed to forestall death in all situations. If the FAP model is to have traction in the current reality of medicine, it must guide us to the wise navigation of limits particularly at the end of life. If immortality is the *telos* of medicine and health care, then perhaps Little's argument holds. But finitude and mortality are still what most of us can expect, and the evidence suggests that we are death denying to the detriment of our patients, particularly in the context of advanced age. Does acceptance of the inevitability of death and the recognition of limits have a place in Little's scheme?

Is a good death part of what it means to flourish as a human? Solon recognised this point well. According to Herodotus, in chastising the vainglorious Croesus, he argued that one cannot be deemed happy until one is dead. One may be fortunate, but fate may alter the course of events. So a life that has truly flourished is assessed in retrospect. Joseph Raz has recently argued that having an influence on the manner and place of death is constitutive of the meaning of a life well led (Raz, 2012). So my final request to Little is to provide an account of flourishing and security that recognises the inevitability of death. Or is survival the truly foundational concept?

Conclusion

I realise that Little could not cover every conceivable nuance of his approach in one essay. My task here has been to stimulate more discussion on what is, without doubt, a most important set of questions related to the nature of medicine and health care that he skilfully explores in his chapter. I suspect encouraging divergent views on these ideas may be part of the motivation behind his writing. While we may not be able to agree on the need for even modest foundations, I do think we would agree on the need for open and honest dialogue about them.

References

Benatar, S. and Upshur, R. (2013) Virtue in medicine reconsidered: individual health and global health. *Perspectives in Biology and Medicine*, in press.

Dostoyevski, F. (1972) *The Brothers Karamazov 1*, translated by Magarshack, D. Harmondsworth: Penguin Books.

Galison, P. (1997) *Image and Logic: A Material Culture of Microphysics*. Chicago, IL: University of Chicago Press.

Horton, R. (1998) The grammar of interpretive medicine. *Canadian Medical Association Journal*, **159**, 245–249.

Peirce, C. S. (1955) The scientific attitude and fallibilism. In Buchler, J. (editor), *Philosophical Writings of Peirce*. New York: Dover Publications.

Poston, T. (2010) Foundationalism. Internet Encyclopedia of Philosophy, www.iep.utm.edu/found-ep/#SSH4aii, accessed 27 March 2013.

Putnam, H. (2004) *The Collapse of the Fact/ Value Dichotomy and Other Essays.* Boston, MA: Harvard University Press.

Raz, J. (2012) Death in Our Life. Oxford Legal Studies Research Paper No. 25/2012; Columbia Public Law Research Paper No. 12–305. Available at SSRN: http://ssrn.com/abstract=2069357 or http://dx.doi.org/10.2139/ssrn.2069357.

Taylor, C. (1989) *Sources of the Self: The making of Modern Identity.* Boston, MA: Harvard University Press.

Taylor, C. (1995) Overcoming epistemology. In *Philosophical Arguments.* Boston, MA: Harvard University Press. Cited from www.marxists.org/reference/subject/philosophy/works/us/taylor.htm.

Upshur, R. E. G. (1999) Priors and prejudice. *Theoretical Medicine and Bioethics,* 20, 319–327.

Upshur, R. E. G. (2000) Seven characteristics of medical evidence. *Journal of Evaluation in Clinical Practice,* 6, 93–97.

Upshur, R. E. G. (2002) If not evidence, then what? Or does medicine really need a base? *Journal of Evaluation in Clinical Practice,* 8, 113–119.

Upshur, R. E. G., VanDenKerkhof, E. G. and Goel, V. (2001) Meaning and measurement: an inclusive model of evidence in health care. *Journal of Evaluation in Clinical Practice,* 7, 91–96.

Values-*based* or values-*informed*? A non-foundationalist argument for the more rational positioning of health care values within a person-centred clinical decision-making framework

Andrew Miles

Introduction

It has been argued that modern medicine does not need a base (Upshur, 2002) and that a more complete understanding of clinical practice is necessary to overcome the current dualism between facts and values in an acknowledgement of the complex interplay between values, perceptions and beliefs that frame how medicine is practised (Miles and Loughlin, 2011; Miles and Mezzich, 2011a, 2011b; Chapter 19). In reviewing the interpretive approach in medicine alongside phenomenological approaches to clinical practice, Upshur is clear that the value of anti-foundationalism in medicine is precisely that it pushes medicine away from simplistic conceptions of the relationship between science and medicine, and in so doing actively prevents incomplete and reductionist models of practice, such as evidence-based medicine (EBM), from prevailing (Upshur, 2002; Chapter 17). Upshur (2002) has argued that scientific evidence is unable to function as the *base* of clinical medicine and that, from the anti-foundationalist stand-point, medicine does not need a single, solid foundation, but can operate well within a dynamic, emergent framework. Real possibilities therefore exist for the integration of categorically different approaches within medicine, so that science and art, fact and value, rather than being held apart as polar opposites, can and should be increasingly yoked together in the service of medicine and humanity (Miles and Loughlin, 2011; Montgomery, 2006; Miles, 2007, 2009a).

In contributing a chapter to the current volume, my purpose is not to support the notion of a values-*based* medicine or practice (VBM/P), but rather to argue against it. Does this mean that I oppose the notion and importance of values in

Debates in Values-Based Practice, ed. Michael Loughlin. Published by Cambridge University Press. © Cambridge University Press 2014.

health care – those of the patient, the clinician(s), the health care system and the 'body politic' of society at large? In short, no – to do so would be manifestly absurd. Rather, I argue that these values are indispensable – indeed inescapable – in the delivery of effective health care, but only when they function as *informing*, not as *foundational*, factors. Values, then, should *inform* clinical decision-making alongside a range of other sources of knowledge relevant to the care of the patient, upon which the clinician can draw variously with direct reference to the unique personal circumstances of the individual clinical case. To assert that values should be ranked in importance above all such other sources of knowledge or that they should represent a preferred foundation for medicine, is to accord them an irrational hegemonic privilege. Such an assertion would be axiomatically misguided and would directly repeat the well-categorised types of epistemological errors committed by the EBM movement over the last two decades of its existence. As modern health care, assisted by profound political change, progressively extricates itself from the reductive epistemic cage of biomedicalism into which the evidence-based medicine movement successfully locked it (Miles *et al.*, 2008) – and where the patient is now being actively returned to the centre of care (Miles, 2013; Miles and Asbridge, 2013) – we must avoid substituting one recommended foundation of medicine, with yet another.

In this chapter, it is not my intention to debate the concept of value – this has occurred elsewhere within this volume at considerable length. My purpose here is to look directly at the concepts of foundationalism, modest foundationalism, anti-foundationalism and relativistic foundationalism in medicine and their relationship to the idea of a values-*based* or values-*informed* medicine or practice. Foundationalism and anti-foundationalism are typically understood as doctrines in the philosophy of knowledge, sharing a common epistemological history. In arguing whether values should function as the base of medicine or simply inform its practice, I found it necessary to examine both systems, reflecting also on the related concepts of 'modest' and 'relativistic' foundationalism. I conclude that the most authentic account of medicine would see it described in non-foundational terms, as primarily a human endeavour which draws necessarily on the multiplicity of medicine's knowledge sources, without being referentially harnessed to any single, privileged foundation.

In posing the question 'If not a values-based medicine and practice, then what?', I describe an alternative approach to the care of those who are ill. 'Person-centred clinical care' (PCCC) has emerged in answer to the philosophical, economic and political crisis in modern medicine and foundationalist confusions occasioned by the rise and fall of the EBM movement (Miles and Mezzich, 2011a; Miles and Asbridge, 2013). I recommend this new approach to clinicians striving to understand and deal with the increasing numbers of people presenting with long term chronic illness and multi-morbid disease, in a world where almost seventy per cent of global deaths now result from illnesses of this nature (Miles and Mezzich, 2012). In concluding, I exhort clinicians, academics and health policy advisers to governments, to reject narrow, foundationalist accounts of the complex clinical, human and moral endeavour that is clinical medicine. Far from extricating a proper consideration of health care values from clinical practice, PCCC acts most assuredly to guarantee it.

Foundationalism in philosophy

Foundationalism has a long and distinguished history within the intellectual tradition. Aristotle, writing in his *Posterior Analytics* (see Harari, 2010), provides a detailed discussion of its tenets, as does Descartes in his *Meditationes de Prima Philosophia* (see Heffernan, 1990). Both philosophers insist that the foundations of knowledge must be irrevocably *certain*. Following Descartes, we see many great minds arguing similarly, including Locke (see Winkler, 1996), Kant (see Guyer and Wood, 1998), Russell (1948), Clarence Irving Lewis (Lewis, 1952) and Roderick Chisholm (see Hahn, 1997), among others. Despite significant differences between different versions of foundationalism, a common thread is the idea that beliefs (particularly if they are to count as knowledge and/or the basis for justified practices) require *justification*. Where justification is inferential in nature, a given belief is justified on the basis of another belief. In such circumstances we are bound to ask how such a supporting belief is itself justified, as our reason for holding the first belief is only as secure as whatever reason there is for holding the supporting belief. In such a train of reasoning, to avoid an infinite regress, either we must come to an arbitrary stopping point, where there is something we 'just believe', groundlessly, or we arrive at some belief that is 'self-evident', such that it makes no sense to question it.

Foundationalism utilises a two-tier structure, employing some types of justification which are non-inferential (which is to say foundational) and other types of justification which are inferential (which is to say non-foundational), positing that they are derived, ultimately, from foundational justification. In defending their theses, advocates of foundationalism typically employ the metaphor of construction, where the foundations of a building need to be laid down in advance of the bricks and mortar that are to be positioned upon them. Sober, for example, asks us to consider what maintains a building upright and prevents it falling over, his answer being a solid foundation and the superstructure attached securely to that foundation (Sober, 2012).

Foundationalism in epistemology has been extensively criticised, and defenders of different versions of foundationalism are frequently in dispute with each other. The strongest form of 'self-evidence', espoused in rationalist versions of foundationalism (most famously that of Descartes), is a proposition whose denial entails a contradiction. But empiricist philosophers deny that any substantive truth could follow logically from a proposition that is 'self-evident' in this sense, and so empiricist versions of foundationalism will appeal to some weaker notion of self-evidence, some basic facts or features of experience that cannot be plausibly denied. Serious problems arise for either form, when it comes to moving from truths of abstract reason or apparently undeniable features of human experience to conclusions about the nature of objective reality and particular situations in the real world. The construction metaphor breaks down here, because we seem to be confronted with an inferential gap between the foundations and the objective claims whose foundation, ground or basis they are presumed to supply. If our beliefs about everyday life and practice really do require a foundation, then it is hard to see how this requirement can realistically be satisfied, leading anti-foundationalists to explore conceptions of justification that do not appeal to the questionable notion of underlying foundations.

Foundationalism in medicine – the example of EBM

In considering whether strong foundations are necessary for medicine and whether they are indeed available, we must ask whether there is any empirical knowledge in this particular context that is so certain that we act in error if we answer in the negative. We know that classical foundationalism insists that strong foundations must exist for any branch of knowledge and that all of our 'other' knowledge – the 'superstructure' (Sober, 2012) – thus rests upon these 'secure' beliefs. But unlike in mathematics or physics or logic, in medicine we have no such assurances that these foundations can or indeed do exist or that they are in fact necessary for an effective clinical practice. To be certain, the care of the sick cannot in any way be directly compared in its epistemology or methodologies with the above sciences or with the premises through which we attempt in philosophy to establish logical proofs. Considerations of this type, however, were either unavailable to (possible) or ignored by (likely) the 'founding fathers' of the evidence-based medicine movement, who have sought, since the early 1990s, to impose upon modern medicine a radically foundationalist account of knowledge and action in clinical practice that, via its scientism (Miles, 2009a; Loughlin *et al.*, 2013a), has occasioned considerable damage to the historic nature, fabric and purpose of the profession of medicine. I consider EBM here for two reasons. Firstly, because EBM provides a highly salutary lesson to those who would argue for foundationalism of any kind in medicine, whether for a foundation represented by scientific evidence or for a foundation represented by values. Secondly, because arguments have been advanced for a 'complementarity' of EBM and VBM, with assertions that they cannot come into conflict and are therefore 'natural partners' within a clinical decision-making framework (cf. the 'two feet' principle, Fulford, 2004).

The term 'evidence-based medicine' was initially employed in 1990, the nomenclature appearing tangentially within the literature in 1991 in advance of a formal proposition published within the *Journal of the American Medical Association* in 1992 (Evidence-based Medicine Working Group, 1992). Employing an appeal to Thomas Kuhn's *The Structure of Scientific Revolutions*, it was asserted that medicine's traditional paradigm had become untenable and that a new model of medical practice had become necessary. Intuition, clinical judgement and experience and pathophysiological reasoning were all collectively de-emphasised and, for the first time within the history of medicine, it was explicitly recommended that medical practice should be fundamentally based on the principles of clinical epidemiology and thus on biostatistical data derived from methodologically limited study designs such as randomised controlled clinical trials (RCTs), meta-analyses, cumulative meta-analyses of RCTs and systematic reviews of the peer reviewed medical literature. Such data were reified as constituting the 'evidence base' of clinical medicine. Startlingly, no empirical evidence was offered by the authors in demonstration of an inherent superiority of the proposed new paradigm over and above the existing one. Indeed, it was admitted that no such evidence existed (Evidence-based Medicine Working Group, 1992).

In affording a primacy in clinical decision-making to scientific evidence derived from epidemiological study designs conducted in rarified trial populations (the so-called 'E' of EBM), the EBM model, via its radical foundationalism, acted to preclude the use within medical practice of the plurality of other sources of clinical knowledge of immediate relevance to the care of patients. It is for this reason that EBM continues to be well described as dogmatic, reductionist and formally scientistic, unable to understand and respond to the human dimension of suffering. Indeed, in insisting that scientific data should provide the singular base of clinical medicine, EBM excluded from primary importance the patient's subjective experience of illness, relegating narrative, values, preferences, cultural background, psychology, emotions, spirituality and psychosocial situation to secondary importance as somehow inferior types and sources of clinical knowledge for decision-making. In exalting objective, quantifiable science and diminishing all of the subjective and qualitative, EBM threatened to denude medicine of its nobility, treating the patient not as a person, but rather as a complex biological machine (Miles, 2012a, 2012b; Miles and Asbridge, 2013). EBM, then, provides the example par excellence of the dangers of foundationalist thought, its limitations having been vividly demonstrated, especially in the context of the inherent and considerable complexity of chronic, multi-morbid illness, the greatest challenge to modern medicine in recent times (Miles and Mezzich, 2012). Is what is needed here the addition or construction of a further 'foundation' (or to use Fulford's preferred expression, another 'foot') for practice (Fulford, 2004), one which uses the term 'values' as a cover-word for all of the human elements of clinical practice EBM served to devalue? Or is it an abandonment of the construction metaphor and thus of the application of ideas derived from foundationalist philosophy to understanding clinical practice? I submit that it is the latter.

It is, perhaps, the recognition of the inescapable complexity of modern clinical practice, coupled with a sustained rejection of the foundationalist doctrine of EBM by large sections of international medicine, coupled again with a major political shift towards the individualisation of care and the return of the importance of the subjective to medicine (Miles, 2012a, 2012b), that is leading EBM away from its radically foundationalist stance in the direction of a more flexible model. But progress in this context has been slow and grudging, leading Charles *et al.* to conclude that, despite its four serial reconstitutions of concept and method, EBM continues to demonstrate a lack of clarity and logic, being inconsistent and incomplete and retaining an ambiguity and incoherence that is the product of a lack of an underlying theoretical basis and the absence of empirical evidence to support its validity (Charles *et al.*, 2011). EBM has always been, and remains, in these authors' view, a belief-based system, devoid of justification and adequate philosophical reasoning. The search for an intellectual justification to defend a position articulated many years previously without one is hardly an approach unknown within intellectual history (Loughlin, 2009), but EBM's retrospective attempts at justification serve to demonstrate how its radical foundationalism ultimately led to its collapse when, on searching for an empirical justification, it failed to find one. Might a more 'modest' foundationalism provide a compromise, a more epistemologically agreeable model?

Modest foundationalism

Foundationalist philosophers cannot but be confronted by the objective limitations of the foundationalist ideal, by the intrinsic limitations of the philosophy itself. How, then, do they deal with such a clearly delineated problem?

In contrast to strong foundationalism, modest foundationalism steps back from requiring the infallibility of basic beliefs. Rather, it views as acceptable the notion that basic beliefs are justified unless evidence to the contrary can be provided. It is foundationalistic because it insists that all non-basic beliefs require ultimate justification by basic beliefs. However, it does not require an infallibility of basic beliefs and recognises inductive reasoning as a permissible form of inference. By its nature, modest foundation-alism accepts adequate justification and does not therefore require the association between perception and reality to be proven.

The version of foundationalism Miles Little defends is a 'modest' form (Chapter 14). Writing in the *Journal of Evaluation in Clinical Practice*, Little (2013) attempts to 'bridge the gap' between a radical foundationalism in medicine and the radical anti-foundationalism that I have proposed as epistemologically and methodologically pivotal to the understanding, application and development of a person-centred medicine. He takes me to task (Little, 2013) for arguing, in defiance of the '... well established philosophical tradition suggesting that all forms of reasoning and rational practice require a base or rational foundation...', that medicine does not have or need a base. My argu-ments were based on those previously articulated by Upshur (2002). On re-reading the papers to which Little takes exception (Miles and Loughlin, 2011; Miles and Mezzich 2011a, 2011b), I find that nowhere did I claim that foundationalist approaches to medical practice were 'fatally flawed' epistemological propositions in medicine. In fact, I agreed with Upshur (2002) that foundationalism, *per se*, could not be '...excluded from a coherent theory of medicine...' and that '...real possibilities exist for the integration of categorically different approaches within medicine' (see Miles and Loughlin, 2011; Miles and Mezzich, 2011b). Of course, a medicine based on science alone is as possible as one based solely on values or one based solely on cultural factors. If patients wish to consult a practitioner of any one of these kinds of medicine then they are as free to do so as they are to consult a practitioner of alternative medicine. The model would be amenable to description and a belief in its superiority to other models could be held, irrespective of an empirical justification. Indeed, the models I have mentioned share with alternative medicine a lack of continuing empirical justification. In the articles to which Little refers, I had intended to make clear that I rejected any such model, because its foundationalism created an irrational hegemony, with such an exclusivity of foundation actively opposing the use of other sources of knowledge vital to a more humanistic account of the care of the sick. In the paper to which Little refers I put it thus:

> There is only one form of medicine, despite the arguments over its base. EBM's initially strident insistence that quantitative scientific data derived from epidemiological and methodologically limited study designs should form the base of clinical practice has been seriously questioned following extensive philosophical argumentation and critique. With such absolutism effectively now defunct, arguments have appeared which commend a 'modest foundationalism' in substitute. These models, however, despite their noble aspirations aimed at philosophical resolution, remain problematic in claiming for medicine largely singular visions predicated upon the specific viewpoints of individual schools of thought. Thus, those colleagues working within narrative theory and practice will argue for narrative-based medicine, while others working within the field of values will argue for values-based care, even others will promote relationship-based practice. We maintain that medicine does not have or need a base, but that it is, in accordance with Montgomery's thinking, a rational practice based on a scientific education and sound clinical experience; in other words, not just a body of scientific knowledge and a collection of well-practised skills, but rather a conjunction of the two: the rational, clinically experienced and scientifically informed care of sick people. Thus, good medical practice remains *informed* by biomedical and technological advance, *enriched* by narrative, *guided* by values and preferences and

centred on the clinician-patient relationship as a dialogue between persons – rather than being trapped in a given epistemic cage and defined by any one particular source of knowledge for decision-making. (Miles and Mezzich, 2011b)

Elsewhere, I argued that:

> In order to participate in the securing of the authentic development of clinical medicine that is person-centred clinical practice, it is difficult to see how EBM can escape the necessity for a fifth reconstitution (beyond its current and fourth metamorphosis), as part of which its vertically ordered hierarchy of evidence is rotated 90 degrees, as it were, to become fully and thus non-hierarchically horizontal. When such a horizontally ordered library of knowledge sources to inform clinical decision-making is created, several additions must be made to it and these will be largely qualitative and person-centred in their nature. None can be given greater weight than another, given that the usefulness of the given knowledge source(s) will depend on the unique circumstances of the individual patient and his/her expected outcomes and goals . . . we have, then, the opportunity to move from an evidence-based to an evidence-*informed* way of 'thinking' and 'doing'. (Miles, 2012b)

Citing the first of these quotations, Little (2013) finds in my position a 'provocative stance, and a dismissal of a long and respectable tradition in the philosophy of knowledge'. He asserts that he and his colleagues at the University of Sydney are 'not advocating absolutism, but attacking it, and seek to make this absolutely clear'. Fair enough. Yet the title of Little's paper states that '. . .Medicine rests on solid foundations', seemingly advocating the very absolutist stance that he has taken care to reject within his paper. Should we forgive Little the rhetorical display of a reactionary entitling of his paper? Or is he not as rejecting of absolutist foundationalism in medicine as he would have the reader believe? After all, in his paper, Little seems to employ 'base' and 'foundation' interchangeably. A closer reading of his paper – and indeed his works within the current volume – might give some clues.

Little (2013) appears to agree with me that classical foundationalism in medicine is 'impossible', yet he seems nervous to dispense with the notion of foundationalism in medicine in the absolutist (anti-foundationalist) manner which I argue is necessary if medicine is to progress. He seems to argue as follows: (1) strong foundations are not available but (2) medicine must have some form of foundation, therefore (3) medicine has to have less than strong foundations, therefore (4) medicine can utilise modest foundations, therefore (5) modest foundations can secure medical theory and practice, so (6) modest foundationalism must be formulated and recommended. I agree with (1) but reject (2) and all the points which follow. In arguing for a 'modest' foundationalism, Little advances a form of *via media*, a middle ground, as it were, that seeks a form of accommodation between what he sees correctly as the polar opposites of foundationalist and anti-foundationalist positions. As I have noted, to seek a synthesis of this type is entirely noble. However, Little's arguments in my view serve only to complicate, not simplify, what has been interestingly – though aptly – described as the 'jungle' of clinical practice. While *viae mediae* can be useful, I believe the compromise Little (2013) proposes to be at the very least a distraction and at the very worst an obstruction to medical progress. Indeed, for me, Little's suggestions 'muddy the waters' and stand in the way of ongoing conceptual clarification and methodological development in the field.

Why do I argue thus? Firstly, I predict that many clinicians will find the concept of a 'modest foundationalism' for clinical practice, in the way Little (2013) presents it, confusing. He does not argue for the establishment of foundations in the strictly Cartesian sense, nor does he argue for moral foundations in the manner in which Kant's categorical imperative clearly does or with reference to Pellegrino's thinking (see Englehardt and Jotterand, 2008). On the contrary, he appears to reject the thinking of these rationalist philosophers by citing, instead, the empiricist, anti-rationalist, sceptic and moral subjectivist that is Hume. Little's reasoning is that there are some things to which human beings 'just do' attribute intrinsic value, notably the examples he gives of 'survival, security and flourishing'. These values are basic (foundational) in that there is no point in questioning why they are valuable, and other values are then 'explained' as being based on them. All social phenomena, including radically differing but sustainable medical practices, can apparently be 'explained' with reference to these values. But what manner of explanation is this? Just as radical foundationalism encountered an explanatory 'gap' when moving from the 'foundations' to the particular facts or phenomena to be explained (or the beliefs to be justified), is there not a similar gap in the case of this 'modest' variety? While, certainly, it is hard to see how a society could be sustainable (i.e. survive) if none of its members valued survival, I do not see how Little can then navigate the 'leap of faith' from this foundational assertion in order to explain these social phenomena in terms of how they instantiate these foundational values. For me, there is a great deal of explanation missing here. I am particularly struck, if not confused, by the examples that Little employs in talking of anti-oppressive movements (and so on) which are highly emotive in nature and surely fail to appreciate that the practices Little deems oppressive, and by implication wrong, may be, in fact, socially sustainable (and therefore every bit as 'based upon' the foundational values as the ones he applauds).

Little's version of foundationalism gives, then, no clear method of resolving any moral question. Indeed, in terms of how different societies have different values, this sociological account seems to tell us nothing of substance at all; only that different societies, with radically different values and ways of treating social problems (including many different and mutually incompatible ways of deciding upon the allocation and organisation of medical treatment), all turn out to be instantiations of the foundational values. A further point to be made here relates to Little's description of his foundational values as 'pre-normative'. How, then, can they serve any justificatory purpose? If I reject the notion that there can be any irreducibly normative truths in a proper 'scientific' account of the world we live in, then, surely, there can be nothing that we just ought to recognise as inherently right or wrong and moral language becomes, in one form or another, just the expression of the way individuals 'feel', providing no way to determine the rightness or wrongness of how they 'feel', other than noting that this is what they do 'feel'. So even if there are some evaluative claims upon which we can all agree (such as the claim that survival – at least for a certain duration, under certain conditions – is good), whenever we find we disagree about any matter of practical significance, appeal to the 'foundations' can 'explain' all possible positions, but cannot explain why we *should* espouse any one position rather than any other. It will be left to how we feel, just as though we had never encountered this explanatory thesis. Modest foundationalism fails, therefore, to provide medicine with a framework via which to advance clinical practices, as there is no non-arbitrary way of bridging the gap between the foundational values identified and specific decisions about real cases. If this is accepted, then what alternatives may exist? Two philosophies immediately come to mind and will be considered here: anti-foundationalism and relativistic foundationalism.

Anti-foundationalism

To anti-foundationalists, foundationalism is, *per se*, an 'odd' reasoning. Rather than an intellectual premise, which seems immediately supportable, foundationalism appears instead as a futile effort to deal with the 'regress' problem of justification within epistemology. As we have seen in the example of EBM, efforts to apply foundationalist thinking to medicine can result in a particular point of view being privileged above others and therefore given a form of 'absolute authority'. In this way, an attempt is made to preclude a collective deliberation. Foundationalist perspectives are, then, *a priori* antagonistic to the fundamental aim of intellectual discourse, aiming to prove, by whatever means, the requisite foundation.

Anti-foundationalism in medicine opposes the hegemonic claims of any particular foundation suggested as the base of clinical practice and posits directly that we cannot identify, less so provide, any one form of knowledge that has secure foundations in either pure experience or pure reason (Rockmore and Singer, 1992; Uebel, 1996; Bevir, 1999). An anti-foundationalist epistemology has many specific implications for health philosophy – some are highly contentious, others less so, but all remain relevant to the ongoing debate. Certainly, anti-foundationalist epistemologies include many that were advanced prior to the appearance of the term itself. One thinks immediately of the post-modernists and post-structuralists as well as the many analytical philosophers who were profoundly influenced by such thinking, such as the pragmatists, most notably Peirce (see Debrock, 1994) (whose fallibilism is a major influence on the anti-foundationalist stance of Upshur) and the substantially influential philosophers Quine (see Gibson, 2004) and Wittgenstein (Wittgenstein, 1974; see also Goodman, 2002).

The anti-foundationalists have defined a variety of epistemologies and these have generated many of the fundamental critiques of the type of positivism and naïve empiricism that has characterised EBM. The aim of this chapter is, nevertheless, not to achieve a form of synthesis of these varying epistemologies, less so to establish a dogmatic definition in the philosophy of medicine. Rather, I aim to espouse the potential benefits for medicine of a pragmatic anti-foundationalism as part of a new model of clinical practice which has been termed 'person-centred clinical care' (PCCC) and to which I will turn prior to concluding. But let us now examine the potential for clashes between scientific evidence of the type espoused by EBM and values as they derive from patients, clinicians, health systems and society as a whole. Does a values-*based* practice invite and make inevitable such a clash? Or is there a sense in which medicine and practice can be based on more than one foundation?

Conflicts between scientific evidence and values and the failed promise of a 'relativistic' foundationalism

In arguing for a clinical practice that is science-based, but *also* values-based, with claims that the two systems cannot enter into a state of irredeemable tension or conflict, Fulford (2004) appears to argue for a relativistic foundationalism. I say 'appears to argue', because Fulford's account of a values-based medicine as compatible with an evidence-based medicine does not achieve an overwhelming clarity, at least for me, on this pivotal point. Fulford's position on philosophical forms of relativism, most notably ethical relativism, is the subject of extensive discussions elsewhere in this volume (see

Chapters 3, 4, 5, 6, 7 and 8) and the reader is referred to those sources for the associated debates. Here, I want to meditate a little on Fulford's apparent proposition, and in doing so I must inevitably return to EBM with its own definition of evidence and how this has changed to include values.

To many philosophers, 'relativistic foundationalism' is oxymoronic and directly contradictory. Followers of the debate in health philosophy will readily recognise that there is a sense in which facts and values can collide. Tonelli, for example (Chapter 19) has cautioned against the simplistic notion (currently extant) that good shared decision-making incorporates 'facts' provided by the physician and 'values' supplied by the patient. This not only demeans physician and patient alike, but leads to an inevitable (and unnecessary) conflict between facts and values, physicians and patients. Any new model of practice proposed to medicine should aim to avoid the collapse of trust within the consultation that would be precipitated by such a clash, and should instead be flexible enough to accommodate such differences. Indeed, it should aim neither to direct the decision, which would be paternalistic, nor merely to provide a 'sea' of treatment options from which the patient is free to select, which would be abandonment. Rather, the clinician should aim to accompany and guide the patient, drawing on the subjective as well as the objective in progressing together towards a mutually acceptable and agreed treatment plan (Miles and Asbridge, 2013).

A key development here of no small importance may be found in EBM's latest metamorphosis. Having previously maintained a radical foundationalism which argued that medicine should be based on data deriving from specific epidemiological study designs and defining 'evidence' accordingly, we find that a major concession has been made. I refer to a notable paper published by Djulbegovic and his colleagues where a re-definition of 'evidence' was advanced, resulting from a certain degree of epistemological 'clarification' of the EBM thesis (Djulbegovic *et al.*, 2009). (While the 'clarification' was in essence a retraction of previous definitions of 'evidence', this is not the immediate point here.) Protagonists of EBM had historically rejected 'unsystematic clinical experience' and the values of patients as not constituting 'evidence' in any sense at all, an observation that is unsurprising, since values do not derive from empirical clinical research studies. However, Djulbegovic's revisionism has led to an important re-definition of EBM's 'evidence'. Indeed, it is now admitted that factors such as clinical intuition, because they are of relevance to decision-making, warrant the description of 'evidence'. I had previously argued that such revisions were inevitable, given a range of socio-political developments and advances in patient-centred care and personalised medicine and that these would force the change noted (Miles *et al.*, 2008). EBM's preparedness to modify the EBM thesis in the face of such developments remains a classical example of cynicism, but such a *volte face* remains of pivotal importance to correcting the defective models of practice that have been spawned by the radically foundationalist EBM ideology. Given that EBM now acknowledges that any type of knowledge, if it is relevant to decision-making, can be described as 'evidence', it is now possible to regard values as evidence within EBM's latest model. Such an accommodation is welcome, illustrating that EBM's radical foundationalism has demonstrated that a 'universal set of rules that govern medical evidence may not be possible to develop'; that 'there are always exceptions to the general rules described in EBM systems' and that 'looking for rules in a world of exceptions' is doomed to failure (Djulbegovic *et al.*, 2009). We see, then, an admission that the results of EBM-approved empirical clinical research (Evidence-based Medicine Working Group, 1992) are now understood as, *ipso facto*, a 'limited source of knowledge and authority in the care of patients' (Miles, 2007). While this is now acknowledged in *theory*, there remain issues of *practice* and the EBM community has been clear that the way in which patient values and preferences are integrated into decision-making remains, for them, 'vexing' (see Miles, 2009b).

Why 'vexing'? Presumably, because Djulbegovic and his colleagues recognise that values can easily come into conflict with scientific evidence, even in a scenario where scientific evidence and values are seen as 'democratically' equal inputs into decision-making. But the global patient-centred care movement has made clear that patient values must always trump scientific evidence. While this leaves the EBM thesis in conceptual ruins, it empowers VBM, affording a certain primacy to values. If this is Fulford's reasoning in arguing for the compatibility of EBM and VBM, then it goes some way in the direction of progress. However, to avoid a new form of foundationalism in medicine, one based on values, the nomenclature of VBM, in employing the word 'based', remains problematic, indeed misnomeric. VBM/P in its current model is hardly *sub specie aeternitatis* – immune from revision. Indeed, EBM has revised itself no less than four times over twenty years and there is little reason why VBM should not change course far earlier, retreating from notions of foundationalism in medicine, to notions of 'informing' and 'guiding', to which status EBM has now been reduced. If commentators had talked about EBM needing to be put 'in its place', then this is that place. VBM should move quickly to occupy the same place in the 'horizontally ordered library of clinical knowledge sources' which enable, not constrain, an effective and fully responsive clinical practice in dealing with the multiple concerns of the patient who is ill and who has approached the clinician seeking help (Miles, 2012a, 2012b; Miles and Asbridge, 2013).

So if not a values-*based* or science-*based* medicine, then what?

When one reflects on the epidemiological transition that has taken place over recent decades in global health care, where acute presentations of disease have been replaced by extraordinarily high levels of long term chronic illnesses of considerable clinical complexity (Miles and Mezzich, 2012), to imagine that only one knowledge source could and should be foundational to the clinical methods required to treat and contain these diseases might seem irrationally optimistic. Indeed, a singular foundationalism prescribing a simple epistemological formula for so complex a human and moral activity as medicine may be thought of as intuitively and immediately suspect. It is in this very context that anti-foundationalism is suggested here to be indispensably necessary to construct a better model of care – one that is far more understanding of and responsive to the realities of a more generalised illness resulting from a specific disease(s) process(es), needing necessarily to draw upon a multiplicity of different knowledge types, sources and 'warrants' for decision-making (see Chapter 19).

Person-centred clinical care (PCCC)

Emerging in the aftermath of the EBM ideology, and with reference to 'many models' clinical practice (exemplified by narrative-based medicine, values-based medicine, preferences-based medicine, relationship-based medicine, cultural sensitivity-based medicine and spirituality-based medicine, etc.), we see the description of a 'person-centred clinical care'. PCCC is in many ways a 'compound' response to a philosophical, economic and political crisis in health care. It rejects the idea of a singular base for medical practice and intervention and instead argues directly for a more complete and reflexive approach to those who are ill. Indeed, PCCC, via its anti-foundationalism, precludes reductionist attempts to describe clinical practice with reference to supposedly objective scientific evidence or other knowledge sources for decision-making, without reference to the relevant understanding of the subjective experience of illness by the patient in all of its complexity. It argues that medicine's wide variety of knowledge sources should be able to form holistic webs in order to build and respond to a clinical picture or 'tapestry'. PCCC concludes, then, that clinical practice consists not of reducing holistic understanding and practical actions to any one particular knowledge base, but rather collects and interprets clinical knowledge from a variety of sources, piecing these together in the gradual formation of the clinical picture (Miles, 2012a, 2012b; Miles and Asbridge, 2013).

The anti-foundationalist nature of PCCC

PCCC, via its anti-foundationalism, draws heavily on traditional understandings in the philosophy of medicine, as exemplified by its holism, constructivism, interpretivism and historicism. This set of characteristics stands in stark contrast to those which define EBM and EBM-influenced clinical medicine, as well as VBM. For this reason, PCCC represents a major challenge to those who would argue for a scientific evidence-based or a values-based model of practice, requiring these colleagues to examine more critically their approaches when recommending a singular foundationalism – or relativistic foundationalism – for medicine. Yet this is not necessarily to ask the authors of these models to revise their theses with undue speed, merely to reflect on them in more intensive depth. On the contrary, ongoing conceptual analysis and data collection from the use of their foundationalist models is a necessary activity, so that the given models can be tested for practical application, durability and clinical and economic outcome. EBM, for example, has in doing so entered a state of increasingly acknowledged conceptual and methodological collapse, conceptual because its definition of evidence has been radically revised and methodological because it lacks methods of incorporating non-scientific evidence with scientific evidence in the making of clinical decisions with (and not in objective isolation from) the subjective individual. It is important that the concept and practice of VBM learns, rapidly and comprehensively, from medicine's two decades of foundationalist tyranny under the EBM ideology (Miles and Loughlin, 2011; Miles, 2012a, 2012b; Miles and Asbridge, 2013).

PCCC, by recognising a values-informed, not a values-based practice, continues to provide intellectual and moral leadership in medicine

For the reasons given above, PCCC has the potential to provide intellectual and moral leadership in medicine. Its strength lies in its non-foundationalism, in what we might term a 'logic of equivalence', in that it attempts to integrate many different traditions within medicine into a single world view, a very particular approach, but one endowed with considerable flexibility. Commonalities are emphasised via the acknowledgement of the fundamental importance of science, values, narratives, etc., as well as assertions that values should trump science if the patient desires so. A new emphasis on the importance of the patient's subjective account of illness and how to respond to it in the clinic and at the bedside is a welcome addition to the highly objective account of illness that has dominated medical discourse in recent years. PCCC rejects the idea that the subjective account of illness is somehow inferior to objective measures of biological dysfunction in decision-making (Loughlin *et al.*, 2013b). Indeed, wise clinicians have always acknowledged the same, and increasingly vocal patients now insist on it. This essential 'interplay' between difference and equivalence, as part of the PCCC discourse, precipitates inevitable hegemonic antagonisms, but ones likely to prove highly productive in refining the conceptually incomplete PCCC model (Miles and Asbridge, 2013). The logic of equivalence is limited by the logic of difference, so that a dominance of any singular proposed foundation for medicine, whether scientific evidence or values, can never become totalising, affording the intellectually necessary space in which counter-hegemonic discourses can emerge. In this way, PCCC has the potential to accommodate and resolve the clashes between facts and values that routinely occur in clinical practice.

Issues of nomenclature

The use of the nomenclature 'person-centred clinical care' or 'person-centred medicine' risks the accusation (as does VBM/P), that such a term represents a further rhetorical addition to the already rhetorically over-burdened nature of health services. It is certainly true (as was and remains the case for 'evidence' in EBM) that the prefix 'person-centred' is invested with a certain degree of rhetorical force, possessing an emotive component as well as a descriptive one (Loughlin, 2002; Miles and Loughlin, 2011). It is (as 'values-based' is in VBM) a pleonasm, a superfluous addition to the word 'medicine', but one which has been employed not for sensationalism or hubris, but rather in the manner of a simple mechanism to remind medicine of its epicentre – the person of the patient. It is beyond the scope of this chapter to provide a detailed account of PCCC, merely to direct the reader to principal sources of study, both those already published (Miles and Mezzich, 2011b; Miles, 2012a, 2012b, 2013) and those imminently to appear in the literature (Miles and Asbridge, 2013) and to confirm that, far from extricating values from clinical practice and health care systems, the new PCCC model of practice most definitively secures them.

Conclusion and an exhortation

Contrary to what some clinician philosophers implicitly assert, arguments for anti-foundationalism in medicine are not obscure, outlandish ideas, to be dismissed as an unsustainable rejection of the idea of a sustainable base for medical practice. Following twenty years of EBM, during which time medicine has collapsed into reductionism, scientism and dehumanisation, the time has come for anti-foundationalism of the type that underpins PCCC to be given serious consideration as a tenable philosophical and methodological approach which represents a major part of the solution of modern medicine's ills, not an additional problem to be contended with. Those who would substitute foundational notions of values for the now collapsed foundationalism of EBM, should consider carefully what they are proposing and the effects that such a substitution is likely to have. Do we need another twenty years of foundationalist argument, this time exalting values, to stand in the way of authentic progress in the care of the sick? The EBM movement has not ended well and neither, I assert, would a movement predicated upon values as the foundation of medicine. The concept of a *base*, while once appealing, has become progressively irrelevant as a function of the move of health care services away from reductive epistemological formulae, towards the patient-centred, 'holistic' model, driven in no small measure by the epidemiological transition from acute medicine to long term chronic illness management (Miles and Mezzich, 2012). The change in understanding of what actually constitutes knowledge for practice and the associated collapse in belief in the EBM 'hierarchy of evidence', surely argues for a radical re-think in medical epistemology and clinical training, not the attempted substitution of one base (scientific evidence) by another (values), however professionally or opportunistically or otherwise attractive such a substitution might be.

Practising clinicians, engaged in the vicissitudes of everyday clinical care, may wonder what the debate in this volume is all about. Discussions of different forms of foundationalism and anti-foundationalism will seem rather alien to everyday patient and professional concerns, representing for these colleagues the preserve and indulgence of academics, subjects of intellectual 'jousting', with little importance for primary, secondary or tertiary care. However, the idea that such arguments have little practical implication for clinical practice would be entirely naïve. The profound importance of such debates is vividly illustrated by the success of EBM ideologues in persuading governments to construct and introduce clinical practice guidelines based on the strong foundationalist perspective of EBM, thereby risking the exclusion of the use of a great deal of other knowledge sources in practice and occasioning great violence to the historic nature and purpose of medicine. The linking of such guidelines to reimbursement contracts and clinician revalidation plans are noteworthy in this very context and demonstrates that philosophical debate is far from tangential to modern medicine. On the contrary, it is in fact *vital*.

Does the anti-foundationalism of PCCC also enable us to realise that our encounters with patients involve practical, moral and political considerations and are by no means all about epistemological or ontological issues? I think that it does. Indeed, the anti-foundationalism of PCCC takes direct account of plurality, difference, 'the way things *really* are'. Pluralism and multiculturalism pose highly specific challenges to modern medicine which cannot be answered by foundationalist philosophies or practices based upon them, such as the notion of a values-based practice. It may be said, indeed, that an effective medicine needs to engage with patients on their own terms, not from the standpoint of foundationalist perspectives easily synthesised in advance via exercises in theoretical medicine. In reality, there is no single base on which medicine can rest. Those academics who attempt to prescribe 'this or that' foundation, increasingly appear, with reference to the complexity of chronic illness management in particular, to be seeking a form of certainty in a field such as medicine which is characterised by inescapable uncertainty. The challenges of dealing with clinical complexity are not solved by such dogmatism (Sturmberg and Miles, 2013). Values, then, those of patients, clinicians, the health care system and of society at large, are indispensable in building effective clinical systems for the twenty-first century – but as *informing*, not as foundational factors. With this said and with reference to what has been written above, I conclude by exhorting clinicians, academics, health care policy-makers and governments to reject narrow, foundationalist accounts of the complex clinical, human and moral endeavour that is clinical medicine and to embrace instead the authentically anthropocentric model of health care that is PCCC.

Acknowledgements

I am indebted to Professor Michael Loughlin for his comments on earlier drafts of this chapter and to Professor Sir Jonathan Asbridge for his insights.

References

Bevir, M. (1999) *The Logic of the History of Ideas.* Cambridge: Cambridge University Press.

Boyd, R. (1991) Realism, anti-foundationalism and the enthusiasm for natural kinds. *Philosophical Studies,* **61**(1–2), 127–148.

Burks, A. W. (1958) *Collected Papers of Charles Sanders Peirce,* 1931–1958 Volumes 1–6, 1931–1935 Volumes 7–8, edited by Hartshorne, C., Weiss, P., and Burks, A. W. Cambridge, MA: Harvard University Press.

Charles, K., Gafni, A. and Freeman, E. (2011) The evidence-based medicine model of clinical practice: scientific teaching or belief-based preaching? *Journal of Evaluation in Clinical Practice,* **17**, 597–605.

Debrock, G. (1994) *Essays Concerning the Epistemology of Charles Sanders Peirce.* Dordrecht: Springer.

Djulbegovic, B., Guyatt, G. H. and Ashcroft, R. E. (2009) Epistemological enquiries in evidence-based medicine. *Cancer Control,* **16**, 158–168.

Englehardt, T. and Jotterand, F. (editors) (2008) *The Philosophy of Medicine Reborn. A Pellegrino Reader.* Indianapolis, IN: University of Notre Dame Press.

Evidence-based Medicine Working Group (1992) Evidence-based medicine. A new approach to teaching the practice of medicine. *Journal of the American Medical Association,* **268**, 2420–2425.

Fulford, K. W. M. (2004) Ten principles of values-based medicine. In Radden, J. (editor), *The Philosophy of Psychiatry: A Companion,* pp. 205–234. New York: Oxford University Press.

Gibson, R. F. (editor) (2004) *The Cambridge Companion to Quine.* Cambridge: Cambridge University Press.

Goodman, R. B. (2002) *Wittgenstein and William James.* Cambridge: Cambridge University Press.

Guyer, P. and Wood, A. W. (1998) *Critique of Pure Reasoning,* translated and edited by Guyer, P. and Wood, A. W. Cambridge University Press: Cambridge.

Hahn, L. E. (1997) *The Philosophy of Roderick Chisholm.* Chicago, IL: Open Court Publishers.

Harari, O. (2010) *Knowledge and Demonstration. Aristotle's Posterior Analytics.* Dordrecht: Kluwer Academic Publishers.

Heffernan, G. (1990) *Meditationes de Prima Philosophia: Meditations on First Philosophy,* edited, translated and indexed by Heffernan, G. Indiana, IN: University of Notre Dame Press.

Lewis, C. I. (1952) The given element in empirical knowledge. *Philosophical Review,* **61**(2), 168–172.

Little, M. (2013) Ex nihilo nihil fit? Medicine rests on solid foundations. *Journal of Evaluation in Clinical Practice,* **19**, 467–470.

Loughlin, M. (2002) *Ethics, Management and Mythology. Rational Decision Making for Health Service Professionals.* Oxford: Radcliffe Medical Press.

Loughlin, M. (2009) The search for substance: a quest for the identity conditions of evidence-based medicine. *Journal of Evaluation in Clinical Practice,* **15**, 910–914.

Loughlin, M., Lewith, G. and Falkenberg, T. (2013a) Science, practice and mythology: a definition and examination of the implications for scientism in medicine. *Health Care Analysis,* **21**, 130–145.

Loughlin, M., Bluhm, R., Stoyanov, D. S. *et al.* (2013b) Explanation, understanding, objectivity and experience. *Journal of Evaluation in Clinical Practice,* **19**, 415–421.

Miles, A. (2007) Science: a limited source of knowledge and authority in the care of patients. *Journal of Evaluation in Clinical Practice,* **13**, 545–563.

Miles, A. (2009a) On a medicine of the whole person: away from scientistic reductionism and towards the embrace of the complex in clinical practice. *Journal of Evaluation in Clinical Practice,* **15**, 941–949.

Miles, A. (2009b) Evidence-based medicine: requiescat in pace? *Journal of Evaluation in Clinical Practice*, **15**, 924–929.

Miles, A. (2012a) Person-centered medicine – at the intersection of science, ethics and humanism. *International Journal of Person Centered Medicine*, **2**(3), 329–333.

Miles, A. (2012b) Moving from a reductive anatomico-pathological medicine to an authentically anthropocentric model of healthcare: current transitions in epidemiology and epistemology and the ongoing development of person-centered clinical practice. *International Journal of Person Centered Medicine*, **2**(4), 615–621.

Miles, A. (2013) Science, humanism, judgement, ethics: person-centered medicine as an emergent model of modern clinical practice. *Folia Medica*, **55**(1), 5–24.

Miles, A. and Asbridge, J. E. (2013) Extending the horizons of 21st century medicine: disease to illness, anonymity to identity, patient to person. *European Journal for Person Centered Healthcare*, **1**(1), in press.

Miles, A. and Loughlin, M. (2011) Models in the balance: evidence-based medicine versus evidence-informed individualized care. *Journal of Evaluation in Clinical Practice*, **17**, 531–536.

Miles, A. and Mezzich, J. (2011a) The care of the patient and the soul of the clinic: person-centered medicine as an emergent model of modern clinical practice. *International Journal of Person Centered Medicine*, **1**(2), 207–222.

Miles, A. and Mezzich, J. E. (2011b) Person-centered medicine: advancing methods, promoting implementation. *International Journal of Person Centered Medicine*, **1**, 423–428.

Miles, A. and Mezzich, J. E. (2012) Person-centered medicine: addressing chronic illness and promoting future health. *International Journal of Person Centered Medicine*, **2**, 149–152.

Miles, A., Loughlin, M. and Polychronis, A. (2008) Evidence-based healthcare, clinical knowledge and the rise of personalised medicine. *Journal of Evaluation in Clinical Practice*, **14**(5), 621–649.

Montgomery, K. (2006) *How Doctors Think*. New York: Oxford University Press.

Rockmore, T. and Singer, B. (editors) (1992) *Anti-Foundationalism: Old and New*. Philadelphia, PA: Temple University Press.

Russell, B. (1948) *Human Knowledge: Its Scope and Limits*. New York: Simon and Schuster.

Sober, E. (2012) *Core Questions in Philosophy. A Text with Readings*. London: Pearson Education.

Sturmberg, J. P. and Miles, A. (2013) The complex nature of knowledge. In Sturmberg, J. P. and Martin, C. M. (editors), *Handbook of Systems and Complexity in Health*. New York: Springer.

Uebel, T. (1996) Anti-foundationalism and the Vienna Circles's revolution in philosophy. *British Journal of the Philosophy of Science*, **47**, 415–440.

Upshur, R. E. G. (2002) If not evidence, then what? Or does medicine really need a base? *Journal of Evaluation in Clinical Practice*, **8**(2), 113–119.

Winkler, K. P. (1996) *John Locke, An Essay Concerning Human Understanding* (abridged and edited with an introduction and notes). Indianapolis, IN: Hackett Publishing Company.

Wittgenstein, L. (1974) *On Certainty*. Oxford: Blackwell Publishing.

Chapter 19

Values-based medicine, foundationalism and casuistry

Mark R. Tonelli

In *Essential Values-Based Practice*, Fulford, Peile and Carroll have endorsed casuistry, a case-based approach to reasoning, as an important tool for clinicians pursuing a values-based practice (VBP) (Fulford *et al.*, 2012). By recognising the value of casuistic (practical) reasoning, values-based medicine (VBM) certainly improves upon evidence-based medicine (EBM), which has advocated a more deductive approach, where the results of clinical research serve as the major premises from which conclusions about particulars are derived. VBM does a great service by focusing on the critical importance of the individual in clinical medicine, compelling clinicians always to ask what makes the patient before them different from others. Such a focus necessitates casuistic reasoning.

Casuistic reasoning begins by asking whether and how a particular case differs from a standard, paradigmatic case, the latter being characterised by general agreement on the best course of action. The more closely related to a paradigmatic case, the more likely the same judgement will apply. Individual differences of any variety, including but not limited to differences in values, will be relevant considerations. The role of casuistry in VBP, however, has been confined to reasoning about values rather than describing medical reasoning as a whole. In their description of VBP, Fulford, Peile and Carroll describe reasoning about values as distinct from reasoning about evidence, with casuistry only applying to the former. Limiting casuistic reasoning in this way is mistaken. Such an approach perpetuates a fact/value dichotomy seemingly necessary to VBM, but which may lead to unfortunate and unnecessary conflicts between judgements based upon facts and judgements based upon values, as well as between the judgements of clinicians and patients. Rather, casuistic reasoning on the part of clinicians can and should incorporate

Debates in Values-Based Practice, ed. Michael Loughlin. Published by Cambridge University Press. © Cambridge University Press 2014.

all factors relevant to a particular case in order to arrive at a recommendation or action, not just the values involved.

VBM also posits that certain values represent core, foundational values (see Chapter 14). But casuistry, while clearly incorporating values, has no particular use for the foundational variety. VBM sees this promiscuous view of values as both a strength and a weakness of casuistry (Fulford *et al.*, 2012). An attempt to place some values above others in a universal fashion, however, undermines the very notion of care focused on the individual.

Casuistry in clinical medicine

Casuistry as a form of moral reasoning has a rich tradition, though one mired in controversy and suspicion. In *The Abuse of Casuistry*, an effort to rehabilitate casuistry, Al Jonsen and Stephen Toulmin each brought their own unique perspectives to the task, perspectives that are critical to understanding casuistry itself as well as to understanding how casuistic reasoning would come to be understood in relation to medical practice (Jonsen and Toulmin, 1988).

Al Jonsen, a theologian and one of the pioneers of the field of bioethics, is perhaps the most clinically focused of those early medical ethicists. He sat through medical school classes, rounded with medical teams and queried physicians on the nuances of diagnosis and treatment, developing an impressive clinical knowledge base. While Jonsen would advance casuistry in the field of medical ethics, developing and promoting a specific (four-box) method of casuistic reasoning for clinical ethics deliberation (Jonsen *et al.*, 2002), it is important to note his assertion that clinical medicine, as a whole, represents a casuistic endeavour.

Stephen Toulmin, a moral philosopher, prior to his collaboration with Jonsen to rehabilitate casuistry, had already proposed and defended a theory of argumentation where presumptive conclusions were reached based upon the specifics of a case (Toulmin, 2003). Toulmin's method of argumentation became the framework for modern casuistic reasoning, defining a rigorous and explicit approach that the authors felt addressed many of the long-standing criticisms of casuistry. A careful and explicit casuistic argument, using the Toulmin framework, avoids the claim that such reasoning is necessarily capricious and arbitrary, the usual criticism of less robust casuistic analyses. His description of practical reasoning did not apply simply to values, but to all factors that would go into supporting a particular conclusion. Toulmin noted, in particular, the complex plurality of what constitutes medical knowledge, recognising the challenge facing the clinician in the era of 'scientific' medicine (Toulmin, 1976).

Toulmin's framework, then, was applied to Jonsen's area of interest, clinical ethics. Debates of casuistry's merits and limitations largely took place within the literature of bioethics. But casuistic reasoning, in fact, provides an excellent description of clinical judgement in general. Jonsen and Toulmin used it as a paradigmatic example of a casuistic discipline (Jonsen and Toulmin, 1988, pp. 36–42). Katherine Montgomery (Hunter) also noted the casuistic nature of clinical medicine prior to the advent of EBM (Hunter, 1989; Montgomery, 2006).

Decision-making for a particular patient is a prudential process. The recognition of the individuality of the patient requires the clinician to start by asking how the patient-at-hand differs from and is similar to other persons with the same condition, in the clinician's experience, in the experience of more expert clinicians, or in the published medical literature. This focus on the case and reasoning by analogy are central to the casuistic process. As we will examine in more detail below, Toulmin's structure of argumentation proves to be an excellent description of and model for casuistic clinical judgement.

VBM and VBP recognise the necessity of casuistic reasoning on the part of clinicians, acknowledging the practical nature of the clinician's task and the importance of viewing each patient as an individual. As proponents of VBP note, reasoning from the case-at-hand must be central to the notion of a person-centred medicine. Currently, however, VBP describes a limited role for casuistic reasoning in clinical practice (Fulford *et al.*, 2012). Practical reasoning is limited by VBP to reasoning about values, a process envisioned to take place 'alongside' of deductive reasoning from evidence. The clinician, in the VBP model, will make an assessment based upon clinical research results and perhaps personal experience and then separately assess the values at play. This dual, but non-parallel, approach, in addition to being unnecessarily complicated, results in the very real possibility of conclusions based upon evidence differing from conclusions based upon values. While proponents of VBM would certainly decide such conflicts in favour of values, such a preference may be less compelling to proponents of EBM. The apparent conflict, however, is merely a result of the dual methodologies applied. A unified approach to considering evidence and values will result in a single, albeit probabilistic, conclusion.

Facts, values and warrants

Certainly the focus of VBM and VBP must be on values. But the distinction between facts and values does not, and should not, need to be made in the practice of clinical medicine. While acknowledging that there is no clear separation of facts and values, the methodology of VBP currently requires clinicians to evaluate values separately. While adopting such an approach may be an effective exercise to demonstrate the importance of values to clinicians, recommending this binary approach for practice is problematic for several reasons. First, any approach that requires clinicians to perform two separate analyses is unlikely to prove particularly attractive to busy clinicians. Second, and as noted above, dual assessments will invariably result in conflicting conclusions, perhaps not infrequently. Finally, by forcing clinicians to consider facts and values separately, the false dichotomy between facts and values is reinforced. So while VBM rightly insists upon clinicians understanding the critical importance of values in the practice of medicine, the current methodology of VBP unnecessarily relegates values assessment to being an 'add-on' to evidence-based practice.

Casuistic reasoning, utilising the form of the Toulmin method of argument, represents an approach to practical reasoning in general, not limited to reasoning about values. Clinicians use casuistic reasoning to arrive at clinical judgements, not only assessments of the values involved (Montgomery, 2006; Tonelli, 2006). The recognition that clinical medicine is a practical enterprise, where judgements and decisions are prudential, personal and probabilistic, seems to have been largely lost in an era of evidence-based medicine. Practical reasoning, to be effective, must take into account all factors relevant to a particular decision, factors that may incorporate facts and/or values.

Practical decision-making must start with the patient-at-hand, one who presents seeking understanding and aid. In order to serve the needs of a patient, the clinician must reach a judgement, or series of judgements, regarding the aetiology of the patient's complaint and what is probably the best way to ameliorate it. The product of this deliberation may be an action or recommendation, but regardless it represents a probabilistic conclusion on the part of the clinician. To get from the case-at-hand to this conclusion the clinician must appeal to warrants in support of the conclusion, warrants that may derive from several topic areas.

Warrants, in Toulmin's framework, serve a necessary explanatory role, providing the step involved in moving from a specific case to a conclusion regarding that case (Toulmin, 2003). For example, Mr Jones has recently had a myocardial infarction and his cardiologist decides to start him on a beta-blocker medication. When asked why, the cardiologist will almost certainly appeal to the warrant: beta-blockers reduce mortality in people who have recently had a myocardial infarction. Since Mr Jones is a particular example of a person who has recently had a myocardial infarction, then it is probably best if he were to receive a beta-blocker. If queried further on how the cardiologist knows the warrant to be valid, she might respond by pointing to a body of medical research, much of it in the form of randomised controlled trials, that demonstrates an improved survival in populations of individuals who received beta-blockers after myocardial infarction compared to those who did not. These research reports serve as backing for the warrant invoked to reach the conclusion that Mr Jones should start taking a beta-blocker.

In this particular example, it may seem almost necessary that Mr Jones be given a beta-blocker. The evidence-based approach to the same case would result in the same conclusion, derived deductively from the evidence that beta-blockers decrease mortality. (Beta-blockers decrease mortality in patients who have had a recent myocardial infarction. Mr Jones has had a recent myocardial infarction. Therefore, the best course of action is for Mr Jones to receive a beta-blocker.) The value of such an intervention seems so self-evident that the fraction of post-myocardial infarction patients in an institution who are receiving a beta-blocker is now used as a metric for assessing overall quality of cardiac care.

Yet a more careful analysis reveals that the warrant relied upon, that beta-blockers reduce mortality in persons who have recently had a myocardial infarction, is alone insufficient to reach the best decision in this, or any other, case. Application of the warrant depends upon an implicit normative assertion that reducing mortality is a worthy goal. That is, the active warrant contains an implicit value judgement, that reduced mortality is beneficial. Not only is this value judgement unspoken, it is likely to go unchallenged even when recognised. All warrants invoked in medical decision-making will contain, implicitly or explicitly, a value element. Beyond the general normative element (that reducing mortality is good), invoking a warrant in a particular case demands that we examine that value-based assertion with regard to that particular patient. Even if improving survival seems generally beneficial, decreasing Mr Jones's risk of death may not be appropriate or desirable. If, for instance, Mr Jones suffered severe and irreversible anoxic brain injury during the arrest that accompanied his myocardial infarction, decreasing his subsequent risk of death does not appear to be clearly beneficial. Similarly, if Mr Jones's previous use of a beta-blocker for hypertension had left him impotent, the appropriateness of a new prescription for him is less clear. As these cases demonstrate, the conclusion that a beta-blocker should be prescribed to a person post-myocardial infarction is a provisional one. The general warrant may not apply to the particular case (as with anoxic brain injury) and under any circumstance it will be subject to rebuttal (as with impotence).

Warrants derived from clinical research, those warrants favoured by evidence-based medicine, are never prescriptive. At best, clinical research produces hypothetical imperatives, of the form: 'If one wants to increase/decrease the chances of A, then do B.' Whether society, the clinician, or the patient sees value in achieving A is central to reaching a conclusion regarding the use of B (Tonelli, 1998). Warrants can also derive from a variety of other sources, including the basic medical sciences and the experiences of clinician and patient. While all warrants contain some value-laden element, some warrants may be primarily value-based. For instance, a patient who refuses blood products for religious reasons introduces a very specific, value-based warrant into a decision around treatment of an upper gastrointestinal bleed. The environment in which medicine is practised, what interventions are available, reimbursed and lawful, may also produce warrants or modify others. Focusing on these specific topic areas can aid clinicians in elucidating all of the warrants relevant to a particular clinical decision (Tonelli, 2006). While the example of Mr Jones is relatively straightforward, more complex clinical decisions require clinicians to weigh a variety of potential warrants, warrants that sometimes conflict. Clinical judgement, then, is the process of establishing the warrants relevant to a particular decision and negotiating between them in order to come to a decision about what is likely to be the best course of action for a particular patient.

For example, a decision regarding the best treatment of a pulmonary exacerbation in a person with cystic fibrosis requires negotiating between multiple warrants, most with both factual and value components. While clinical research provides a few general warrants (antibiotics are likely to help), pathophysiologic reasoning may be used to guide specific antibiotic choices (based upon the sputum culture results). The strength of warrants related to the duration and location (inpatient or outpatient) of antibiotic therapy will be affected by patient and clinician experience and values (an inpatient stay is likely to jeopardise the patient's employment status and intravenous antibiotics given four times a day are difficult to manage at home). The decision-making process in such a case should not constitute two parallel evaluations, one evidence-based and the other value-based. Such a methodology will produce conflicts when the evidence-based and value-based conclusions do not coincide. (For instance, if the evidence-based approach results in a conclusion that two intravenous antibiotics in an inpatient setting would be best while the values-based approach results in conclusion that combined oral and inhaled antibiotics in an outpatient would be best.) Such conflicts are unnecessary. When all relevant warrants are considered in a single casuistic analysis, a decision regarding what is likely to be the best choice for a particular patient follows.

Casuistic reasoning in clinical medicine will result in variability in practice. No demonstrable best course of action follows from the application of empirical evidence to every particular example of any diagnosis. The provision of a beta-blocker is best for a person with a recent myocardial infarction except when it is not. Determining whether clinical practice guidelines apply to individual patients is a hallmark of sound medical practice. Such a determination requires understanding how the individual is similar to and differs from others with the same malady. While differences in goals and values must be considered, so must differences in physiology. The right choice of action for one patient, then, may be very different from the right choice for another patient with the same disorder. While EBM has attempted to decrease variability in medical practice, variability will be a hallmark of person-centred medical care.

Casuistry and foundations

In the field of medical ethics, casuistry has been viewed in opposition to principlism, the attempt to solve specific ethical problems via direct application of a fundamental principle. So it might appear that values-based medicine, specifically when appealing to foundational values, would have little use for casuistry. Yet casuistry, as we have seen, has been embraced by VBP as a tool for incorporating values into clinical decision-making, allowing for care to be individualised. How, then, do foundational values relate to casuistic reasoning?

Casuistic disciplines, by their very nature, do not need foundations. (Though in practice it is more straightforward when there are shared values.) The particular case provides the basis for the argument and subsequent claim, with warrants supporting that conclusion deriving from a variety of sources, none of which holds any special status relative to others. Any particular value, foundational or otherwise, may or may not be relevant to a particular medical decision. Warrants supported by or based upon any particular value may be the most compelling; warrants stemming from foundational values have no special worth.

In his chapter dealing with foundational values in medicine, Miles Little advocates for three such values: survival, security and flourishing (Chapter 14). As he acknowledges explicitly, these foundational values have little to do with clinical reasoning and medical decision-making. Rather, he asserts, all health care is grounded in these values, while how the foundational values are made manifest in any particular society or system will vary. On a day-to-day basis, derivative values and axioms will play a more active role in medical policy and practice. Appeals to foundational values will only be implied. Such an understanding anticipates the very limited role of foundational values in casuistic medical reasoning.

The foundational values proposed by Little often serve the role of providing a very general rationale for invoking warrants of a particular variety. In our example of beta-blockers, the warrant noting decreased mortality in post-myocardial infarction patients can be seen as relevant to the discussion because survival (with regard to an individual as well as the species) is seen as something to be valued. In fact, clinical research studies choose to measure survival not because it is a 'hard' endpoint, but for the same reason that Little proposes it as a foundational value: without survival little else of value seems possible. Similarly, the focus of a large percentage of clinical research studies on some aspect of 'quality of life' can be viewed as a recognition of the importance of flourishing, another of Little's foundational values. While flourishing itself does not lend itself well to quantitative analysis, the more practical notion of quality of life has spawned many thousands of different tools that purportedly measure some aspect of health-related flourishing (Garratt et al., 2002). Little's foundational values, then, can be seen as providing general normative weight for many warrants derived from clinical research. But this general normative support is only general, making foundational values relatively meaningless for decisions involving individuals.

Non-foundational values, the axioms that Little notes tend to dominate discussions regarding policy and practice, will also dominate casuistic analyses. Using the example of Mr Jones again, the question of whether to give him a beta-blocker after he has suffered a severe anoxic brain injury does not come down to valuing survival in general, but to whether it is right to provide supportive medical care to a person in a persistent vegetative state. Deliberation is likely to invoke a wide variety of non-foundational values, values dealing with the appropriate allocation of resources and what it means to respect persons. In the circumstance of beta-blockers causing impotence to an otherwise functional Mr Jones, the decision requires some deliberation regarding the values around sexual functioning compared to a statistical likelihood of living longer. In other words, it is not surviving or flourishing that matter to clinicians and patients, but surviving and flourishing in particular ways. In the first case, a particular axiom that asserts we should not utilise health care resources on individuals who will never again be conscious could be invoked, trumping the general warrant invoked for using a beta-blocker. In the second, Mr Jones is likely to have his own axioms related to the value of sexual functioning, values that would need to be elicited in order to arrive at a recommendation regarding re-instituting beta-blockade. Here again, it is important to note that the clinician's judgement and subsequent recommendation must incorporate Mr Jones's values not as a separate consideration, but as integral to the decision itself.

Casuistic reasoning, in starting with the case, will deal almost exclusively with mid-level, specific or personal values, axioms that are held by the clinician and/or the patient. Appeals to foundational values are not only unnecessary, but are likely to prove distracting.

Summary

VBM and VBP have rightly emphasised the centrality of values to clinical decision-making. Yet insisting that facts and values should be dealt with separately and in different manners represents an epistemic error by VBM. Yoking an independent values assessment to an evidence-based decision-making process complicates the clinician's work and, ultimately, may serve to devalue values. In an era when data have become the currency of the health care realm, driving not only care decisions but allocation of scarce resources and reimbursement, even suggesting that data and evidence can be evaluated in a value-free fashion is not simply wrong, it is dangerously wrong. Rather than attempting to tease out values for separate analysis, VBM and VBP would be best served by describing the manner by which all factors, value-laden facts and factually burdened values, can be considered and incorporated into clinical decision-making. VBP is right to embrace casuistry, but needs to broaden the role of casuistic reasoning in clinical medicine. Casuistic reasoning allows clinicians to evaluate all potential warrants relevant to a decision for a particular patient, not simply those that are value-based. Making values explicit, as VBM has so strongly encouraged, in turn improves the quality of casuistic reasoning, which has been faulted for not recognising bias and allowing for prejudice (Kopelman, 1994). A formal model of casuistic analysis along the lines of Toulmin's description of argumentation will make such reasoning not only more robust, but open to rebuttal.

Casuistry does not depend upon foundational principles or values. Whether there are shared values that serve as a foundation for medical practice remains largely irrelevant to clinicians and patients. Most casuistic reasoning will utilise mid-level values as normative backing for warrants invoked in support of a conclusion. Foundational values will generally be too far removed, and far too non-specific, to aid in clinical decision-making.

VBM and VBP rightly recognise the inadequacy of current EBM models of clinical decision-making and have done a great service to the practice of medicine by focusing on the critical importance of values. By adopting a broader understanding of casuistic reasoning, VBP could recognise that values are interwoven into all potential warrants relevant to a particular decision, including the warrants derived from clinical research and privileged by EBM.

References

Fulford, K. W. M., Peile, E. and Carroll, H. (2012) *Essential Values-Based Practice: Clinical Stories Linking Science with People.* Cambridge: Cambridge University Press.

Garratt, A., Schmidt, L., Mackintosh, A. and Fitzpatrick, R. (2002) Quality of life measurement: bibliographic study of patient assessed health outcome measures. *British Medical Journal*, **324**, 1417.

Hunter, K. (1989) A science of individuals: medicine and casuistry. *Journal of Medicine and Philosophy*, **14**, 193–212.

Jonsen, A. R. and Toulmin, S. (1988) *The Abuse of Casuistry.* Berkeley, CA: University of California Press.

Jonsen, A., Siegler, M. and Winslade, W. (2002) *Clinical Ethics.* New York: McGraw-Hill.

Kopelman, L. (1994) Case method and casuistry: the problem of bias. *Theoretical Medicine*, **15**, 21–37.

Montgomery, K. (2006) *How Doctors Think.* New York: Oxford University Press.

Tonelli, M. R. (1998) The philosophical limits of evidence-based medicine. *Academic Medicine*, **73**, 234–240.

Tonelli, M. R. (2006) Integrating evidence into clinical practice: an alternative to evidence-based approaches. *Journal of Evaluation in Clinical Practice*, **12**, 248–256.

Toulmin, S. (1976) On the nature of physician's understanding. *Journal of Medicine and Philosophy*, **1**, 32–50.

Toulmin, S. (2003) *The Uses of Argument.* Cambridge: Cambridge University Press.

Values-based medicine and patient autonomy

Robyn Bluhm

Respect for patient autonomy is central to bioethics and to health care. This importance is reflected in the numerous attempts to give patients a greater say in medical decision-making; these include shared decision-making, patient-centred medicine, and evidence-based patient choice. Yet the fact that there *are* diverse approaches indicates that it is not clear how best to incorporate the patient's perspective. Moreover, among bioethicists, there has been criticism of the tendency to equate patient autonomy with informed consent, or even informed choice. One key reason for this is that focusing on choice does not give a broad enough understanding of the way that patients' autonomy may be important in health care.

Bill Fulford and Miles Little have each proposed theories that aim to clarify the important role of values in health care. Each theory is called 'values-based medicine' (VBM) (Fulford's is also known as 'values-based practice'), but the two VBMs are very different. Little suggests that they are compatible, but does not say much about why or how the two VBMs fit together. This chapter aims to evaluate the implications of the two VBMs for patient autonomy. My central claim is that Little's version of VBM can provide a grounding and focus for Fulford's version that can help the latter to avoid criticisms about its ability to accommodate patient autonomy. Conversely, though, Little's approach needs to be fleshed out in order to clarify how it applies specifically to health care.

I will begin with a discussion of autonomy in health care, briefly sketching an approach to patient autonomy that goes beyond the dominant understanding of autonomy in terms of informed consent or informed choice. I next outline Fulford's version of VBM and argue that it poses problems for patient autonomy. I then turn to

Debates in Values-Based Practice, ed. Michael Loughlin. Published by Cambridge University Press. © Cambridge University Press 2014.

Little's VBM, which aims to identify certain universally shared, fundamental values and I argue that these values mesh nicely with the approach to autonomy that I developed in the first section. Little's VBM also provides Fulford's version with the resources to address the problems I identified and to promote patient autonomy. In summary, the theories are compatible; Little's VBM emphasises values that are central to patient autonomy and that can provide a much-needed focus to Fulford's VBM, while Fulford's work provides health care providers with skills that can help to promote it.

Autonomy in bioethics

The importance of respecting patient autonomy has been emphasised by bioethicists, in response to worries about explicit coercion of patients/research participants, and also, more subtly, in response to worries about paternalism in health care. Susan Sherwin notes that, because health care providers have technical expertise that patients lack, they may all-too-easily come to believe that they 'are better able to judge what is in the patient's best interest than is the patient' (Sherwin, 1998, p. 20). Sherwin goes on to describe the dominant conception of patient autonomy as one that protects the choice of a competent patient by ensuring that she is given sufficient information to make a choice among a range of available options and is free of explicit coercion toward or away from a particular choice. Yet, she argues, this understanding of autonomy obscures the ways in which oppressive social practices can affect autonomy.

Susan Dodds has, like Sherwin, raised doubts about the adequacy of this view of autonomy, arguing that patient autonomy must be understood as more than just a matter of choice or of rational decision-making. She draws on work by Diana Meyers to show that many health care decisions are not just isolated choices that are best understood as answering the question 'What do I want to do now?', but are in fact broader questions more relevant to the question 'How do I really want to live my life?' (Dodds, 2000, p. 227, referring to Meyers, 1989, p. 48). Dodds emphasises that illness may threaten autonomy: 'the suddenness and significance of some health care crises force a radical reassessment of one's self-understanding, which may effectively derail a person's autonomy competency' (p. 230).

Dodds emphasises the short term effects of a health crisis on autonomy, but I have added to this that many chronic health conditions require a longer period of adjustment or periodic re-evaluation of the question of how best to live one's life (Bluhm, 2009, 2012). On this view, patient autonomy is best understood in terms of the way that health care decisions can promote or constrain patients' overall life goals and plans, rather than in terms of the freedom of specific decisions themselves. While a short term health crisis may temporarily 'derail' an individual's autonomy, learning to live with a chronic health condition may involve changing one's life goals and plans.

In the next section, I will outline Fulford's approach to VBM. Because he has such an inclusive sense of the term 'values', his theory has the potential to address the type of autonomy that I have just described; however, there are some serious problems with the theory as it stands that prevent it from fulfilling this potential.

Fulford's VBM

Fulford's version of VBM starts from the observation that all decisions are informed by both facts and values. While there are certain key values that are generally accepted (such

as respect for autonomy and acting in a patient's best interests), the increasing technological complexity of medicine, as well as changes within society as a whole, mean that
value conflicts are becoming increasingly common. The challenges raised by these conflicts are made more complex because values are often not made explicit and people may
assume that their values are shared when they are actually not. Moreover, when broad
values are shared, 'differences at other levels may become obscured' (Petrova *et al.*, 2006,
p. 704); for example, a physician and her patient, or two members of a health care team,
may agree that whatever actions are taken should be in a patient's best interests, but may
disagree about what those best interests are, or about the best way to promote them.

Fulford's VBM thus aims to promote awareness of values and value conflicts, as well as
to equip health care providers with the skills required to manage these conflicts. He
contrasts VBM with bioethics, characterising the latter as taking a 'quasi-legal' approach
that emphasises the development of rules to ensure good *outcomes*. By contrast, VBM is
intended to provide 'a less prescriptive and more local approach' than bioethics (Petrova
et al., 2006, p. 706). It focuses on 'good *process*, in the form particularly of improved
clinical practice skills' (Petrova *et al.*, 2006, p. 706). These skills are supposed to allow the
individuals concerned to balance diverse sets of values, rather than dealing with universally accepted values.

The development of these skills is a central contribution of VBM. Using them,
clinicians should be better able to clarify and make explicit both their own values and
those of their patients. By careful attention to the things that their patients and colleagues
say, clinicians can become more aware of the values that are held, perhaps subconsciously,
by the various people involved in a clinical decision. They can also come to recognise
better their own values and the way that their values can influence their own preferences in
caring for patients. Fulford suggests that a variety of tools are available, from both
philosophy and empirical social sciences, to help clinicians to become more aware of,
and to balance, conflicting values.

Fulford intends the concept of 'values' in VBM to be very inclusive. He emphasises that
'values are wider than ethics, extending to needs, wishes, preferences, indeed to any and all
of the many and diverse ways in which people express, directly or indirectly, negative or
positive evaluations and value judgments' (Fulford, 2011, p. 976). In addition, the values
of a number of *people* are relevant, adding to the proliferation of values in VBM. Certainly,
the patient's values are important, but so, too, are the values of the health care providers
(from various disciplines) involved in his care, his family and other informal carers, 'and
indeed the manager and policy maker' (Fulford, 2013, p. 538). Because of this, Fulford says
that VBM 'goes beyond patient autonomy' (Fulford, 2013, p. 538), which he understands
as synonymous with 'freedom of patient choice' (Fulford, 2011, p. 976). But given that
values, on Fulford's view, go beyond choices, one can possibly put patients' values first
without claiming that choice is the only thing that matters. VBM might be able to
accommodate the richer view of autonomy that I outlined in the previous section.

Yet even when clearly discussing values, Fulford is not clear on *whose* values are
central. He outlines ten principles of VBM, two of which are particularly relevant to the
role that values should make in promoting patient autonomy. These two principles,
however, are in tension with each other. The 'patient perspective' principle says that
'VBM's "first call" for information is the perspective of the patient or patient group
concerned in a given decision' (Fulford, 2004, p. 206), but the 'multi-perspective principle'
says that 'In VBM, conflicts of values are resolved primarily, not by reference to a rule

prescribing a "right" outcome but by processes designed to support a balance of legitimately different perspectives' (Fulford, 2004, p. 206). Fulford describes VBM as relying on dissensus rather than consensus, which means that 'the values of those concerned, instead of being subordinated one to another, remain in play to be balanced according to the circumstances presented by a given decision' (Fulford *et al.*, 2012, p. 165). Again, these perspectives include not only the patient's, but also those of anyone who is 'concerned (directly or indirectly) in a given situation' (Fulford, 2013, p. 541).

How should we understand the idea that everyone's values should count? Not only is the doctor's office beginning to look a little crowded, with all of the policy-makers and family members, but it is also not clear at all that everyone's values *should* count in making decisions about the care of a patient. While respect for patient autonomy should not mean that *anything* the patient says goes, neither should the preferences of health care providers or other individuals determine the care a patient receives. More needs to be said about how to balance conflicting values once they have been recognised.

Tim Thornton has suggested that in trying to avoid the 'quasi-legal' approach of bioethics, VBM replaces the idea that there is a single, correct answer to a specific kind of problem with the idea that there is a single, correct process for solving all problems. He claims that, on VBM, 'Fundamentally, all and any values deserve a hearing. All and any can be valued if they survive the right process' (Thornton, 2011, p. 991). In replying to Thornton, Fulford says, first, that not *all* values deserve a hearing. For example, racism and other forms of discrimination are simply not legitimate and so need not be considered when diverse values are being weighed and balanced.

More important, perhaps, is Fulford's second response, which is that 'while people's values are highly diverse, they are not chaotic' (Fulford, 2013, p. 539). Instead, he says, VBM starts from the fact that, in practice, there will be a framework of shared values within which diversity and disagreement occur, so that a group of stakeholders can find enough in common to permit discussion. Yet the mere appeal to such a framework is not sufficient to solve the problem of how to balance values. For one thing, as noted above, Fulford is well aware that agreement about 'broad' values can coexist with disagreement about how to best make decisions that align with these values. For another, the type of framework Fulford has in mind is very broad. He cites the National Institute for Mental Health in England (NIMHE) as an example of a framework of shared values. This framework requires the recognition of the importance of values, a commitment to raising awareness of values and their effect on health care practice, and respect for the diversity of values. It therefore does not guarantee that any of the specific values that might affect a clinical decision are actually shared.

Furthermore, Fulford acknowledges that a shared framework is not sufficient to resolve problems; he notes that within such a framework, 'a process is needed to support balanced application of shared values' (Fulford, 2013, p. 539). Although he acknowledges the importance of both tacit knowledge and individual judgement in making clinical decisions (Fulford, 2013, p. 542), Fulford still does not explain what such a process would look like. A similar point has been made by Bob Brecher, who says that Fulford's emphasis on recognising the diversity of values that may be encountered 'leaves unrecognized, let alone answered, the question of who is going to do what with this "diversity," of who is going to "incorporate" it and how, and of how and by whom the conflicts that Fulford [rightly] recognizes are going to be resolved' (Brecher, 2011, p. 997). Brecher worries that either the choice will be made by a clinician or manager who insists on solving the conflict their own way, or the patient will be 'saddled' with the choice and blamed for anything that goes wrong. I suggest, though, that it is inevitable that clinicians will end up being the decision-makers in clinical settings. After all, VBM is itself an effort to develop skills for health care providers, for those who provide care, rather than those who receive it. This is why it is necessary to stipulate that those who practise VBM must be careful to adopt the patient's perspective.

In summary, my discussion so far has raised two key problems for the ability of Fulford's VBM to promote patient autonomy. First, two of the principles of VBM raise the question of both how to put patients' values first and how to balance all legitimate perspectives. Yet basic concern for patient autonomy would mean that it is important also to recognise when it is legitimate to consider the values of anyone other than the patient. After all, the whole point of emphasising respect for autonomy at all comes from the realisation that health care providers may be tempted to think that they know better than the patient what is best for them. Second, VBM does not provide clear guidance for 'balancing' various parties' values once they have been elicited – and there is reason to think that, by default, it puts this responsibility (and power) in the hands of clinicians. Taken together, these problems raise the worry that patients' values will be lost in the process of 'integration'. In the next section, I begin to show that Miles Little's approach to VBM can be used to develop a solution for these problems by giving a focus to the values that Fulford's VBM has elicited.

Little's VBM

Miles Little's VBM is very different from Fulford's. For one thing, Fulford's VBM is practical, focusing on skills that can improve the practice of medicine, whereas Little's is largely a theoretical endeavour that seeks to provide a foundation for medicine. According to Little, examining human societies can lead us to an understanding of the basic (foundational) values that guide all human activity. He identifies three such values: survival, security and flourishing. Survival is straightforwardly understood; it is the preservation of a life, which Little and his coauthors suggest is probably instinctive. Security is necessary because we can only tolerate a certain amount of disorder and unpredictability and still be able to live our day-to-day lives. Flourishing refers to individual and social development. While there are many ways for an individual to flourish (Little *et al.*, 2011), all human beings seem to have a need to transcend their day-to-day lives and to engage in activities that are meaningful to them. Little argues that these values are descriptive and 'prenormative' in that they appear to be necessary and valued in all societies. In fact, he goes so far as to suggest that a society that did not share these foundational values would not be recognisably human (see Chapter 14, p. 174).

Little's discussion, however, is focused on the values underlying *all* human activity and much remains to be said about how medicine, and health care more generally, contribute to the satisfaction of these values. In one paper, Little and his colleagues note that their version of VBM explains why we have health systems, as well as why particular health systems have evolved in the specific (and different) ways that they have, and that it also provides a basis for a critique of health systems 'at all levels', from individual patient encounters to their bureaucratic background (Little *et al.*, 2011). They suggest that attention to these fundamental values, and the different ways in which they may be understood by people involved in a particular situation, can help us to understand disagreements. (Here they echo Fulford, who also recognises that situations in which values conflict, or at least appear to, have much to teach us.)

Little and colleagues explicitly contrast their version of VBM with Fulford's, describing the latter as emphasising 'patient preferences and teachable clinical skills – that is, the acquired and developed skills to recognize and act upon patient preferences' (Little *et al.*, 2012, p. 1020). Yet elsewhere, Little suggests that the two versions of VBM are compatible, and that the only real difference is that his model incorporates foundational values that, presumably, ground preferences (Chapter 14). In the next section, I discuss what Fulford's theory might look like, and the implications for patient autonomy, if Little's foundational values are included.

VBM and patient autonomy

Little and colleagues do not address the practical question of *how* medicine can and should contribute to fulfilling these three values, though they do suggest (and I agree) that these goals do underlie clinical practice. That medicine contributes to survival is relatively clear, and while much could be said about how far medicine should go in attempting to reach this goal (particularly in the context of end-of-life decision-making), I will not consider these issues here. Instead, I will focus on the other two foundational values, security and flourishing. In particular, I will consider the relationship between these two values, as well as their relationship with autonomy, health and illness.

To begin with, note that there is an interesting relationship between security and flourishing as Little describes them. Security is necessary to our day-to-day function, while flourishing requires that we transcend the (merely) day-to-day in order to create a meaningful life, whatever that might be for a particular individual. One possibility is that security is necessary for flourishing, for example in the way suggested by Maslow's hierarchy of needs, on which lower level physical and social needs must be satisfied before an individual can begin to address her need for self-actualisation. Another is that some lack of security is compatible with, or even necessary for, flourishing, in the way that artists and writers may create their art in response to suffering or that (for the rest of us) an experience of loss of security can prompt us to re-evaluate the kind and sources of meaning we want in our lives. Either way, it seems that some level of security (most of the time) is required for an individual to flourish; nobody can do so if they completely lack security.

I mention this because illness is an important source of insecurity. Even relatively trivial illnesses – a bout of flu, or an injury such as a broken bone or a burn – interrupt our sense that we are secure and safe. This suggests that an important goal of medicine should be to restore a patient's sense of security, in part by addressing the physical problem and, where possible, restoring the patient to health, but in cases where the health issues will be long term or permanent, it is equally important that health care providers help a patient to develop a renewed sense of security that is compatible with their state of injury or illness. Similarly, in order to be successful, health care must be able to help patients who have learned to cope with a chronic health problem in their day-to-day lives to flourish, to create a life that is responsive to their new health circumstances, but that is meaningful (in whatever specific form that takes for that individual).

This brief description, I think, shows that understanding the goals of medicine in terms of the contribution of health care to a patient's security and flourishing is compatible with the account of autonomy that I sketched at the beginning of the chapter. If patient autonomy is understood in terms of the question 'How do I want to live my life (given the conditions and constraints imposed by my illness)', then medical decisions that contribute to a patient's sense of security and ability to flourish will help to answer that question.

With this in mind, we can return to the relationship between Fulford's VBM and Little's. As I have discussed above, critics of Fulford's view, including Little, have worried that it gives too much weight to (mere) preferences, that any values at all are eligible to influence health care decision-making. I worry, in particular, that because Fulford does not specify how the values that different people bring to a decision are to be balanced, and because it seems that it is up to physicians to do the balancing, Fulford's version of VBM might fail to contribute appropriately to patient autonomy.

I now suggest that Little's version of VBM has the potential to ground Fulford's, or even, in the terms that Fulford himself uses, to provide a shared framework of values that can direct decision-making. If the goal of health care decisions is to use available treatments and services in a way that promotes patients' sense of security and/or their flourishing, this addresses Thornton's criticism, and also Brecher's worry that responsibility for decision-making will ultimately fall to one party at the expense of other views. Because decision-making will be directed to a shared goal, incorporating Little's fundamental values into VBM will require the participation of patients, so even if health care providers remain responsible for *using* the skills of VBM, they must do so in a way that is directed toward the patient's needs and desires.

Importantly, focusing on security and flourishing does not mean that anything a patient wants should be done. People can be wrong about what will contribute to these goals in their own lives. This is particularly true when their lives have been dramatically changed by illness and they must, as a result, rethink their personal values and goals. Health care providers can help a patient to understand what it will be like to have a health problem, or to undergo a particular treatment, in order to help her to make better decisions about what she wants and how best to try to achieve it. At the same time, only the patient can judge how well her own life is going, so the success of a particular decision can only be judged by the patient.

In summary, Fulford's version of VBM focuses on eliciting values from patients and other parties to health care decision-making, but it does not provide a clear process for using these values to guide decision-making. Little's, by contrast, does not provide practical guidance, but does identify several foundational values that are basic to health care. Together, the theories provide a framework that focuses decisions on patients' needs and equip health care providers with skills that allow them to address these needs. This combined approach may help patients to maintain (or to regain) their autonomy in the face of a serious illness.

Acknowledgements

Thank you to Michael Loughlin and to Mona Gupta for their comments on earlier drafts of this chapter.

References

Bluhm, R. (2009) Evidence-based medicine and patient autonomy. *International Journal of Feminist Approaches to Bioethics*, **2**(2), 134–151.

Bluhm, R. (2012) Vulnerability, health, and illness. *International Journal of Feminist Approaches to Bioethics*, **5**(2), 147–161.

Brecher, B. (2011) Which values? And whose? A reply to Fulford. *Journal of Evaluation in Clinical Practice*, **17**, 996–998.

Dodds, S. (2000) Choice and control in bioethics. In Mackenzie, C. and N. Stoljar, N. (editors), *Relational Autonomy: Feminist Perspectives on Autonomy, Agency, and the Social Self*, pp. 213–235. New York: Oxford University Press.

Fulford, K. W. M. (2004) Ten principles of values-based medicine. In Radden, J. (editor), *The Philosophy of Psychiatry: A Companion*, pp. 205–234. New York: Oxford University Press.

Fulford, K. W. M. (2011) The value of evidence and evidence of values: bringing together values-based and evidence-based practice in policy and service development in mental health. *Journal of Evaluation in Clinical Practice*, **17**, 976–987.

Fulford, K. W. M. (2013) Values-based practice: Fulford's dangerous idea. *Journal of Evaluation in Clinical Practice*, **19**, 537–546.

Fulford, K. W. M., Peile, E. and Carroll, H. (2012) *Essential Values-Based Practice: Clinical Stories Linking Science with People*. Cambridge: Cambridge University Press.

Little, M., Lipworth, W., Gordon, J., Markham, P. and Kerridge, I. (2011) Another argument for values-based medicine. *International Journal of Person Centered Medicine*, **1**, 649–656.

Little, M., Lipworth, W., Gordon, J., Markham, P. and Kerridge, I. (2012) Values-based medicine and modest foundationalism. *Journal of Evaluation in Clinical Practice*, **18**, 1020–1026.

Meyers, D. T. (1989) *Self, Society and Personal Choice*. New York: Columbia University Press.

Petrova, M., Dale, J. and Fulford, K. W. M. (2006) Values-based practice in primary care: easing the tensions between individual values, ethical principles, and best evidence. *British Journal of General Practice*, **56**, 703–709.

Sherwin, S. (1998) A relational approach to autonomy in health care. In *The Politics of Women's Health: Exploring Agency and Autonomy*, pp. 19–47. The Feminist Health Care Ethics Research Network. Philadelphia, PA: Temple University Press.

Thornton, T. (2011) Radical liberal values-based practice. *Journal of Evaluation in Clinical Practice*, **17**, 988–995.

Responses to contributions, suggestions and critiques

Miles Little

In this chapter, I respond to those who have been kind enough to write chapters that either use the foundations-axioms-practices (FAP) model or critique it. Lipworth and Montgomery (Chapter 15) and Montgomery and Lipworth (Chapter 16) have used the model to explore issues in empirical ethics and the sociology of medicine respectively. Bluhm (Chapter 20) has examined both the FAP model and Fulford's model to see how, singly and together, they measure against the standards of autonomy. Tonelli (Chapter 19) has used casuistry as a benchmark against which to test the claims of the FAP construction. Upshur, in Chapter 17, undertakes a thoroughgoing deconstruction of my arguments from both philosophical and practical perspectives, as does a very severe Miles in Chapter 18.

Lipworth and Montgomery have used the AP portion of my model alone as a framework in an empirical ethics project that explores the expressions of virtue in qualitative interviews with representatives of the research and medical arms of pharmaceutical companies in Australia. The foundational values added little to their interpretation of the data, just as Tonelli predicts in Chapter 19. Lipworth and Montgomery, however, did find the AP combination useful as a heuristic that recognised strong valuations of virtuous agency in the interviewees, and a commitment to the achievement of wisdom in the practice of their roles. Interviewees expressed a desire to achieve balance between their commitment to the interests of the firm and the public interest. The pharmaceutical industry is much criticised for its attitudes and practices, and it is refreshing to read that there are people in the industry who have clear views about ethics and an understanding of the ethical quandaries they face. These findings suggest that the FAP model is productive

Debates in Values-Based Practice, ed. Michael Loughlin. Published by Cambridge University Press. © Cambridge University Press 2014.

to use, although I am not sure that a similar finding could not have been achieved by other methodologies.

Montgomery and Lipworth in Chapter 16 have used the FAP model to explore the social reasons behind the persistence of medicine as a profession and the persistence of its perceived importance in most societies. Their paper is more theoretically oriented, and develops a way of examining the problem at the levels of individuals, interactions and communities. It employs the whole FAP model to explain the persistence and standing of medicine as a social practice. It works out the implications of the FAP model in considerable detail, and it acknowledges the evolutionary component. Finally, it concludes that the FAP model can draw together the two most common explanations for medicine's persistence and status, the functionalist and power-oriented theories. Theirs is a more detailed exploration than anything I have done to date, and I am reassured to see that there were fresh insights to gain for such experienced academics.

Bluhm (Chapter 20) uses autonomy as her yardstick to assess the contribution that the FAP model might make to an understanding of medicine's functions and practices. Having sketched out her conception of autonomy, she concludes (p. 250) 'that understanding the goals of medicine in terms of the contribution of health care to a patient's security and flourishing is compatible with the account of autonomy that I sketched at the beginning of the chapter.' And she links autonomy and the achievements of security and flourishing more explicitly when she adds: 'If patient autonomy is understood in terms of the question "How do I want to live my life (given the conditions and constraints imposed by my illness), then medical decisions that contribute to a patient's sense of security and ability to flourish will help to answer that question.' Bluhm goes further by linking Fulford's conception of VBM with mine: 'In summary, the theories are compatible; Little's VBM emphasises values that are central to patient autonomy and that can provide a much-needed focus to Fulford's VBM, while Fulford's work provides health care providers with skills that can help to promote it.' She concludes that the two programmes can be integrated to achieve practical ends: 'Together, the theories provide a framework that focuses decisions on patients' needs and equip health care providers with skills that allow them to address these needs. This combined approach may help patients to maintain (or to regain) their autonomy in the face of a serious illness.'

Tonelli (Chapter 19) uses casuistry to measure the strengths and weakness of my version of VBM.[1] He concedes that my foundational values 'can be seen as providing general normative weight for many warrants derived from clinical research.' But he claims that these foundational values are 'relatively meaningless for decisions involving individuals'. I understand what he means, but must disagree. In clinical situations, there remain underlying drives to keep patients alive, secure and flourishing as individuals. They are never irrelevant, though they may often be implicit. Tonelli picks up the non-foundational values (axioms and practices) as being relevant to his preferred casuistry, and I agree that

---

[1] The use of 'my' at this point is definitely ungenerous, but signals that what is being written here is my responsibility. The 'Sydney VBM' is the product of many minds, including those of Wendy Lipworth, Kathleen Montgomery, Jill Gordon, Pippa Markham, Ian Kerridge, Lucie Rychetnik and Claire Hooker. I know they would never agree unreservedly with what I write, and so I acknowledge their contributions with gratitude, and absolve them of blame for my shortcomings and cognitive errors.

this is the level of clinical action and of much casuistic reflection. The foundational values sit there, sustaining our practices and reflection, without necessarily impinging on consciousness. But they are always there, and it does no harm to acknowledge their justifying presence.

At another point, Tonelli accuses VBM of separating facts and values, thereby committing an 'epistemic error'. I disagree strongly with this claim. VBM, in either construction, sees facts as playing out against a background of values that help us to assess the relevance and applicability of evidence. The fact/value distinction may be argued over by epistemologists, but facts and values are firmly co-located within VBM.

Tonelli's devotion to casuistic reasoning provides him with a strong grounding for his critique, but I fail to see where the argument really lies. VBM does not exclude casuistry, but in my own version it situates casuistry within the broader domain of wide reflective equilibrium. Wide reflective equilibrium incorporates previous moral experience, ethical learning, intuition, the details of context and the formal use of ethical structures (including casuistic reasoning) as fuel for reflective consideration. We are not in disagreement over the value of casuistry. As my own Chapter 14 concludes, 'We all have values. The more we know about them, recognise them, discuss them and acknowledge how sustaining they are, the better our medical and social discourse is likely to be. VBM is another reflective means to add to the repertoire of wide reflective equilibrium.'

Ross Upshur (see Chapter 17) has written a deeply thoughtful analysis of my arguments. The rest of this chapter is mainly a response to his objections. I value them highly, but I think that he and I are much closer in our positions than a reader of both chapters might assume. I must acknowledge with respect his 'training in mathematics and logic', but I suspect that much of the apparent dispute has a semantic origin. We are in accord, for example, on fallibilism, the evaluation of evidence-based medicine, the importance of temporal and spatial context in epistemology, the orneriness of human nature and the desire of some humans to promote their interests at the expense of others. We agree on the inevitability of death (Little, 1999), and on the need to define personhood and freedom. We disagree about what is *implied* by 'modest' foundationalism, about normativity, about the usefulness of 'soft' science and about the need to distinguish between the processes of evolution and the imperfections of human nature. And we disagree about whether I am writing about epistemology. He seems to think I am, but I claim to be writing about the evolution of social humanity. What follows sometimes endorses what he writes, and sometimes respectfully disagrees.

Foundationalism and fallibilism

Upshur's most serious criticism is directed against the whole concept of foundationalism, which he links to his arguments against any need to provide a basis for knowledge as it translates into medical practice. But from the outset he faces problems, the first of which is consistency. Despite his sustained attack on foundationalism, he seems unable to avoid falling back on foundationalist arguments and language. I am generally suspicious of *tu quoque* arguments, but in this case Upshur's apparent dilemma is logically important. We see his difficulty on p. 214, where he counsels that 'Rather than looking for the foundation, we should trace back the multiple strands of science and ethics that have informed and shaped modern medicine.' We are entitled, I think, to ask what tracing back implies. To the anti-foundationalist, there is no point in tracing back, since that exercise would lead us nowhere. On p. 212, he is even more explicit when he rejects foundation-alism 'by seeking foundations in a framework deriving and adapting arguments from Hilary Putnam, Charles Taylor and Peter Galison'. Here is an anti-foundationalist invoking foundations. Surely this illuminates a semantic problem, rather than any substantive disagreement. Upshur has his grounding (foundations?) in logic and mathematics; mine are – to some extent – based in qualitative social research, but this does not mean that either of us can do away with foundations at some level, and Upshur seems to concede this. The meanings of terms like 'foundations' are constrained by those disciplines. They are used in my chapters as entropy is used in informatics, as metaphors, if you like, demarcated by stipulative definitions. Upshur has his own meaning for 'emergent', which I respect now that he has explained it. But his use of the word unexplained led to misunderstanding. I have tried to define my terms as I went along, in the full knowledge that I was using contestable labels for contestable concepts, because I could think of no other words that came close to what I wanted to describe. But more on that later.

There are many similar instances where the differences between his fallibilism (to which I subscribe) and my aetiological foundationalism seem to collapse. On p. 213, for example, he poses a question:

> I think this definition coheres with what Little espouses, but it remains unclear to me how a modest foundationalism improves accepting a non-foundational form of fallibilism that I have argued for elsewhere. Is there a psychological or normative advantage to come from wedding language about foundations or bases to an account of what it means to be engaged in medicine?

I confess that I fail to see the point. Fallibilism seems to acknowledge that 'frameworks' are defeasible, and frameworks seem to act as starting points – as logic and mathematics do. The real sticking point seems to be 'language about foundations'. I am perfectly happy to endorse fallibilism in the epistemological domain. All that I seek is an *explanation* for the persistence of and the public devotion to the complex, barely comprehensible and very expensive practice of medicine, a project realised in some detail by Montgomery and Lipworth in Chapter 16. I think Upshur is quite understandably focused on medical practice and its normative regulation, which is logically posterior to the foundational concepts that I am postulating. I cheerfully concede that practice is where the action is, but I ask *why* it exists and why it persists. This in no way questions the importance or intellectual validity of his concerns. But I must ask if he sees a *disadvantage* to the use of this kind of rather reticent foundationalism? Chapters in this volume by Montgomery and Lipworth (Chapter 16) and Lipworth and Montgomery (Chapter 15) show that the FAP model can be used as a means to examine other, broader issues related to health. VBM of this kind underpins reflective equilibrium (Daniels, 1980, 1996; DePaul, 2001) as a mode of ethical deliberation, and acknowledges Tonelli's casuistry as an essential component of contextual ethics (see Chapter 19). Bluhm (Chapter 20) sees problems with my formulation, but also acknowledges that it can provide a basis and justification for Fulford's form of VBM.

Epistemology

Let me confront another set of powerful objections, based on the perceived epistemological weakness of my position. The following quote is from p. 213:

Charles Taylor, in his paper 'Overcoming epistemology' argues how strategies rooted in attempts to ground knowledge in secure foundations fail because the knower and the known are intimately intertwined. As he argues:

> But once we take this point, then the entire epistemological position is undermined. Obviously foundationalism goes, since our representations of things – the kinds of objects we pick out as whole, enduring entities – are grounded in the way we deal with those things. These dealings are largely inarticulate, and the project of articulating them fully is an essentially incoherent one, just because any articulative project would itself rely on a background or horizon of non-explicit engagement with the world. (Taylor, 1995, p. 6)

I have no difficulty in agreeing with Taylor and Upshur because I am not trying to use an epistemological manoeuvre. This is a misinterpretation. The foundations I am talking about are not epistemological, but very persistent *social* reference points, and I am trying to make sense of values and the ways in which they translate into action or behaviour in different contexts and different cultures. The foundations are vulnerable, as wars, GFCs, mad gunmen and natural disasters regularly demonstrate, but freedom movements, resistance to oppression and resilience in the face of natural disasters remind us that they do endure. They offer partial understanding of the ways in which humans respond to all kinds of experience, whether of joy, contentment, disaster or suffering. They are clearly stated to underpin evolutionary social processes, not knowledge. Axiology is not the same as epistemology.

There is a further point of criticism that is paradoxical. Having disposed of foundationalism *tout court*, Upshur then disposes individually of survival, security and flourishing as not being foundational anyway. To take one example, on p. 216 Upshur states 'Similarly, security would not be foundational in my account. It may be desirable, but from a fallibilist perspective, "epistemic insecurity" is constitutive of human existence.' That is certainly true, but my interpretation of insecurity extends well beyond the epistemic to cover existential insecurity – which is not necessarily desired by the insecure, nor good for them. I do not for a minute think that the Syrian civilians caught in the current cross-fire want to be where they are, nor do I believe that their plight should be a standard constituent of human existence. They explicitly seek to survive and to be secure, to escape toward places where security is more assured and survival perhaps possible. Epistemic insecurity is a small part of their problem.

Social research and social axioms

Much of the apparent gap between Upshur and myself, therefore, seems to be semantic, and some of it seems to reflect a supposition that I am talking about epistemology rather than social evolution. It also reflects a different evaluation of the validity and justification for social science and qualitative research. Upshur's pointed questions about 'social axioms' illustrate the problem clearly (p. 217):

> So a question I would ask is what is the meaning of axiom in this context? These generalised beliefs as stated in the quotation are expansive enough to cover virtually anything, and given the admitted variability of these axioms, they seem to do no specific work.

In qualitative and social research, the work goes on in open systems, unlike the work of mathematics and logic. Their 'sciences' operate differently. In qualitative research, there are no determinate results, but only tendencies, explanations, understandings. Of course, something similar can be said of much public health research, where statistical probability is regarded as an authoritative result, even though it simply indicates a tendency. Only laboratory science, like mathematics, can claim to work with determinacy within closed systems. Social axioms are useful as concepts because they *tend* to indicate what certain groups of people do and how they judge, just as the results of controlled trials indicate the *tendency* (although seldom the certainty) of a treatment to do something useful or desirable. Despite their indeterminism, qualitative results are valuable just because they increase our understanding of human history, experience and culture. And they are often the basis of quantitative studies that use the categories developed by qualitative researchers.

Value-laden words

The other semantic gap that I think causes trouble is one of my own making, the deployment of value-laden, semantically complex words – survival, security, flourishing – to 'code' complex concepts that emerged from empirical qualitative investigations. This *might* have been avoided if, for example, I had called them Primordial Factors I, II and III, and explicated them one by one. As it is, Upshur cannot see them as pre-normative, and I understand that difficulty. He writes on p. 216: 'I find it hard to understand survival, security and particularly flourishing as pre-normative.' This, I think, conflates the concepts with the long historical discourse about them. The fact that they are so much discussed emphasises their primordial status. I am asking readers to perform an *epoche*, to remove the semantic history attached to the axiomatic and practical side of the values continuum, and to consider the F-values as something essentially human like opposable thumbs. They are a given. We are stuck with them. Because we cannot avoid them – or rather, their culturally determined expressions – in one form or another, we transfer normativity to the *words* themselves, unable to perform the bracketing required to regain an understanding of their inescapable evolutionary presence – as inescapable as opposable thumbs. Once again, would it help to call them 'Primordial Factors I, II and III'? Not much, I suspect, because the explication would inevitably use words also charged with history, meaning and significance. I am reminded of the remark made by the nineteenth century cleric Sydney Smith, who observed two women arguing violently from upper story windows on either side of a narrow Edinburgh lane. 'They will never agree', he said, 'for they argue from different premises.'

Andrew Miles's chapter is hostile in many ways to what I have written, and it too obviously argues from different premises to mine. I am chastened by many of his criticisms, but confused by others. His very clear demolition of foundationalism in any form in an epistemological sense is a fine and clear statement of a very similar set of misgivings set out by Upshur, and my answers remain the same. I am not trying to construct a rigid base or foundation for medicine's *knowledge*, nor for the details of its practice, nor its bioethics. My foundations (whether rightly named or not) are *explanatory* in an aetiological or evolutionary sense. They are not prescriptive. We have and we maintain a medical enterprise because we want to survive and feel secure, and we want to be able to construct a narrative of our lives which tells of our flourishing. These are evolutionary programmes we seem to have built into our stone-age brains because we are relatively weak and slow, have less refined instincts than many other animals, need to be open to a wide world, have language and reason, and are self-protectively social – claims that owe much to readings of Fichte, Herder and Gehlen's philosophical anthropology. I am making (modest) claims in the domains of social interaction and anthropology, not within the territory of epistemology.

Miles is at pains to dismiss the need for foundations in most of our endeavours, but at times he too seems to pose problems for himself. He writes, for example on p. 221,

> I conclude that the most authentic account of medicine would see it described in non-foundational terms, as primarily a human endeavour which draws necessarily on the multiplicity of medicine's knowledge sources, without being referentially harnessed to any single, privileged foundation.

This is a strong, but puzzling statement, and I am not sure what it implies. Does this mean that medicine does not even need to value human life in quantity and quality? That all the effort and expense put into public health and healing are committed without reason? I am unable to answer those questions from within Miles's declared set of beliefs.

Miles is also dismissive of my version of foundationalism because it drifts (in his view) into a loose relativism, in which norms are created by what people 'feel' (p. 227):

> If I reject the notion that there can be any irreducibly normative truths in a proper 'scientific' account of the world we live in, then, surely, there can be nothing that we just ought to recognise as inherently right or wrong and moral language becomes, in one form or another, just the expression of the way individuals 'feel', providing no way to determine the rightness or wrongness of how they 'feel', other than noting that this is what they do 'feel'. So even if there are some evaluative claims upon which we can all agree (such as the claim that survival – at least for a certain duration, under certain conditions – is good), whenever we find we disagree about any matter of practical significance, appeal to the 'foundations' can 'explain' all possible positions, but cannot explain why we *should* espouse any one position rather than any other. It will be left to how we feel, just as though we had never encountered this explanatory thesis.

But my 'values' are avowedly *pre-normative*, which is to say that they do not dictate how a society will evolve its ethical norms. What they do predict is that every surviving society will develop systems that allow their members to survive in some measure of security and to flourish according to the perceptions and beliefs developed during the evolution of that society. It is precisely *verstehen* that they offer, an understanding of the pluralist practices that Miles appeals to in order to justify his preference for person-centred medicine or care. The three foundational 'values' (whatever you may want to call them yourself) do not prescribe how you shall behave. Instead, they suggest how you may understand, and how you may establish some grounds for understanding of and even respect for practices that seem otherwise puzzling or even unintelligible. It is only when we come to the evolutionary level of establishing social axioms and translating them into practice that norms emerge.

For these, and many other, reasons, I am especially puzzled by Miles's concluding statements (p. 233):

> I conclude by exhorting clinicians, academics, health care policy makers and governments to reject narrow, foundationalist accounts of the complex clinical, human and moral

endeavour that is clinical medicine and to embrace instead the authentically anthropocentric model of health care that is PCCC.

I can find no claim that I have made that the sort of VBM set out in this book does not 'embrace ... the authentically anthropocentric model of health care that is PCCC'. It seems to me that this rhetorical flourish undermines the real opportunity for us to develop further what is already major common ground – although the strength of Miles's language and his consistently negative critique might suggest to the reader that he and I came from vastly different commitments.

Conclusion

The critiques of both Upshur and Miles have given me pause, and stimulated a good deal of thought, and I am immensely grateful that they took the time and trouble to engage with work that they clearly found flawed. I suffer from no illusion that the FAP model of values-based medicine will produce a revolution in medical thinking, policy or practice. It is unlikely even to affect medical education in the form that I commit to. Fulford's is a more practical approach than mine, and I endorse his campaign to teach skills that will encourage recognition of and respect for person-hood, individuality and cultural difference. My contribution, I hope, will simply add a justification for Fulford's privileging of preferences, and some further insight into what it is that preferences actually express. This is the point that is persuasively argued by Bluhm in Chapter 20 in this book. The two approaches to VBM comple-ment one another.

You might, then, legitimately ask how this form of VBM would translate into medical education. Fulford has set out his axioms, and developed a teaching programme for medical students (Fulford, 2004). I support what he has achieved and endorse his recommendations. My own work leads us to suggest a more discursive mode of advice that might lead medical students to think about foundational values and their deployment in medical knowledge, enculturation, ethical quandaries, decision-making, medical virtues and the processes of education. The following section shows how our formulation, based on the corpus of work that emerged from our VBM study (Little, 2002, 2012; Little et al., 2011a, 2011b, 2011c, 2012; Gordon et al., 2012, Lipworth et al., 2012), might translate into educational terms.

Advice for people entering the medical course

Medical education aims to help strongly motivated people to become doctors. That sounds pretty obvious and straightforward, but the process is, of course, a very complex one.

Values

Medicine is based neither on science nor on evidence. Neither of these provides justifica-tion for the immense amount of money, time and effort devoted to the practices of health care. Medicine is certainly patient-centred, because it would cease to exist if there was no illness, and therefore no patients. But why does medicine exist at all? Why should ill people not be allowed to suffer and die without societies providing so much for their support and relief?

It seems that societies cannot function without acknowledging three foundational needs or values – the need to survive, the need to feel secure, and the need to flourish by transcending the day to day demands of life. Each culture will play out systems to support security and allow for flourishing in very different ways. Some ways we may find unacceptable from a Western liberal standpoint, but each society will have systems of health, law, education, welfare, worship, entertainment and so on, designed to enhance or protect the fundamental values. Thus, health services help people to survive, to feel secure in the face of illness, and to flourish or regain a capacity to flourish by providing rehabilitation, aged care, reconstructive surgery and so on.

It is these foundational values that provide a justification for health care services. Evidence in medicine is valuable because it provides a rationale for certain kinds of practice, but the practice itself is only justified if we refer beyond evidence to the foundational values.

So what will you encounter in a medical course?

Knowledge

The most obvious need you have is for *knowledge*. Even that is not as straightforward as it seems. People tend to think that medicine is scientific – meaning that it is based on experiments and developments in subjects such as chemistry and physics, and in laboratory work with bacteria, viruses and cells, and in clinical trials where treatments are examined for their effects. Those disciplines work with objective data, and the results of their investigations can be reported and read by doctors and other health workers, and by the general public, so that everyone will know the 'best' way to treat someone with an illness.

In practice, however, medical knowledge is far less certain than laboratory science. Laboratory science works with more or less closed systems – which is to say that most components of any system can be 'controlled' so that only one component is studied. You can do this with a system of chemical reactions, or the behaviour of bacteria, but you cannot do the same with humans. A human 'system' has so many components, all functioning at the same time and interacting with one another, that a scientist cannot really isolate any one component completely for study. Even the act of studying a biological system is likely to alter the system itself or inter-related systems. These are open systems, subject to continual minute-to-minute changes and to influences that cannot be 'controlled out'. Furthermore, there are social and psychological forces that act on parts of the human complex of systems in highly significant ways, and there are individual genetic and developmental influences that make for important individual variations.

So we can distinguish between at least three kinds of knowledge that are important for students and practitioners of medicine to gain, to examine critically, and to use to benefit others. The first is *determinate knowledge*, the kind generated by bench-top science under controlled conditions – the kinds of chemical laws, for instance, that allow pharmaceutical scientists to synthesise new drugs. The second is *bio-knowledge*, the tendencies that can be documented for disease outcomes with and without treatment, or the epidemiological observations that come from controlled trials. Bio-knowledge is essentially probabilistic; it gives an indication of what will happen to groups of people with the same pathology, or is happening to groups of people with similar biochemical profiles. Finally, *life-world knowledge* has special standing in medicine. Doctors are presumed to be wise about the ways that people react psychologically to stress and bereavement, to know how to communicate bad news, to be able to deal equably with people with whom they have nothing in common.

Medical knowledge changes all the time, which means that medical practice is constantly changing. Peptic ulcers were once believed by the best informed doctors to result from too much gastric acid secretion. Now we believe that most are caused by infections. Knowledge is subject to constant revision, and today's 'knowledge' is really today's 'warranted assertability'. Knowledge in clinical medicine is essentially pragmatic. We regard as true what works in practice, or seems to work best in practice.

Enculturation

Gaining the knowledge is only a part of medical education. Knowing what doctors know does not mean that you will automatically think and act like a doctor. Learning to do that involves becoming *encultured* into the discourse community of medicine, and its more specialised sub-communities. This will mean acquiring modes of perceiving people and their illnesses in ways that may seem initially unfamiliar and strange. You will of course bring your own values and ways of responding to others as you enter the medical course. These habits of response probably explain why you chose to do medicine. The medical course will teach you to develop a medical 'gaze' that looks beyond the common-sense observations that you might make as you enter medicine, and to appreciate mechanisms and responses that may seem strange and even threatening to others. You will learn to handle the distress of others, while protecting your own mental equilibrium. You will have to find your own ways of doing that, but those around you will be serving as role models that you want to follow or to reject. The learning process extends well beyond the formal teaching programme, but your own natural reactions will generally be modified by experiences and the culture of medical practice into which you will progress further and further with time.

Enculturation is good in some ways, dangerous in others. It works well in indicating ways to handle medical problems in approved ways, but it can also interfere with your own critical reasoning. It is easy to fall back into familiar patterns of practice and reasoning, and to overlook the demands of context, to forget that an individual may have special beliefs and perceptions that should be respected, to ignore the signals of distress that you would probably pick up as an early medical student. You may stop noticing or feeling critical of the brusque or insensitive behaviour of colleagues, or even your own brusque and insensitive behaviour. Enculturation is a resource, but it is also a threat to your own natural compassion and empathy.

Ethical quandaries

One of the distinctive features of medical practice is the nature of its ethical *quandaries*. As a doctor, you must deal in any specialty with vulnerable people, and you must do so within cultural and social contexts. People's beliefs and needs will clash with your own beliefs and needs. Bureaucratic rules will repeatedly interfere with your ability to enact the judgements you make about what would be best for this or that patient; resource constraints will mean that some treatments or diagnostic tests will not be available when they might be safer or more reassuring. At times, the law will determine what you can or cannot do, and this may clash with what you and your patient might want.

Ethics in medicine is largely concerned with these quandaries, which develop because of a complex of demands between yourself as a doctor, your patient and her values and beliefs, the complex of rules and institutional requirements that define medicine as a discipline, the culture in which the medical encounter takes place, and the distinctive context of the encounter between individuals with illnesses and the medical practitioners.

You will learn to apply your specialised knowledge, including practical skills, to these quandaries, and you will learn from formal teaching of ethics, but, far more importantly, from the experiences of seeing others handling quandaries and handling them yourselves.

Decisions

Your enculturation, your continuing education and your identity as a doctor will all depend very greatly on your making decisions. Your decisions will be made in the worlds of bio-knowledge and the life-world. You will make them about your own career and your own desire to do good and to avoid regret, and you will make them about the lives and welfare of others. In your student days, you will practise decision-making and you will watch others making clinical decisions, and you will learn something about decision theory and evidence-based medicine. The further you progress, the closer decision-making comes to the core of your identity as a doctor. You will see the effects of your decisions, and learn what it is like to live with their consequences, whether they are beneficial or not. You will develop a style of decision-making that reflects fundamental beliefs about hope and resignation, about when to intervene and when to wait. You will find that you will become more aware of the contexts – social, cultural, personal and medical – that may change your actions and judgements to respond to particular aspects of any given case.

Reflecting on decisions is a major educational enhancement. To recognise regret for what it is, to understand its relationship to risk, to confront its lessons, are all signs of maturity and of a desirable medical virtue.

Virtues

A good decision is one that saves life, provides some certainty or security to the ill, or restores or enhances the capacity of people to flourish. That is the function of medicine, to ensure the foundational needs or values. You will find that you will perceive among your mentors, teachers and colleagues acts that strike you as particularly effective in promoting the foundational values, or that disturb you because they seem to devalue them. Practising doctors recounting their careers speak repeatedly in terms of the *virtues* of doctors they have encountered during their student days and practising lives.

Virtues have a rather sanctimonious ring to their name, but they have a reality that resonates with doctors. The old cardinal virtues, including courage, justice and temperance, are all valued, but there are two meta-virtues that attract the most praise. These are *phronesis*, which is practical wisdom, the virtue of doing good, or beneficence, and *prudence*, which is the virtue of avoiding doing harm. Doctors reflecting on their careers praise these virtues of judgement and action above all others. They admire the capacity of the wise practitioner to make decisions that avoid harm and produce what is perceived to be the best possible outcome within the context of the case. Medical education begins in medical school, but it goes on into the post-graduate years and never stops throughout a practising lifetime, because the acquisition of wisdom depends on repeated reflection on the experiences and decisions of a practising life.

Education

You will be taught the knowledge-base you need to become a doctor, but you will also learn something about the philosophy of medicine. You will be encouraged to apply this basic philosophy to each component of the medical course, so that you can repeatedly critique what you are learning, and put it into the changing contexts of Australian and global cultures. Hopefully, this will encourage you to reflect on the medical habits, institutions and practices to which you will be repeatedly exposed for your whole practising lifetime. We do not aim to produce a generation of medical philosophers, but we do hope to help you to become reflective practitioners who understand something about

- the values that justify the complex discipline of medicine,
- the nature of the knowledge that is indispensable to skilled medical practice,
- the processes of enculturation into the medical discourse community,
- the formative role of decisions in establishing your medical style and reputation,
- the nature of the ethical quandaries that doctors face each day,
- the virtues that mark the good practitioner, and
- the role and nature of reflection in your continuing education.

It takes a working lifetime to become a wise doctor, but the effort is worthwhile for those with beneficent motives and a desire for practical wisdom. Medicine is a way of life, a good and useful way.

References

Daniels, N. (1980) Reflective equilibrium and Archimedian points. *Canadian Journal of Philosophy*, **10**, 83–103.

Daniels, N. (1996) *Justice and Justification: Reflective Equilibrium in Theory and Practice.* Cambridge: Cambridge University Press.

DePaul, M. R. (2001) *Balance and Refinement: Beyond Coherence Methods of Moral Inquiry.* London: Routledge.

Fulford, K. W. M. (2004) Ten principles of values-based medicine. In Radden, J. (editor), *The Philosophy of Psychiatry: A Companion*, pp. 205–234. Oxford: Oxford University Press.

Gordon, J., Markham, P., Lipworth, W., Kerridge, I. and Little, M. (2012) The dual nature of medical enculturation in postgraduate medical training and practice. *Medical Education*, **46**(9), 894–902.

Lipworth, W., Kerridge, I., Little, M., Gordon, J. and Markham, P. (2012) Meaning and value

in medical school curricula. *Journal of Evaluation in Clinical Practice*, **18**, 1027–1035.

Little, M. (1999) Assisted suicide, suffering and the meaning of a life. *Theoretical Medicine and Bioethics*, **20**(3), 287–298.

Little, M. (2002) Humanistic medicine or values-based medicine? What's in a name? *Medical Journal of Australia*, **177**(6), 319–321.

Little, M. (2012) The precarious future of the discourse of person-centered medicine. *International Journal of Person Centered Medicine*, in publication.

Little, M., Gordon, J., Markham, P., Lipworth, W. and Kerridge, I. (2011a) Making decisions in the mechanistic, probabilistic and scientific domains of medicine: a qualitative study of medical practitioners. *International Journal of Person Centered Medicine*, **1**(2), 376–384.

Little, M., Gordon, J., Markham, P., Rychetnik, L. and Kerridge, I. (2011b)

Virtuous acts as practical medical ethics: an empirical study. *Journal of Evaluation in Clinical Practice,* **17**, 948–953.

Little, M., Lipworth, W., Gordon, J., Markham, P. and Kerridge, I. (2011c) Another argument for values-based medicine. *International Journal of Person Centered Medicine,* **1**(4), 649–656.

Little, M., Lipworth, W., Gordon, J., Markham, P. and Kerridge, I. (2012) Values-based medicine and modest foundationalism. *Journal of Evaluation in Clinical Practice,* **18**, 1020–1026.

Walking the VB-talk: concluding reflections on models, methods and practical pay-offs

K. W. M. (Bill) Fulford and Miles Little

Our first reaction when Michael Loughlin suggested an edited collection covering our two very different approaches to working with values in health care was mixed. On the one hand we are both fully paid up members of the 'more than one tool in the tool kit' club. But we had concerns about coverage and coherence.

We should not have worried! Skilled and experienced editor that he is, Michael has done a wonderful job in assembling a diverse range of commentators from all of whom whether severe critic or critical friend we have gained many new insights. We have separately thanked our respective commentators. We want to take this further opportunity to say a joint thank you both to the contributors to this book as a whole and to Michael for all his hard work and harder diplomacy in building what amounts to a new community of ideas on values in contemporary health care practice.

So where does all this leave us? Where does the relationship between our two models of values-based health care stand in the light of the community of ideas represented by the commentaries? How should we build on this community of ideas? And what might be the practical pay-off for health care practitioners?

VBP and FAP

Our first point straight off the bat is that our two models are complementary. Robyn Bluhm (Chapter 20) says just this in relation specifically to autonomy: 'Little's VBM' as she puts it (p. 245) 'emphasises values that are central to patient autonomy and that can provide a much-needed focus to Fulford's VBM, while Fulford's work provides health care providers with skills that can help to promote it.' Thus, she

Debates in Values-Based Practice, ed. Michael Loughlin. Published by Cambridge University Press. © Cambridge University Press 2014.

continues, 'this combined approach may help patients to maintain (or to regain) their autonomy in the face of a serious illness.' Generalising Bluhm's point we have: FAP (Little's VBM, based on foundations, axioms and practices) focuses on answers while VBP (Fulford's VBM) focuses on the skills and other process elements involved in getting answers; the combined approach thus adds up to 'answers and how to get them'. Simple!

This way of characterising the relationship between our two models is helpful in a number of respects. Importantly, it avoids the equal and opposite stereotypes of VBP as an 'anything goes' process-only approach and of FAP as laying down 'what goes' in an authoritarian way insensitive to context. Both models are about balanced decision-making in the challenging circumstances created by the increasing complexity of contemporary health care practice. Yes, there are differences of emphasis: this after all is why FAP and VBP are complementary. But the differences in question are just that, differences of emphasis. FAP does have built-in foundational values but these F-values, of survival, security and flourishing (which anyway are only 'modestly foundational', see below), have to be taken as part of the full package that includes A (contextually focused bridging axioms) and P (practices that deliver on FA in day-to-day individual decision-making). VBP, similarly, although indeed focusing more than FAP on processes for practical delivery (the P in VBP), has to be read with its own guiding values as expressed in its premise (of mutual respect) and the locally agreed frameworks of shared values within which balanced decisions are taken on individual cases. There is indeed a rough equivalence here (and it is only rough, see below) between on the one hand the F-values of FAP and the premise of VBP, and, on the other hand, the A-values of FAP and the frameworks of shared values of VBP.

Both the similarities however and the differences between our two models run deeper than this. We return to the differences below. But among the further similarities between FAP and VBP are:

(1) shared (implicit) epistemic values – as Gideon Calder (Chapter 9, p. 118) rightly notes these include 'openness towards outcomes [and] sensitivity to context';
(2) a shared debt to David Hume – the F-values in FAP are modestly foundational values in being derived as limiting steps in Hume's method of iterative enquiry; the premise of VBP is derived from the is-ought debate with its origins in Hume's (paraphrased) dictum 'no ought from an is';
(3) a shared shift in our respective methods of values-enquiry from substantive to analytic ethics, respectively axiology in FAP and philosophical value theory as an ordinary language informed meta-ethics in VBP ('axiology' and 'meta-ethics' are widely used as synonyms);
(4) a recognition in this shift to the analytic that the very term 'values' and its denotation in health care carries a complex and variable range of meanings covering not only such familiar (in health care) categories as needs, wishes and preferences but also less familiar though no less relevant values such as aesthetic values;
(5) for this if for no other reasons, both models seek starting points (a better term perhaps than either 'foundations' or 'premise') that are in one way or another pre-normative (albeit contestably so, as we both recognise this to be); and with these pre-normative starting points particularly in mind,

(6) FAP and VBP have the shared practical objective of supporting balanced decision-making (represented respectively by the 'reflective equilibrium' of FAP and the 'dissensus' of VBP) on individual cases in the particular circumstances presented by the contingencies of day-to-day health care practice.

A values alphabet?

A further important similarity between FAP and VBP is that both self-identify as partners not merely one with the other but also with the wide range of further decision support tools available for working not only with values but also with evidence in health care. Other value-support tools include, in addition to law and the many varieties of substantive ethics, decision analysis, health economics, and various areas of the humanities, not to mention the resources of empirical research disciplines such as psychology, ethnography and anthropology. Evidence-support tools include not only the resources for meta-analysis of quantitative data represented by evidence-based practice, but also corresponding resources for working with qualitative evidence (in the social sciences) and indeed first-personal narratives.

We welcome in particular among these other decision support tools the growing importance of first-personal narratives as a return to the traditional observational basis of medicine in individual case histories. One manifestation of this is the emerging movement in person-centred medicine. Andrew Miles (Chapter 18) as a prominent figure in this movement sees FAP as inconsistent with its person-centred aims. We recognise his concerns. But they are concerns that apply equally to VBP as to FAP if either becomes reduced through over-simplification to cut-price versions. Such cut-price versions would indeed be inimical to person-centred medicine not just in its evaluative but also in its scientific aspects (the evaluative aspects of person-centred medicine being concerned with e.g. preference-unique individuals, its scientific aspects being concerned with e.g. genetically unique individuals). As we have argued earlier in this book, such risks should be taken seriously. The greater risk currently, however, as we see it, is of person-centred medicine itself becoming reduced to a cut-price version in which the personal in medicine is not merely re-established but is inflated to the point that it eclipses the communal – a medicine in which 'Me medicine' eclipses 'We medicine' as the ethicist and philosopher Donna Dickenson (2013) has graphically put it. This is a risk that as we discuss further below (in relation to the challenges of global health) FAP and VBP taken together could play a key role in averting.

A further manifestation of medicine's return to its roots in individual case histories is the rise of casuistry or case-based reasoning in clinical ethics as reflected in a number of the commentaries in this book. Casuistry is both integral to and enhanced by VBP (see Chapter 13) and bears a similar two-way relationship with FAP. Rather less well developed but crucial to decision-making no less in We-medicine than in Me-medicine is the irreducible role of clinical judgement and its dependence (its critical dependence) on tacit as well as explicit knowledge. Tim Thornton although focusing in this book on the premise of VBP (Chapter 4), has elsewhere started to map out some of the specifically philosophical resources for a deeper understanding of the role and importance of individual clinical judgement and tacit knowledge in health care (Thornton, 2006). We welcome work in these areas as providing vital additional resources in our shared task of countering the 'cut-price' uses of both ethics and evidence-based practice that are so widely prevalent in contemporary health care.

In all these respects then, neither FAP nor VBP offers a *sine cure* to working with values. Both models claim modest contributions as decision support tools to be used always in partnership with other approaches. This is why as we put it earlier we are both fully paid up members of the 'more than one tool in the tool kit' club. It is important in this respect to recognise further that even within the values-based part of the tool kit there is a variety of tools. VBC (values-based commissioning, Heginbotham, 2012) is one such tool that takes values-based approaches beyond the individual to the collective, a move the importance of which is emphasised here by Sridhar Venkatapuram (Chapter 11). There is also in the UK a similarly motivated (by diversity of values) development drawing on health economic theory called value-based pricing (VBP, www.2020selection.co.uk/images/pdfs/value-based-pricing.pdf). The philosopher David Seedhouse has developed an approach to values-based decision-making (VBD) that is the basis of a powerful web-based training tool called the 'values exchange' that is already being used in a number of medical schools around the world (see for example http://vxcommunity.com and http://warwick.vxcommunity.com).

So with a veritable alphabet of values-based approaches already in play and no doubt more on the way it is reasonable to ask (as Gupta asks of VBP in Chapter 7) just what exactly are our two particular 'VB tools' good for. We have responded to this question separately in our respective contributions to this book. Here we respond together and to the question as aimed specifically at the need for both Fulford and Little versions of VBM. The question thus limited might be put thus: 'If FAP and VBP are as you (Fulford and Little) have suggested so similar, why do we need both? You tell us that FAP with VBP together give us 'answers and how to get them'; fine, so why should we not simply merge your two models and get two for the price of one?' To answer this question we need to turn from the similarities to a key difference between FAP and VBP.

A key difference between FAP and VBP

A key difference between Fulford-VBP and Little-FAP is in what we called earlier our respective starting points. The difference is evident to a first level of approximation in the way we describe these starting points: Fulford describes VBP as starting from the premise of mutual respect for differences of values; Little describes FAP as starting from the F-values (foundational values) of survival, security and flourishing. Thus expressed, however, it might seem that our different ways of describing our starting points reflect no more than or can be understood as a further difference between us merely of emphasis. We resist this. We believe our respective starting points represent a radical and possibly in principle irreducible difference between us. We believe further that it is in virtue as much of this radical difference as of any similarities between us that our two models provide complementary resources for balanced clinical decision-making. To see this, however, we need to go behind the philosophical scene, as it were, to look at how we get to our starting points. For of course any starting point is always at the same time the end of some other journey.

The journey in question, as we have indicated, takes both of us, although in different ways, to Hume. But as we journey in different ways with Hume so we end up on different sides in the is-ought debate that Hume started. We are well aware that at this point we will immediately be in trouble with those among our philosophical colleagues who believe that the is-ought debate as such is over; or at any rate that the debate is otiose in the sense that (post-Quine) 'is' and 'ought' are now seen to be not sufficiently different for there to be a debate about the relationship between them (like arguing about the relationship between 'nought' and 'zero'). We do not have space here to enter into the debate about the debate. Sufficient for our present purposes – of explaining the difference between us and its implications for practice – is that the distinction between 'is' and 'ought' persists in ordinary (including health care) language (as indeed we would add it persists in philosophical language). In what follows then (and borrowing from Putnam, 2002) we will be concerned with the distinction between 'is' and 'ought' without implying still less relying on there being a dualism between them.

So understood then, Fulford's journey takes him to the *non-naturalist* 'no ought from an is' side in the is-ought debate while Little's journey takes him to a *qualified naturalist* 'some oughts from some is'. Fulford's non-naturalist journey is evident in his original *Moral Theory and Medical Practice* (Fulford, 1989) and intellectual debt to the non-naturalist R. M. Hare: he (Fulford) is persuaded by the argument (originally from G. E. Moore) from non-contradiction. Little's naturalist journey by contrast is evident in the contingent derivation of his F-values based on Hume's observation of an actual if not necessary end to iteratively asking 'why?': he (Little) is persuaded by his observation that iteratively asking 'why be healthy?' ends up rather quickly with the F-values of FAP.

There is of course much more that could be said here: Fulford might argue that it is not self-contradictory to deny that even survival (one of Little's F-values) is good; Little might reply that it would be if not actually self-contradictory at any rate evolutionarily self-defeating in the sense that without survival we would not be here to engage in the debate at all; Fulford could counter that the contingencies of evolution cut both ways, that if 'we' meant 'we Dodos' the survival of 'we humans' would not be even a modestly foundational value; to which Little could counter with 'flourishing' since implicit in the value of survival is that there is something (literally) worth surviving for, which the progressive destruction of our planetary life-support system represented by the (apparently) remorseless extermination of species puts very much at risk; and Fulford would then say 'fine' but by the same contingencies the 'security' F-value of FAP has arguably the wrong valence since a little more *insecurity* might be essential if we are to prevent our evolutionarily driven instincts from driving us not to survival but to extinction; and . . .

At this point, practitioners listening in on this debate might feel some impatience with the philosophical issues at stake. 'Come back to us' the busy practitioner might reasonably exclaim 'when you have sorted yourselves out!' But the point is precisely the opposite. The technical niceties of the is-ought debate are not for every practitioner – no more (and no less) are the technical niceties of corresponding debates in the sciences for every practitioner. What matters to the busy practitioner is translation of research (of whatever kind) into practice. And it is translation that matters here. For it is precisely the open and unresolved nature of the is-ought debate underpinning equally VBP and FAP that translates via their respective starting points into their complementary practical roles as decision support tools in clinical care. Too firm and final a belief in the possibility of foundations leads all too easily via the belief that 'we' have found such foundations to the abuses of absolutism. Too firm and final a belief in the impossibility of foundations leads all too easily via the belief that 'so anything goes' to the equal and opposite abuses of relativism. Between us our two models, underpinned as they are by the two sides in the is-ought debate, embody a balance between these two extremes. The balance for as long as the is-ought debate itself remains unresolved is a dynamic and open balance. It is this dynamic and open balance that provides a robust theoretical underpinning for the complementary practical roles of FAP and VBP in supporting the 'balanced decision-making under the conditions of uncertainty' required of today's health care practitioners.

The pay-off for practice

Just where and how FAP and VBP and indeed other tools from the tool kit are used in practice will depend on the particular demands of a given situation. But that both tools, both FAP and VBP, are needed is clearly illustrated by the challenges of global health highlighted by Sridhar Venkatapuram (Chapter 11) in this book. Sridhar generously indicates the potential of VBP for global health. But as noted in Chapter 13, he points out that the particular focus of VBP's skills-based approach on individual clinical decision-making puts it out of kilter with the growing epidemiological and public health evidence suggesting that the drivers of mortality and morbidity are predominantly not at the level of the individual but of the collective. And in the face of manifest health injustice on a global scale he challenges the process-emphasising VBP to 'take a position' on relevant substantive values.

With just VBP in the tool kit Sridhar's challenge is not readily met. As Fulford indicates (Chapter 13) there are shifts in values-based thinking towards the collective (such as the now well-established programmes in values-based commissioning). But VBP is not designed to 'take a position' beyond locally agreed frameworks of shared values and the limitations imposed by its premise of mutual respect. So used on its own the VBP 'tool' would be less than a good fit to Sridhar's hand. Whereas the FAP tool by contrast suggests a rather good fit. Its starting-point F-values actually include a value embraced by Sridhar, 'survival', and it seems likely that the other FAP F-values of 'security' and 'flourishing' would also be entirely to the point. VBP though would not now be redundant: to the contrary it would be the first tool out of the tool kit when it comes to the 'local initiatives' to which Sridhar points. And as Fulford indicated there have been relevant developments at the local level such as the education and training initiatives developed by Ed Peile and David Davies in Malawi. And Werdie van Staden's early work on *batho pele* (a collective-VBP based on African concepts) offers a possible bridging approach. So both VBP and FAP will be needed and are available to respond to Sridhar's challenge as will other tools including of course his own cutting edge work bringing together moral philosophy and health economics in a new model of health justice.

Walking the VB-talk

Our aim in these concluding comments has been to deliver a values-based message but also to deliver this message by modelling a values-based method. Our values-based message is that models such as FAP and VBP have complementary roles to play alongside other clinical decision-making support tools in the health care tool kit. The challenge for health care whether at the individual or collective level is the ever-growing complexity of both the evidence-base and the values-base of clinical decision-making. Faced with such complexity, health care decision-making risks becoming caught between the *Scylla* of cut-price rule-book simplifications and the *Charybdis* of becoming 'paralysed by hesi-tancy' (as Russell, cited by Fulford, Chapter 13, put it). As contributions to the growing alphabet of values-based approaches, FAP and VBP have a role to play in avoiding these twin extremes by supporting balanced decision-making under conditions of uncertainty at all levels of health care engagement from the individual to the collective.

Some among our philosophical colleagues may find this too anodyne a conclusion. 'Where' we can hear some say 'are the fire and fizz of argumentative debate that we expect of philosophical exchange?' The point is fair. This particular exchange, however, is not between philosophers alone but between philosophers in conversation with practitioners. It is here we believe that the values-based method we have adopted in these concluding comments is itself part of the message. As values-based models, FAP and VBP, as we have said, aim to support balanced health care decision-making under conditions of uncertainty. Used separately, FAP supports balanced decision-making through 'reflective equipoise' achieved by cashing out modestly foundational values through locally derived axioms into practice. VBP on the other hand supports balanced decision-making through a clinical skills-based process of 'dissensual decision-making' within locally agreed frameworks of shared values. What is required in practice though (as illustrated above by the challenge of global health) is what might be called a meta-VB approach in which VBP and FAP are both available as distinct but complementary tools in the practitioner's tool kit. And this meta-VB approach we believe depends on those involved in developing VB tools themselves modelling their own VB practice.

We should not wish to be misunderstood here. VB practice in philosophy is entirely compatible with sharp critical exchange. It is indeed among the roles of philosophy in practice to avoid premature closure on complex problems: this is a key role of philosophy in mental health for example. And as we have indicated here, the complementary roles of FAP and VBP as decision support tools depend precisely on the differences rather than on any similarities between them. Philosophers moreover, like any other group, are vulnerable to plain 'spats'. And perhaps behind our own study doors and between consenting experts, 'winning' is as respectable a motivation in philosophy as in any other field. But to the extent that philosophers seek to engage with practical disciplines there is scope for less point-scoring and more point-making aimed not at 'winning' but at that reflective philosophical equipoise that underpins reflective practice. This is what we have tried to model in these concluding comments. And it is this that we hope will be among the pay-offs for practitioners from the new community of ideas brought together by Michael Loughlin in this book.

References

Dickenson, D. (2013) *Me Medicine vs. We Medicine: Reclaiming Biotechnology for the Common Good.* Columbia, NY: Columbia University Press.

Fulford, K. W. M. (1989, reprinted 1995, 1999) *Moral Theory and Medical Practice.* Cambridge: Cambridge University Press.

Heginbotham, C. (2012) *Values-Based Commissioning of Health and Social Care.* Cambridge: Cambridge University Press.

Putnam, H. (2002) *The Collapse of the Fact/Value Dichotomy and other Essays.* Cambridge, MA: Harvard University Press.

Thornton, T. (2006) Tacit knowledge as the unifying factor in EBM and clinical judgement. *Philosophy, Ethics, and Humanities of Medicine,* 1, 2doi:10.1186/1747-5341-1-2.

Index

Page numbers followed by 'n' refer to notes.